Evidence-Based Orthodontics

Evidence-Based Orthodontics

Edited by Kaley Ann

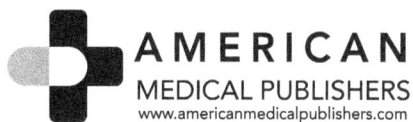

AMERICAN
MEDICAL PUBLISHERS
www.americanmedicalpublishers.com

American Medical Publishers,
41 Flatbush Avenue,
1st Floor, New York,
NY 11217, USA

Visit us on the World Wide Web at:
www.americanmedicalpublishers.com

ISBN: 978-1-63927-054-5

Cataloging-in-Publication Data

Evidence-based orthodontics / edited by Kaley Ann.
    p. cm.
Includes bibliographical references and index.
ISBN 978-1-63927-054-5
1. Orthodontics. 2. Dentistry. I. Ann, Kaley.
RK521 .E77 2022
617.643--dc23

Table of Contents

Preface

In my initial years as a student, I used to run to the library at every possible instance to grab a book and learn something new. Books were my primary source of knowledge and I would not have come such a long way without all that I learnt from them. Thus, when I was approached to edit this book; I became understandably nostalgic. It was an absolute honor to be considered worthy of guiding the current generation as well as those to come. I put all my knowledge and hard work into making this book most beneficial for its readers.

Orthodontics is a discipline of dentistry that focuses on the diagnosis, prevention and correction of malpositioned teeth and jaws. It is majorly used to treat malocclusions and the control and modification of facial growth. The majority of orthodontic appliance therapy is done using fixed appliances and removable appliances. There are two main types of orthodontic appliances: active and functional. Active appliance is the tool that is used to apply forces to the teeth in order to change its relation. Functional appliances can be used to correct the occlusion when there is a maxillary over jet and class II occlusion. Aesthetics, oral health, stability and function are some aspects that should be kept in mind while planning treatment for a patient. The book studies, analyzes and upholds the pillars of orthodontics and its utmost significance in modern times. It presents researches and studies performed by experts across the globe. This book will prove to be immensely beneficial to students and researchers in this field.

I wish to thank my publisher for supporting me at every step. I would also like to thank all the authors who have contributed their researches in this book. I hope this book will be a valuable contribution to the progress of the field.

Editor

Premaxilla: up to which age it remains separated from the maxilla by a suture, how often it occurs in children and adults, and possible clinical and therapeutic implications: Study of 1,138 human skulls

Mariana Trevizan[1], Paulo Nelson Filho[2], Solange de Oliveira Braga Franzolin[3], Alberto Consolaro[1,4]

Objective: To evaluate topographic and temporal aspects of premaxillary bone and premaxillary-maxillary suture, since they are fundamental anatomical elements little explored clinically. **Methods:** 1,138 human dry skulls were evaluated, of which 116 (10.19%) of the specimens were children, and 1,022 (89.81%) were adults. The skulls were photographed and the percentage of premaxillary-maxillary suture opening was determined. Subsequently the data were tabulated and submitted to statistical analysis, adopting a level of significance of 5%. **Results:** The progression of premaxillary suture closure from birth to 12 years of age was 3.72% per year. In 100% of the skulls up to 12 years, the premaxillary-maxillary suture open in the palatal region was observed, while 6.16% of adults presented different degrees of opening. **Conclusions:** The premaxilla exists in an independent way within the maxillary complex and the presence of the premaxilla-maxillary suture justifies the success of anteroposterior expansions to stimulate the growth of the middle third of the face, solving anatomical and functional problems.

Keywords: Premaxilla. Maxillofacial development. Maxilla. Sutures.

[1] Universidade de São Paulo, Faculdade de Odontologia de Ribeirão Preto, Programa de Pós-Graduação de Odontopediatria (Ribeirão Preto/SP, Brazil).
[2] Universidade de São Paulo, Faculdade de Odontologia de Ribeirão Preto, Departamento de Clínica Infantil (Ribeirão Preto/SP, Brazil).
[3] Universidade do Sagrado Coração, Departamento de Odontologia (Bauru/SP, Brazil).
[4] Universidade de São Paulo, Faculdade de Odontologia de Bauru (Bauru/SP, Brazil).

» The authors report no commercial, proprietary or financial interest in the products or companies described in this article.

Alberto Consolaro
E-mail: consolaro@uol.com.br

INTRODUCTION

The premaxilla and the upper lip are formed between the fourth and seventh weeks of intrauterine life[1,2]. After that, the embryo's head elevates and no longer touches the cardiac prominence.[3] The mandible then grows, which creates room for the tongue to move down, at the same time that the palatine processes proliferate and elevate toward midline in a hinge movement,[4] to join and form the secondary palate[1,2] after leveling.

Around the seventh month of intrauterine life, there is a change in blood supply to the face at a critical time for the development of the face and the palate. The premaxilla begins to ossify at this stage,[5] and the center of ossification is separate from the actual maxilla.[6] In the anterior region, it levels with the primary palate, preserving the incisive foramen and canal in the midline, which are derived from the primary and secondary palates and contain vessels, nerves, glands and segments or remnants of the nasopalatine duct.[7]

In the first years of postnatal life, cranial growth predominates over facial growth.[8,9] During this period, mandibular growth is exuberant, while the growth of the maxillary complex is limited. The maxillary complex grows toward the anterior and inferior region[10] in a predominantly horizontal movement in the first decade of life and a vertical movement in the second decade. The morphological and clinical therapeutic descriptions of the maxillary complex hardly ever mention the anterior segment,[11] although it is an independent bone that only later overlaps into a semi-independent bone.

The premaxilla, where the four maxillary incisors are,[12,13] develops from the primary palate[5,14] and is closely related to the development of the human face.[12] The limits of the premaxilla are defined by a suture that goes from the incisive foramen to the region between the lateral incisors and canines, with a variable position between these teeth.[15] This gives shape to what has formerly been called the incisive bone.[5] This suture goes down from the junction of the maxillary and premaxillary growth centers, close to the lower portion of the pyriform aperture, to the alveolar margin in the region of the canine, crossing the palate to the incisive foramen.[16]

Four parts of the premaxilla may be identified: 1) its body, which is continuous with the maxilla; 2) its alveolar portion, which holds the teeth; 3) the palatine process; and 4) the stenonianus (infravomerine) process, which fuses with the cartilage of the nasal septum and vomer.[6]

The anatomy of the premaxillary area has not been fully described[17]. The time in its growth and development when the suture between the premaxilla and the maxilla fuses, so that they become a single bone, has not been determined.[18] Abnormal growth in this region may be correlated with malformations, such as prognathism, deep bite and protrusion.[12]

Comprehension of the mechanism of formation and the causes of orofacial developmental disorders requires full knowledge of embryology and anatomy.[7] The understanding of premaxillary development and how it is associated with the maxilla may:

1) Help to understand the etiology of cleft lip and palate and its subsequent effects on craniofacial growth, so that more refined and pertinent treatments of these developmental disorders may be planned

Initial facial development is not associated in any way with the ossification centers, which form later than the embryonic processes that give origin to facial tissues and components. Bone sutures are not the places where the embryonic processes touched each other. These are two independent phenomena, especially in relation to the time when they occur.[7]

Cleft position does not always coincide with the premaxillary-maxillary suture,[12,15,19] because bone development does not match primary facial development. Face formation lines are not identical to those where bone growth centers meet in all sutures, including the premaxillary-maxillary suture. Bilateral cleft lip and palate produce a premaxillary protrusion, which includes the soft tissue below the nose and the teeth in these region.[20] Treatment follows several stages, such as alveolar bone grafting, with a graft that may be autogenous or synthetically manufactured[22] and is used to fix the cleft. The existence of a premaxilla as an independent bone makes it possible to move it[18] to reduce the cleft before grafting and to place it at a more favorable position.

Premaxilla: up to which age it remains separated from the maxilla by a suture, how often it occurs in children...

3

2) Establish the principles and promote the development of new treatments for the changes in development and growth of the maxillary complex and the midface using the anteroposterior expansion of the maxilla

Orthodontic appliances may lead the premaxilla to a more beneficial anterior position[23,14] by stimulating the maxillary sutures.[23] The stimulation of the premaxillary-maxillary suture results in the development of this region[18,23-25] by means of inflammation and repair that culminates in remodeling the maxillary complex,[26] which may be used for the non-surgical protraction of the maxillary complex following, for example, the Ertty Gap III® protocol.[27] Therefore, the suture between the premaxilla and the maxilla may be the adequate biomechanical point for interventions in cases of Class III malocclusion, in which the diagnosis indicates insufficient maxillary complex development. The existence of a premaxilla as an independent bone allows for sutural movement and periosteal bone growth to correct certain malocclusions, with a reduction of risk and severity and even eliminating the need for surgery.

3) Establish and promote existing and new treatments for cases of nasal obstruction of newborns due to congenital pyriform aperture stenosis

Nasal obstruction in infants is a potentially serious condition[28], as it may lead to respiratory failure of the newborn[29]. One of its causes is congenital pyriform aperture stenosis, with a narrowing of the anterior third of the nasal fossa caused by excessive growth of the medial nasal process of the maxillary complex.[30] The intermaxillary bone, or premaxilla, is the main limit of the pyriform apertures, and parts of this bone may be occasionally seen lateral to the pyriform apertures up to about the fifth year of life, together with the nasal bone, which closes the pyriform aperture and touches the frontal bone.[12] The existence of the premaxilla as an independent bone makes it possible to move it[18] and thus remove airway obstructions.

Knowledge of all the aspects of the premaxillary bone and premaxillary-maxillary suture is essential and fundamental for clinical and therapeutic uses. Therefore, the objectives of this study were:

» To determine the frequency of an open premaxillary-maxillary suture in dry human skulls of children and adults.

» To analyze the topography of the premaxillary-maxillary suture to understand its function and relevance in the craniomandibular skeleton.

» To estimate the time of premaxillary-maxillary suture closure in human development.

» To evaluate the implications of these results for treatment options for situations, conditions and diseases that affect this anatomic region.

MATERIAL AND METHODS
Ethical issues

This project was submitted to and approved by the Ethics in Research Committee (ERC) of the *Faculdade de Odontologia de Ribeirão Preto, Universidade de São Paulo* (FORP-USP, under code CAAE 61308316.0.0000.5419), as well as by the ERC of the *Faculdade de Odontologia de Piracicaba, Universidade de Campinas* (FOP-UNICAMP, under code CAAE 61308316.0.3002.5418), and the ERC of the *Escola Paulista de Medicina, Universidade Federal do Estado de São Paulo* (EPM-UNIFESP, under code CAAE 61308316.0.3003.5505). This study used skulls of the Discipline of Anatomy of the *Faculdade de Odontologia de Bauru, Universidade de São Paulo* under permission from the professor responsible for its anatomic collection. Informed consent for the use of skulls was waived, but there was explicit authorization from the people responsible for the use of these specimens in each institution participating in the study.

Sample

Skulls were included in the study regardless of sex, ethnicity or age. Exclusion criteria were the impossibility to examine the site of the premaxillary-maxillary suture visually, cranial deformities and skulls of individuals that had syndromes.

Determination of age

Age was determined by evaluating the approximate phase of deciduous and permanent tooth eruption, as described by Schour and Massler (1941), and confirmed using the method described by Rai et al[31] (2014). Age groups were classified into scores, as described in Table 1. The determination of approximate age was not performed for adult skulls.

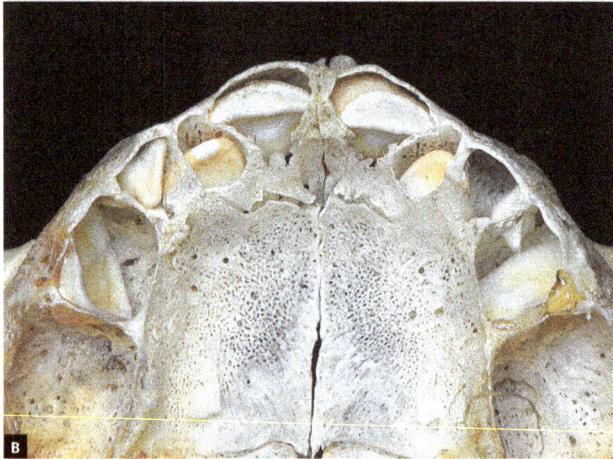

Figure 1 - A) Facial region; **B**) palatal region. Note the greater width of the premaxillary-maxillary suture, and its linear shape, perpendicular to the mid-palatal suture.

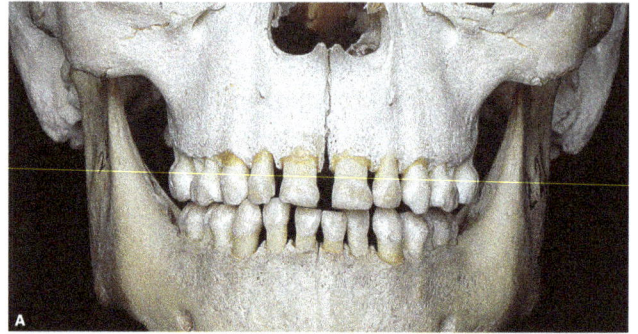

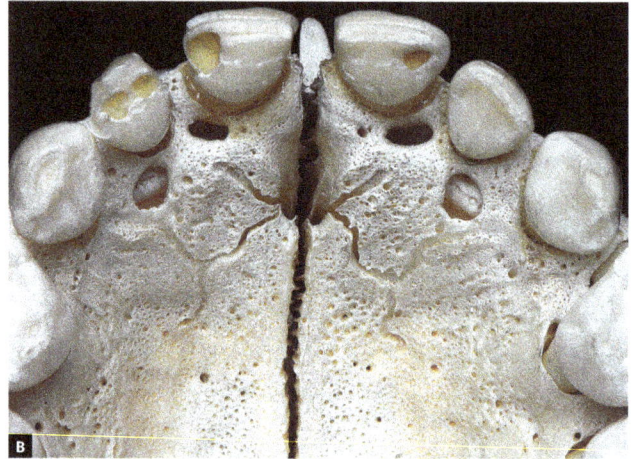

Figure 2 - A) Facial region; **B**) palatal region. Exuberant and serpiginous aspect of premaxillary-maxillary suture.

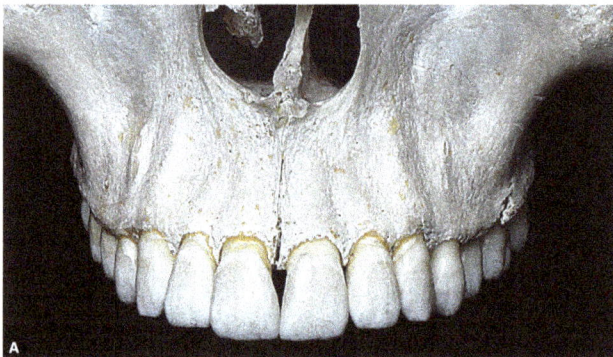

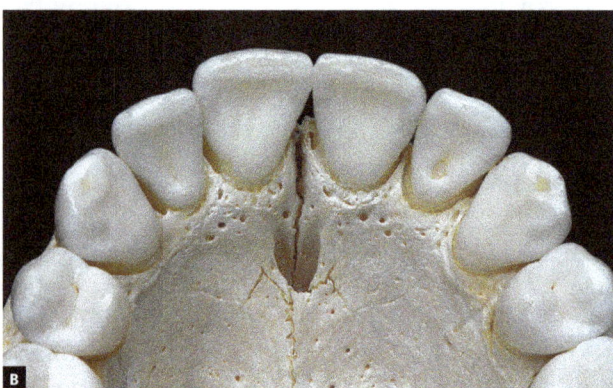

Figure 3 - A) Facial region; **B**) palatal region. Simple and linear aspect of premaxillary-maxillary suture.

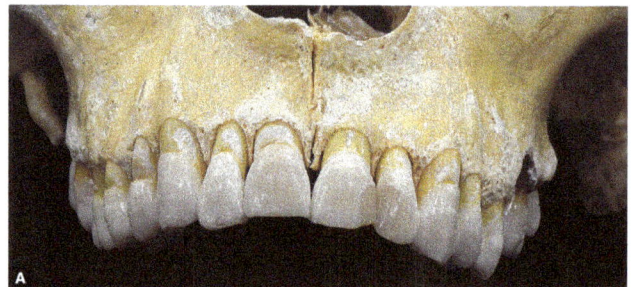

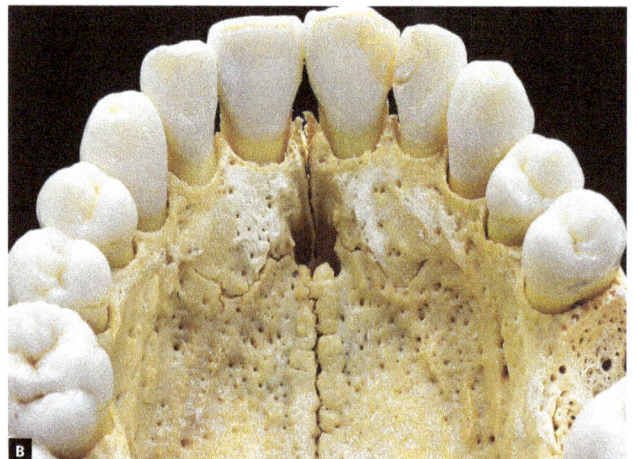

Figure 4 - A) Facial region; **B**) palatal region. Smaller width and origin in lateral wall of incisive foramen.

Table 1 - Scores for approximate age.

Score	Age group
0	Up to birth
1	0 to 3 years
2	3 to 6 years
3	6 to 9 years
4	9 to 12 years
-	Older than 12 years

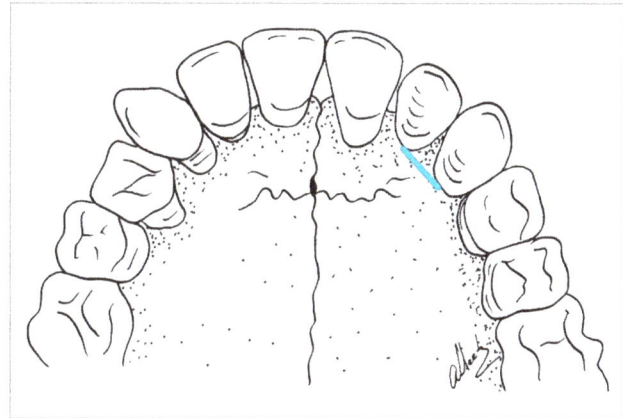

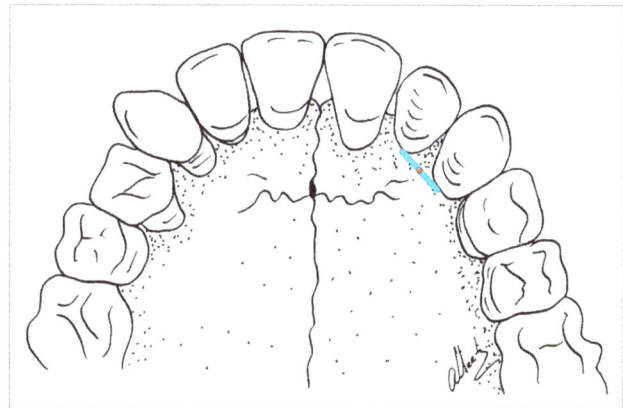

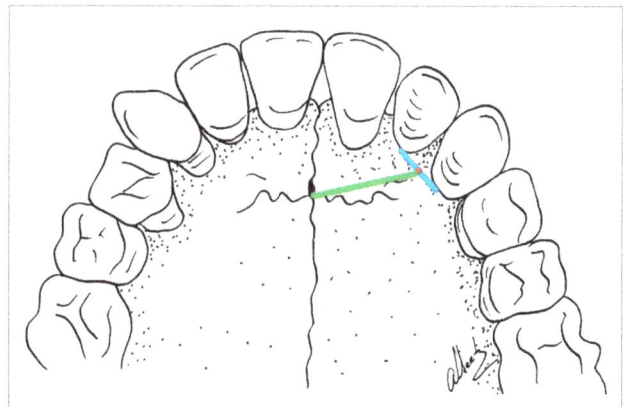

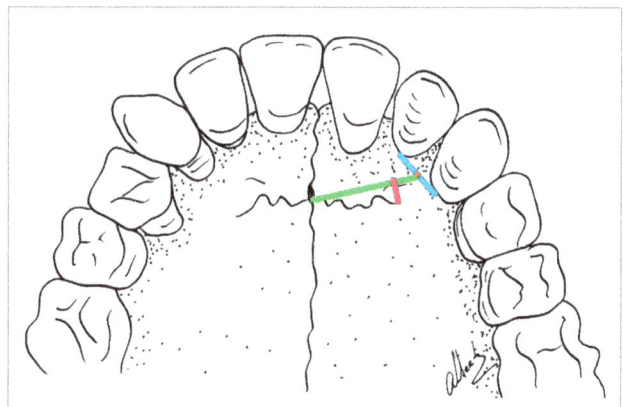

Determination of premaxillary-maxillary suture presence

All skulls were visually examined by two observers. The analyses were conducted following the different topographic regions on buccal and palatal views (Figs 1, 2, 3 and 4) because this bone does not develop uniformly or symmetrically in all regions. All skulls of individuals under 12 years of age were photographed. The skulls of older individuals were photographed only in cases of previous visual confirmation of the existence of the premaxillary-maxillary suture.

Determination of the opening/closing ratio of the premaxillary-maxillary suture

To determine the percentage of opening of the premaxillary-maxillary suture, two observers independently identified the side on which the suture had the longest opening and traced a straight line from the incisive foramen to the middle point between the maxillary lateral incisor and the maxillary canine in the palatal region. The end of the suture was projected orthographically onto this straight line, and the percentage of opening was calculated according to the ratio between the length of the open segment projection and the total segment length. The evaluation of suture opening percentage considered that 100% open were those sutures that reached the end of the straight line, and 0%, those that did not extend from the incisive foramen, as shown in Figure 5.

Figure 5 - Sequence to determine the percentage of premaxillary-maxillary suture opening/closure.

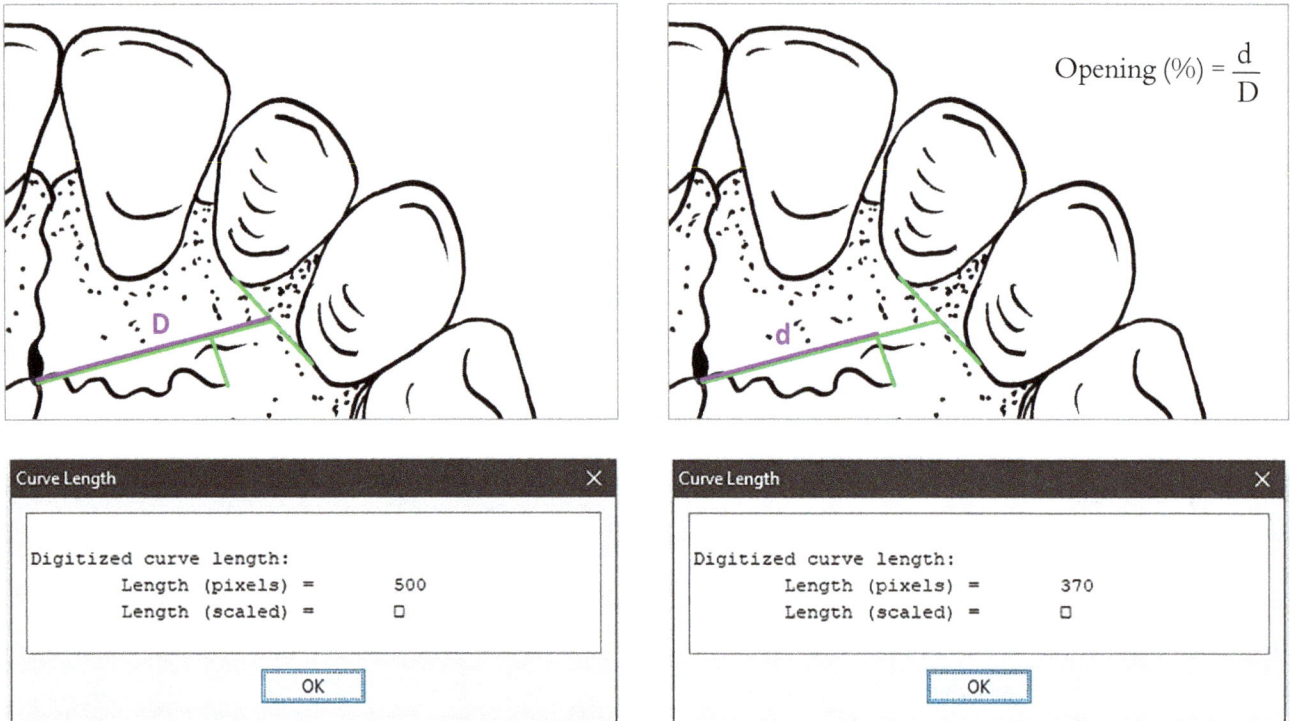

$$\text{Opening (\%)} = \frac{d}{D}$$

Figure 6 - Sequence to measure premaxillary-maxillary suture opening in pixels.

Statistical analysis

The data collected were tabulated using Microsoft Excel 2013 software. The segments described in the last section were measured using the software Plot Digitizer v. 2.6.8, which provides distances between two selected points in pixels (Fig 6). After that, data were analyzed using PAST software (Paleontological Statistics Software Package for Education and Data Analysis, National University of Ireland, Galway, Ireland). The Pearson correlation test was used to analyze the percentage of premaxillary-maxillary suture opening and the number of deciduous and permanent teeth, age and age scores. The level of significance was set at 5%.

RESULTS

Of the 1,138 specimens evaluated, 116 (10.19%) skulls were of infants and children, and 1,022 (89.81%), of adults. Of the infant and child skulls, 13 were of individuals in intrauterine life and 103, extra uterine life, as shown in Table 2 and illustrated in Figure 7.

The 13 skulls in the intrauterine life group had a gestational age of four to five months. They all had 100% opening of the premaxillary-maxillary suture on the palatal view, a finding that was repeated for all the

Table 2 - Number of specimens according to age groups.

Age group	Number of specimens	% of specimens
Intrauterine life	13	1.14%
Score 0	22	1.93%
Score 1	60	5.27%
Score 2	15	1.31%
Score 3	3	0.26%
Score 4	3	0.26%
Total no. of children	116	10.19%
Adults	1,022	89.81%
Total	1,138	100%

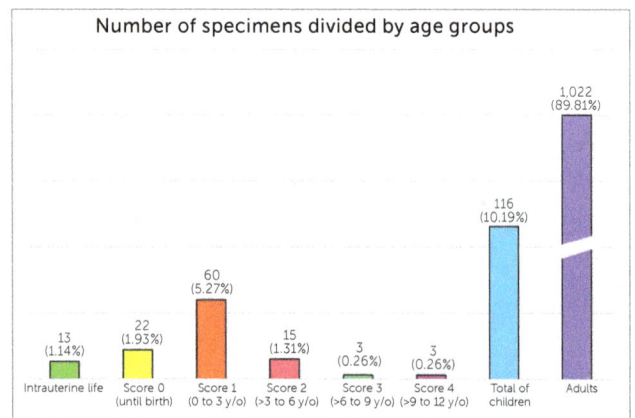

Figure 7 - Number of specimens divided by age groups.

Table 3 - Distribution of skulls of children according to mean premaxillary-maxillary suture opening and closure, and mean number of deciduous and permanent teeth according to age scores.

Age score	Number of skulls	Mean opening (%)	Mean closure (%)	Mean number of deciduous teeth	Mean number of permanent teeth
0	22	100	0	0	0
1	60	96.09	3.91	6.07	0
2	15	83.59	16.41	10	0.93
3	3	65.04	34.96	7.3	4.67
4	3	56.04	43.96	0.67	11.33
Total	103				

22 skulls of stillborns. An open suture was not identified on the frontal view of any of these specimens.

The 81 skulls of the extra uterine and not stillborn group belonged to children 6 months to 12 years old. The greatest frequency, 60 skulls, had score 1, that is, zero to three years of age; and 54% of them had 100% opening of the premaxillary-maxillary suture; the other 6 had openings ranging from 34.35% to 86.4%, with a standard deviation of 23.10% (Fig 12).

Table 3 shows skull distribution, mean premaxillary-maxillary suture opening percentage and mean number of deciduous and permanent teeth according to age scores. Closure percentage was recorded as the difference from the opening percentage (100% – opening%).

Figure 8 replicates the data in Table 3, but shows them as percentage of deciduous teeth, considering 20 teeth as complete deciduous dentition (100%), and percentage of permanent teeth, considering 28 teeth (100%) at age 12 as complete permanent dentition. The correlation between percentage of permanent teeth and premaxillary-maxillary suture was negative for opening and positive for closure.

The Pearson correlation test was used to quantify the correlation of premaxillary-maxillary suture closure and number of permanent teeth, number of deciduous teeth, age and age score. Results and p values are shown in Table 4.

The highest correlation coefficient was that between the mean number of permanent teeth and the percentage of premaxillary-maxillary suture closure ($r = 0.9177$), at a test power of $\alpha=1.0$ (Fig 9).

The analysis of number of permanent teeth revealed a value of $r=0.5294$ ($p= 8.95E-09$), which indicates a moderate positive correlation. The linear regression equation was $y= 0.0711x + 0.1064$. Figure 10 shows the regression line, the line equation and the values of r^2 and r. Figure 11 gives an example of the association between age in months and percentage of premaxillary-maxillary suture closure.

According to data for the skulls in the zero-to-12 years group and using the line equation and age in years, we found a projection of premaxillary-maxillary suture closure of 3.72% per year.

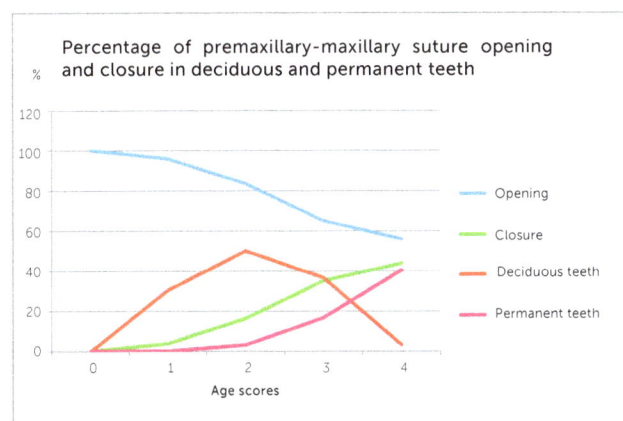

Figure 8 - Mean percentage of premaxillary-maxillary suture opening, mean percentage of deciduous teeth and mean percentage of permanent teeth according to age score.

	Closure of premaxillary-maxillary suture (%)	p value
No. permanent teeth	r= 0.5294	8.95E-09
No. deciduous teeth	r= 0.2907	0.0028976
Age	r= 0.6142	5.18E-12
Age score	r= 0.5550	1.17E-09

Table 4 - Pearson correlation between premaxillary-maxillary suture closure percentage and number of deciduous and permanent teeth, age and age scores.

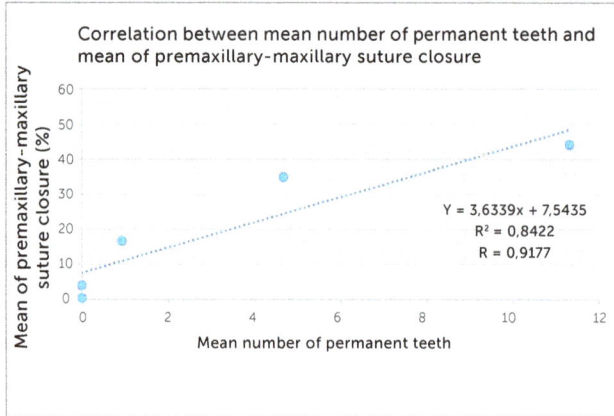

Figure 9 - Correlation between percentage of premaxillary-maxillary suture closure and mean number of permanent teeth.

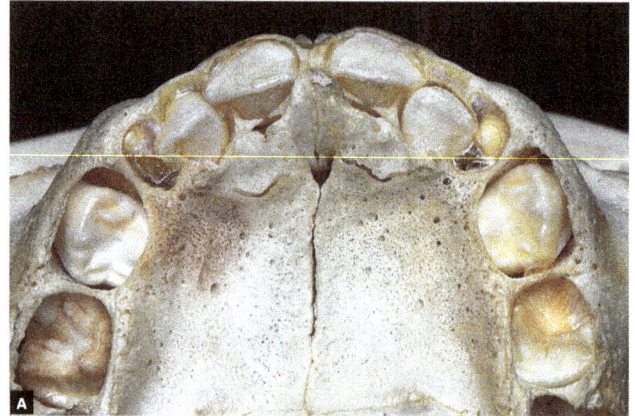

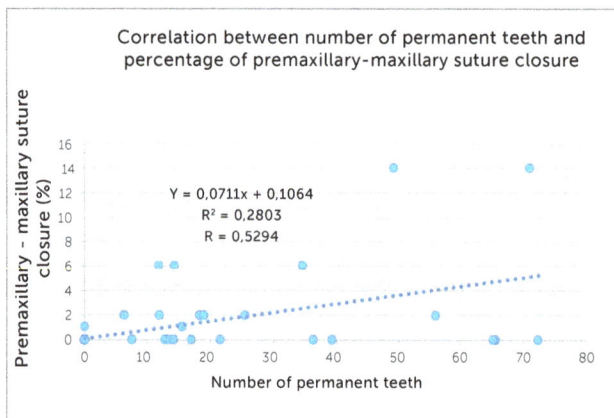

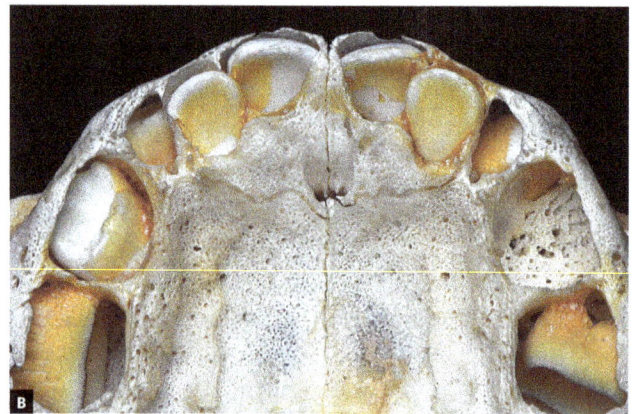

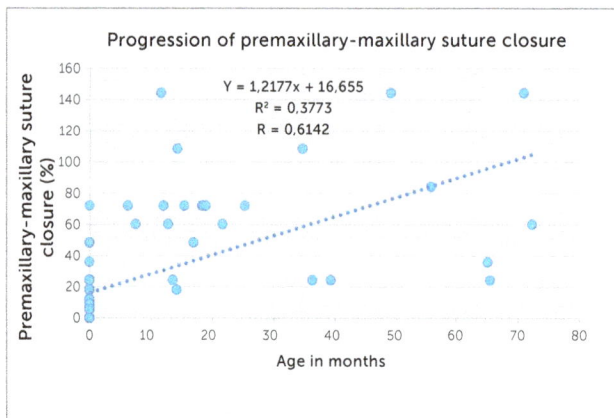

Figure 10 - Correlation between percentage of premaxillary-maxillary suture closure and number of permanent teeth.

Figure 11 - Correlation between age in months and percentage of premaxillary-maxillary suture closure: progression of premaxillary-maxillary suture closure.

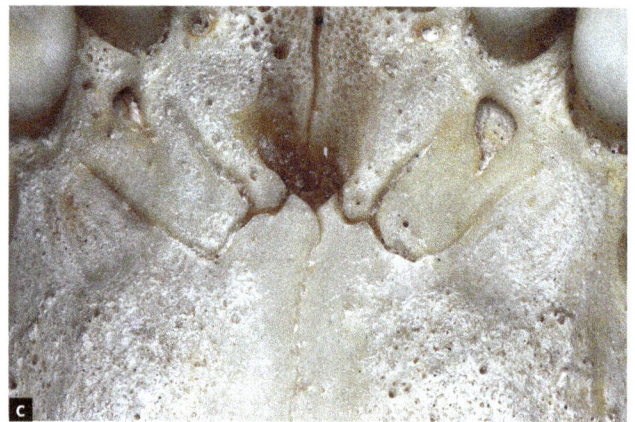

Figure 12 - Morphological patterns of premaxillary-maxillary suture in children, with irregular shapes that are simple or complex, but always greatly variable.

Of the 1,022 adult skulls, 959 (93.84%) had a completely closed suture, that is, there was no suture, whereas 63 (6.16%) had different percentages of open and partially open sutures (Figs 13 and 15).

Mean percentage of premaxillary-maxillary suture opening in the 63 skulls with a opening suture was 41.11%, with a standard deviation of 25.28%, a minimal value of 10%, a maximal value of 90%, and a median value of 30%. Figure 14 shows a boxplot with the minimal and maximal values, median value and quartiles.

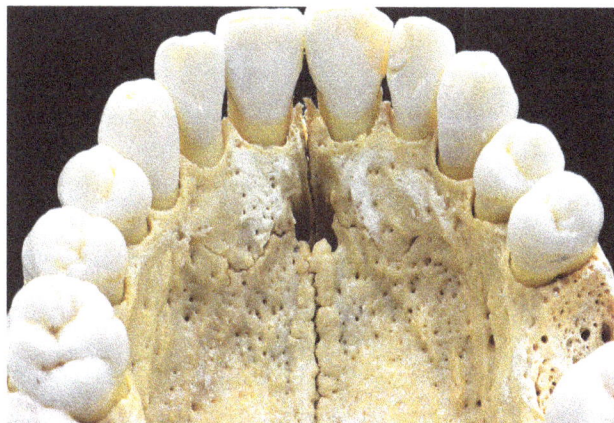

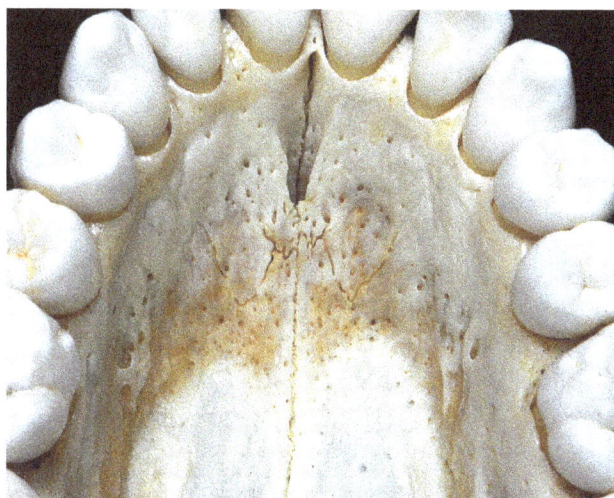

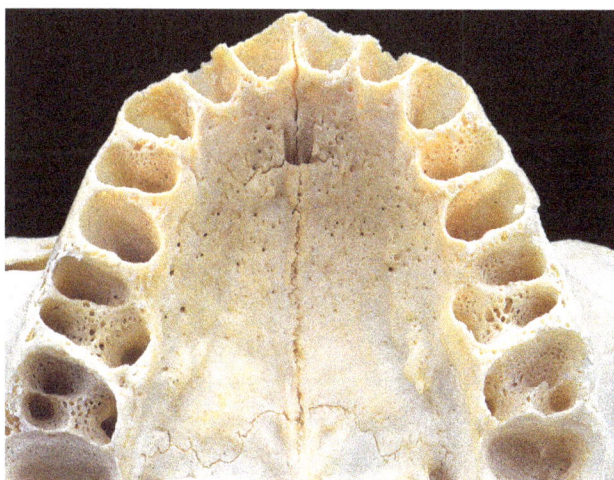

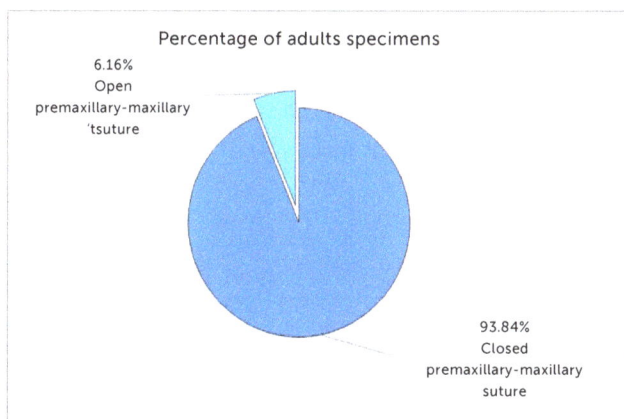

Figure 13 - Prevalence of adult skulls with open premaxillary-maxillary suture and closed premaxillary-maxillary suture.

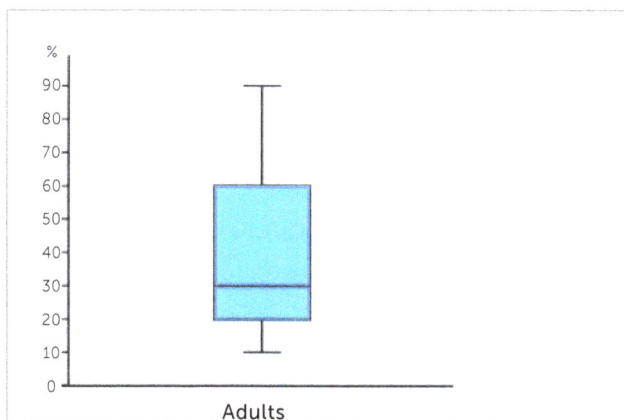

Figure 14 - Boxplot of the percentage of open premaxillary-maxillary sutures in adult skulls.

Figure 15 - Morphological patterns of premaxillary-maxillary suture in adults: note great morphological variability.

DISCUSSION

Neglected and still denied today by many scholars, the existence of the premaxilla offers treatment options to promote the growth of the mid third of the face, which may be a solution for some severe anatomical and functional problems.

In several areas of human development, no other element has raised as much controversy and discussion as the premaxilla. However, these facts do not justify its absence or little importance in innumerable Anatomy, Orthodontics and Odontopediatrics textbooks, among others,[13,16,32,33] especially when its relevance is taken into consideration.[6,18] Classified as a transient osseous element, with certain proper ossification centers, and subsequently unified to the maxilla,[6,13,18,34-36] denying its existence is a basic conceptual mistake.[33,38-41]

The resistance to its recognition probably results from its early closure in the facial region,[16,42-44] that is, in the alveolar part with facial process, which supposedly occurs in the first trimester of prenatal life.[16] The earliest age found in this study was for a specimen of 16 weeks of intrauterine life, in which no opening of the suture was seen on the frontal view. Therefore, its closure in this region occurred at four months of intrauterine life.

The absence of a suture on the facial side results from the fusion of the nasal and incisive bone processes of the maxilla, which, however, remains patent in the palatal region during all early childhood.[13,45] Despite that, it may sometimes persist into adulthood, as demonstrated in this study. This is an indication of the development of the human face, as the human premaxilla is similar to that of other mammals in shape, sutural limits, ossification, place and function, except for its absence on the facial side in certain stages of development[6]. In the newborn skull, sutures are widely open to allow for bone growth. Before they grow, a large number of bones, over 300, are independent, but that number goes down to 206 in adults because of the unification of several bones.[46]

In 2015, Botti et al[47] reported that premaxillae are difficult to identify in studies of human anatomy, but argued that denying the existence of premaxillary bones would be incompatible with the successive development of the primary and secondary palates, as well as with the persistence of the incisive canal as a vestige of its articulation to form the hard palate.

The agenesis of the premaxillary bone in some diseases[48,49] makes its existence and autonomy obvious, because the bone posterior to the premaxillary-maxillary suture, the maxillary bone, is present and functional.

Variability in suture obliteration time may be one more of the reasons that make the premaxilla a singular bone that is so rarely studied or used for treatments. These findings have been confirmed in this study by the innumerable time differences in suture obliteration, which suggest that premaxillary-maxillary suture closure in the palatal region occurs as age advances. This process is similar to that of formation and growing of permanent teeth, which are also associated with age, as reported previously.[50] The analysis of Figure 8 reveals a similarity between the curves of increase in the number of permanent teeth and increase in closure of the suture under study.

The morphological disappearance of the premaxillary-maxillary suture, at an earlier age or in adults, may be assigned to the vertical growth of the maxillary complex and, in consequence, of all hard palate. The growth of the vertical maxillary complex has been described in Embryology textbooks that report growth as craniomandibular[33]. This vertical growth makes palatal bone remodeling and reshaping more dynamic and constant, so that it responds to new functional and anatomical demands of craniomandibular growth. As this growth is constant and moves the hard palate down and forward, inevitably the premaxillary-maxillary suture tends to disappear, because is no longer submitted to functional demands after a certain period.

Sex and nutritional status affect the time of appearance of both the ossification centers in an individual and, consequently, bone development,[51-53] which may justify the large variation in the times of premaxillary-maxillary suture closure found in the present study. However, on the palatal side, this suture often remains patent during all early childhood. We found 100% opening of the premaxillary-maxillary suture in 54 (52.42%) specimens aged zero to three years, and three (20%) of those aged three to six years. No specimens aged more than six years had 100% opening.

The present results suggest that the premaxillary-maxillary suture closes earlier on the facial side, but remains open at different rates in the palatal region during childhood and, sometimes, into adulthood.

This opening may be a biomechanical point for orthodontic and orthopedic action that may lead to favorable results both esthetically and anatomically.

At 12 years of age, the premaxillary-maxillary suture may remain open, as three (100%) skulls in that age group had an open suture in this study. The age group of specimens of older individuals could not be determined at a minimally accurate level.

According to the approximate estimation of premaxillary-maxillary suture closure from birth to 12 years defined in this study, closure occurs at a rate of 3.72% per year. Therefore, the earlier the intervention, the easier and more flexible is bone movement, and the greater are the chances of success.

A suture is the connection between two bones, a narrow band of dense fibrous connective tissue that forms an immovable joint.[26,54] Sutures unite bones and play an important role in growth, as they are remodeled by stimulation,[26,54] which is the case of the sutures in the maxillary complex,[23] including the premaxillary-maxillary suture.

The maxillary complex is composed of membranous, highly malleable bones whose sutures act as growth sites[12] when stimulated to proliferate,[55,56] that is, when the bones that are joined by these sutures are submitted to traction. The premaxillary-maxillary suture, called incisive suture in the past, outlines the palatine process of the premaxilla and the palatine process of the maxilla,[6] and, therefore, generates growth in these areas when stimulated. Therefore, the manipulation of the premaxillary-maxillary suture may correct deficiencies in the horizontal development of the maxillary complex before bony bridges are created, in which case surgical expansion is necessary. This is the case of median palatal expansion, in which failure is associated with the skeletal maturation of the patient.[23,56-58] In 1982, Schwartz[56] found an association of success and failure of orthopedic protraction of the maxillary complex with premaxillary-maxillary suture closure.

The use of the Ertty Gap III® protocol had excellent results in maxillary complex protraction in children up to 13 years of age. It is simple, has a low cost, and its esthetic results are satisfactory when compared with other appliances for the same purpose. With an intraoral system, there is greater collaboration by the patient, and the continuity of force application promotes better results than intermittent forces, which is usually the case of other appliances.[27]

In relation to the maxillary complex, which is divided into anterior, middle and posterior, the premaxillary bone is usually included in the maxilla. However, the present authors suggest that the term maxilla should refer only to the portion derived from the embryonic maxilla,[6,13] and should not include the premaxillary bone, because the anterior, premaxillary segment is autonomous during a certain time of human development and extremely valuable anatomically and functionally. Moreover, the term premaxilla should remain in use for human beings, even after the incomplete or complete closure of the premaxillary-maxillary suture.[13]

In adults, some remnants of the suture in the palatal region may be seen, which is in agreement with other findings.[12,43,50] In Germany, Kadanoff et al[59] found the premaxillary-maxillary suture or its remnants in 11.1% of the adults. In our study, in Brazil, we found it in 6.16% of the specimens, but it was not possible to accurately determine the geographic origin of each specimen. The premaxilla tends to disappear in adulthood.[12] Therefore, expansion attempts to correct problems associated with positioning should be approached in childhood, and chances of success are greater at earlier ages because of bone development and maturation (Fig 16).

The association between premaxilla and maxilla has also been the focus of discussions and disagreement and is hard to understand.[32] Some authors argue in favor of a "fusion theory", in which there is the unification of the two bones,[16,60-62] whereas others defend a theory of "excessive growth", in which the premaxilla would be "embraced" by the maxilla.[13,42,63] Shepherd and McCarthy,[6] in 1955, however, demonstrated that the concepts above are not sufficient to describe the correlation between bones, and that what in fact occurs is resorption and replacement: while the premaxilla undergoes resorption, the maxillary trabecular bone fuses into the premaxillary bone. These three concepts are complementary and progressively explain the association between bones from the beginning to the end of the process. The growth of the maxillary complex generates several pressure and tension forces that direct its enlargement and growth and determine its final bone shape: these forces are called growth vectors. The explanation that we have for this anatomical continuity between the premaxilla and the maxilla claims that it occurs due to accelerated bone remodeling and re-

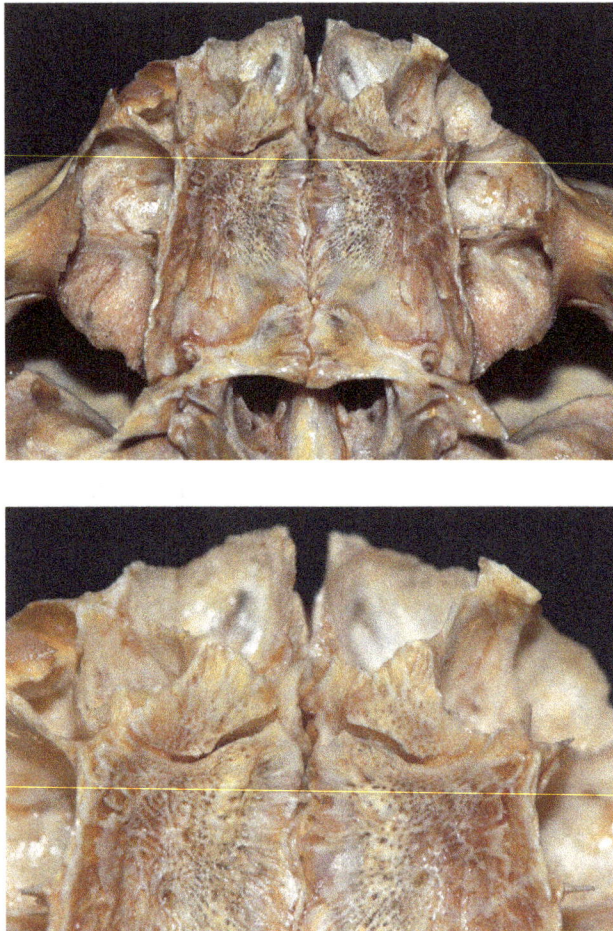

Figure 16 - Early development of premaxillary-maxillary suture, about six months postnatally. Distribution of trabecular bone associated with sutures and cortical bone, probably due to growth vectors.

shaping in the palatal region to respond to vertical growth of the face, as previously mentioned. Bone remodeling and bone reshaping in the entire skeleton respond to functional demands, and their continuity eventually eliminates the premaxillary-maxillary suture when the functional demands for the premaxilla no longer exist. Therefore, the bone structures of both parts unite, and the suture tends to disappear without any perceptible sign in most human beings. Its most clarifying evaluation should be conducted using imaging studies. Occasionally it appears on occlusal radiographs of patients in the first decade of life, but it is thin and narrow, which makes its visualization difficult on conventional imaging studies.[23] The attempt to visualize the suture on both conventional and digital occlusal radiographs of randomly selected skulls was not successful, as it was not possible to identify it in pilot studies carried out before

this study. The use of CT may enable its visualization and measurement, but the efficiency and pertinence of tests and protocols should be evaluated before they are used. The use of CT scans in pediatric patients should be carefully evaluated and considered because of the latency of side effects for individuals with a longer life expectancy, such as children, who form a group at a greater risk than adults.

This study confirmed once more the existence of the premaxillary-maxillary suture and its frequency, and this confirmation supports the use of treatment strategies for the anteroposterior expansion of the maxillary complex.[27] However, as mentioned before, this depends on skeletal maturity, and consultations and diagnoses at an early age are essential because treatment success is inversely proportional to development.

The simplicity of the fact that the premaxillary-maxillary suture explains a difficult concept, the anteroposterior expansion of the maxillary complex, may excite the sensitive nature of researchers. There is no better theory to explain the clinical results obtained.[55] The movement of the premaxilla offers new opportunities for Orthopedics, Orthodontics and surgeries of this anatomical region to treat craniomandibular development and growth disorders.[18] The resolution of conditions, such as the reduction of cleft lip and palate, the removal of nasal obstruction in congenital stenosis and correction of prognathism due to deficient development of the maxillary complex (Ertty Gap III[27]), involves several areas of knowledge in Dentistry and, therefore, their associations and prognoses are complex. Moreover, several correlations should be defined in future studies:

1. Identify, limit and evaluate premaxillary-maxillary suture closure using imaging studies, including 3D reconstructions, as planning and prognosis parameters of orthodontic and orthopedic maxillary treatments.

2. Correlate premaxillary-maxillary suture closure and midpalatal suture closure[65]. Late closure with opening of the midpalatal suture may be associated with the same phenomenon for the premaxillary-maxillary suture.

3. Investigate the association between premaxillary-maxillary suture closure or its prolonged opening with facial patterns or occlusion Classes I, II or III.[50] Early or late closure of the premaxillary-maxillary suture may affect facial type.

4. Study the interference of midpalatal expansions using different appliances, such as Haas, Hyrax and MARPE, in the premaxillary-maxillary suture, as the anterior screws of the MARPE appliance are placed at the level of the third palatine rugae, very close to the premaxillary-maxillary suture. The effect that it may have on maxillary process movement should be studied, because these screws may not be located in the maxilla in all cases — and if the premaxilla with a suture is still present, results may be different.[11,66]

5. Study premaxillary-maxillary suture opening or closure and the intensification of childhood oral habits and how they may be associated.

The existence of the premaxilla was used as a reference point at the time of Goethe to distinguish human beings from other mammals,[46] as unusual as it may seem to be today. At that time, the premaxilla was seen as one of the characteristics that differentiated animals from human beings. When Goethe detected and described the human premaxilla to the scientific community, a taboo was broken and, at the same time, placed him in history as one of the precursors of Darwin's theory of evolution. However, still today we find texts that deny the independent existence and identity of this anatomical and functional structure. The present results in a study of 1,138 dry human skulls allow us to argue that the premaxilla does exist!

CONCLUSIONS

The results of this study suggest that:

1. The progression rate of premaxillary-maxillary suture closure from birth to 12 years of age was 3.72% per year.

2. All pediatric skulls up to 12 years of age had an open premaxillary-maxillary suture in the palatal region, at different opening percentages.

3. Adults may have an open premaxillary-maxillary suture.

4. The percentage of adults with an open premaxillary-maxillary suture was 6.16%.

5. The presence of a premaxillary-maxillary suture explains the success of anteroposterior expansion of the maxillary complex.

6. The existence of the premaxillary-maxillary suture supports the use of treatments for the growth of the middle third of the face to solve anatomical and functional problems.

Acknowledgements

We thank professors Ana Claudia Rossi, PhD, Eduardo Cotecchia Ribeiro, PhD, Jesus Carlos Andreo, PhD, and Simone Cecilio Hallak Regalo, PhD.

Author's contribution (ORCID ⓘ)

Mariana Trevizan (MT): 0000-0002-7582-1167 ⓘ
Paulo Nelson Filho (PNF): 0000-0001-8802-6480 ⓘ
Solange de O. B. F. (SOBG): 0000-0002-6396-2886 ⓘ
Alberto Consolaro (AC): 0000-0002-5902-5646 ⓘ

Data acquisition, analysis or interpretation: MT, PNF, SOBG, AC. Critical revision of the article: MT, PNF, SOBG, AC. Final approval of the article: MT, PNF, SOBG, AC.

REFERENCES

1. Lubit EC. Fissura labial palatina. Quintessência. 1978;512(3):1-7.
2. Pashley NR, Krause CJ. Cleft lip, cleft palate, and other fusion disorders. Otolaryngol Clin North Am. 1981 Feb;14(1):125-43.
3. Ferguson MW. Developmental mechanisms in normal and abnormal palate formation with particular reference to the aetiology, pathogenesis and prevention of cleft palate. Br J Orthod. 1981 July;8(3):115-37.
4. Tuchmann DH, Haegel PH, Solère M. Embriología cuadernos prácticos. 2ª ed. Barcelona: Toray-Masson; 1969.
5. Sperber GH. Craniofacial embryology. 2ª ed. Chicago: Year Book Medical Publishers; 1976.
6. Shepherd WM, Mc Carthy M. Observations on the appearance and ossification of the premaxilla and maxilla in the human embryo. Anat Rec. 1955 Jan;121(1):13-28.
7. Consolaro A, Trevizan M, Consolaro RB, Oliveira IA. Mecanismos de formação da face: o que ocorre é nivelamento, e não fusão, dos processos. Rev Clin Ortod Dental Press. 2017;15(5):96-110.
8. Bishara SE. Textbook of Orthodontics. San Louis: WB Saunders; 2000.
9. Bishara SE. Ortodontia. 2ª ed. São Paulo: Ed. Santos; 2004.
10. Bjork A, Skieller V. Growth and development of the maxillary complex. Inf Orthod Kieferorthop. 1984;16(1):9-52.
11. Suzuki HM, Previdente LH. Suzuki SS, Garcez AS, Consolaro A. Expansão Rápida da Maxila Assistida com Mini-implantes / MARPE: em busca de um movimento ortopédico puro. Rev Clin Ortod Dental Press. 2016;15(1):110-25.
12. Barteczko K, Jacob M. A re-evaluation of the premaxillary bone in humans. Anat Embryol (Berl). 2004 Mar;207(6):417-37. Epub 2004 Feb 4.

13. Woo JK. Ossification and growth of the human maxilla, premaxilla and palate bone. Anat Rec. 1949 Dec;105(4):737-61.

14. Revelo B, Fishman LS. Maturational evaluation of ossification of the midpalatal suture. Am J Orthod Dentofacial Orthop. 1994;105(3):288-92.

15. Lisson JA, Kjaer I. Location of alveolar clefts relative to the incisive fissure. Cleft Palate Craniofac J. 1997 July;34(4):292-6.

16. Noback CR, Moss ML. The topology of the human premaxillary bone. Am J Phys Anthropol. 1953 June;11(2):181-8.

17. Hafkamp HC, Bruintjes TD, Huizing EH. Functional anatomy of the premaxillary area. Rhinology. 1999;37(1):21-4.

18. Trevizan M, Consolaro A. Premaxilla: an independent bone that can base therapeutics for middle third growth! Dental Press J Orthod. 2017 Mar-Apr;22(2):21-6.

19. Delaire J. Lateral limits of the os incisivum. Fortschr Kieferorthop. 1965;26(4):391-5.

20. Baxter DJ, Shroff MM. Developmental maxillofacial anomalies. Semin Ultrasound CT MR. 2011 Dec;32(6):555-68.

21. Precious DS. A new reliable method for alveolar bone grafting at about 6 years of age. J Oral Maxillofac Surg. 2009 Oct;67(10):2045-53.

22. Hallman M, Thor A. Bone substitutes and growth factors as an alternative/complement to autogenous bone for grafting in implant dentistry. Periodontol 2000. 2008;47:172-92.

23. Haskell BS, Farman AG. Exploitation of the residual premaxillary-maxillary suture site in maxillary protraction. An hypothesis. Angle Orthod. 1985 Apr;55(2):108-19.

24. Vardimon AD, Graber TM, Voss LR, Verrusio E. Magnetic versus mechanical expansion with different force thresholds and points of force application. Am J Orthod Dentofacial Orthop. 1987;92(6):455-66.

25. Witzig JW, Spahl TJ. The clinical management of basic maxillofacial orthopedic appliances. St. Louis: C.V. Mosby; 1987.

26. Consolaro A, Consolaro MFM-O. Protocolo semanal repetitivo de expansão rápida da maxila e constrição alternadas e técnica da protração maxilar ortopédica efetiva: Porque? Como?. Rev Clin Ortod Dental Press. 2007;6(6):110-1.

27. Silva E, Meloti F, Pinho S, Gasque CA. Correção da Classe III esquelética em pacientes jovens – Ertty Gap III®. Orthod Sci Pract. 2017;10(39):244-64.

28. Faust RA, Phillips CD. Assessment of congenital bony nasal obstruction by 3-dimensional CT volume rendering. Int J Pediatr Otorhinolaryngol. 2001 Oct 19;61(1):71-5.

29. Brown OE, Myer CM, Manning SC. Congenital nasal pyriform aperture stenosis. Laryngoscope. 1989;99(1):86-91.

30. Tagliarini JV, Nakajima V, Castilho EC. Congenital nasal pyriform aperture stenosis. Braz J Otorhinolaryngol. 2005;71(2):246-9.

31. Rai V, Saha S, Yadav G, Tripathi AM, Grover K. Dental and skeletal maturity - a biological indicator of chronologic age. J Clin Diagn Res. 2014 Sept;8(9):ZC60–4.

32. Carmody KA, Mooney MP, Cooper GM, Bonar CJ, Siegel MI, Dumont ER, et al. Relationship of premaxillary bone and its sutures to deciduous dentition in nonhuman primates. Cleft Palate Craniofac J. 2008 Jan;45(1):93-100.

33. Ten Cate AR. Histologia Bucal : Desenvolvimento Estrutura e Funcao. 5ª ed. Rio de Janeiro: Guanabara Koogan; 2001.

34. Kraus BS, Decker JD. The prenatal inter-relationships of the maxilla and premaxilla in the facial development of man. Acta Anat. 1960;40:278-94.

35. Kvinnsland S. Observations on the early ossification of the upper jaw. Acta Odontol Scand. 1969;27(6):649-54.

36. Mooney MP, Siegel MI. Developmental relationship between premaxillary-maxillary suture patency and anterior nasal spine morphology. Cleft Palate J. 1986;23(2):101-7.

37. Mooney MP, Siegel MI, Kimes KR, Todhunter J. Premaxillary development in normal and cleft lip and palate human fetuses using three-dimensional computer reconstruction. Cleft Palate J. 1991;28(1):49-53.

38. Wood NK, Wragg LE, Stuteville OH. The premaxilla: embryological evidence that it does not exist in man. Anat Rec. 1967 Aug;158(4):485-9.

39. Wood NK, Wragg LE, Stuteville OH, Oglesby RJ. Osteogenesis of the human upper jaw: proof of the non-existence of a separate premaxillary centre. Arch Oral Biol. 1969 Nov;14(11):1331-9.

40. Vacher C, Onolfo JP, Lezy JP, Copin H. The growth of the maxilla in humans. What place for the premaxilla? Rev Stomatol Chir Maxillofac. 2001 June;102(3-4):153-8.

41. Jacobson A. Embryological Evidence for the Non-Existence of the Premaxilla in Man. Angle Orthod. 1957;27(4):199-201.

42. Wood-Jones F. The Fate of the Human Premaxilla. J Anat. 1938 Apr;72(Pt 3):462.

43. Behrents RG, Harris EF. The premaxillary-maxillary suture and orthodontic mechanotherapy. Am J Orthod Dentofacial Orthop. 1991 Jan;99(1):1-6.

44. Macklin C. The skull of a human fetus of forty-three mm greatest length. Contribution to Embriology. 1921;48(10):57-103.

45. Sejrsen B, Kjaer I, Jakobsen J. The human incisal suture and premaxillary area studied on archaeologic material. Acta Odontol Scand. 1993;51(3):143-51.

46. Consolaro A. A pré-maxila e a evolução do homem!. Jornal da Cidade. 2018 [2018 20 Out];(25). Disponível em: https://www.jcnet.com.br/Ciencias/2018/10/a-premaxila-e-a-evolucao-do-homem-por-alberto-consolaro.

47. Botti S, Rumeau C, Gallet P, Jankowski R. Vomero-premaxillary joint: a marker of evolution of the species. Eur Ann Otorhinolaryngol Head Neck Dis. 2017 Apr;134(2):83-7.

48. Chen CP, Huang JP, Chen YY, Chern SR, Wu PS, Su JW, et al. Chromosome 18p deletion syndrome presenting holoprosencephaly and premaxillary agenesis: prenatal diagnosis and aCGH characterization using uncultured amniocytes. Gene. 2013 Sept 25;527(2):636-41.

49. Savastano CP, El-Jaick KB, Costa-Lima MA, Abath CM, Bianca S, Cavalcanti DP, et al. Molecular analysis of holoprosencephaly in South America. Genet Mol Biol. 2014 Mar;37(1 Suppl):250-62.

50. Maureille B, Bar D. The premaxilla in Neandertal and early modern children: ontogeny and morphology. J Hum Evol. 1999 Aug;37(2):137-52.

51. Pryor JW. Difference in the Ossification of the Male and Female Skeleton. J Anat. 1928 July;62(Pt 4):499-506.

52. Francis CC. Factors influencing appearance of centers of ossification during early childhood: II. A comparative study of degree of epiphysial ossification in infancy under varying conditions of diet and health. Am J Dis Child. 1940;59(5):1006-12.

53. Christie AU, Dunham EC, Jenss RM, Dippel A. Development of the center for the cuboid bone in newborn infants: a roentgenographic study. Am J Dis Child. 1941;61(3):471-82.

54. Consolaro A, Consolaro MFM-O. Expansão Rápida da Maxila e Constrição Alternadas (ERMC-Alt) e técnica de Protração Maxilar Ortopédica Efetiva: extrapolação de conhecimentos prévios para fundamentação biológica. Rev Dental Press Ortod Ortop Facial. 2008;13(1):18-23.

55. Spahl TJ. More on premaxillary-maxillary suture. Am J Orthod Dentofacial Orthop. 1991;100(6):19a-23a.

56. Schwartz JH. Dentofacial growth and development in Homo sapiens: evidence from perinatal individuals from Punic Carthage. Anatomischer Anzeiger. 1982;152(1):1-26.

57. Wertz RA. Skeletal and dental changes accompanying rapid midpalatal suture opening. Am J Orthod. 1970;58(1):41-66.

58. Wertz R, Dreskin M. Midpalatal suture opening: a normative study. Am J Orthod. 1977;71(4):367-81.

59. Kadanoff D, Mutafov S, Jordanov J. Anthropological and anatomical characteristics of the bony palate. Gegenbaurs Morphol Jahrb. 1969;114(2):169-76.

60. Chase W. The early development of the human premaxilla. Am Dent Assoc. 1942;29(17):1991-2001.

61. Piersol GA. Human Anatomy. 9th ed. Philadelphia: Lippincott; 1930.

62. Scaeffer JP. Morris' Human Anatomy: a complete systematic treatise. 10th ed. Philadelphia: The Blakiston; 1942.

63. Ashley-Montagu MF. The Premaxilla in the Primates. Quarterly Rev Biol. 1935;10(1):32-59.

64. Brenner DJ, Doll R, Goodhead DT, Hall EJ, Land CE, Little JB, et al. Cancer risks attributable to low doses of ionizing radiation: assessing what we really know. Proc Natl Acad Sci U S A. 2003 Nov 25;100(24):13761-6. Epub 2003 Nov 10.

65. Ennes JP. Consolaro A, Ortis MFM, Velloso TRG. O periósteo e a ortopedia dos maxilares. Rev Dental Press Ortod Ortop Facial. 2001;6(4):77-89.

66. Consolaro A. Reabsorções dentárias nas especialidades clínicas. 3ª ed. Maringá: Dental Press; 2005.

2

Perception of midline deviations in smile esthetics by laypersons

Jamille Barros Ferreira[1], Licínio Esmeraldo da Silva[2], Márcia Tereza de Oliveira Caetano[3], Andrea Fonseca Jardim da Motta[3], Adriana de Alcantara Cury-Saramago[3], José Nelson Mucha[4]

Objective: To evaluate the esthetic perception of upper dental midline deviation by laypersons and if adjacent structures influence their judgment. **Methods:** An album with 12 randomly distributed frontal view photographs of the smile of a woman with the midline digitally deviated was evaluated by 95 laypersons. The frontal view smiling photograph was modified to create from 1 mm to 5 mm deviations in the upper midline to the left side. The photographs were cropped in two different manners and divided into two groups of six photographs each: group LCN included the lips, chin, and two-thirds of the nose, and group L included the lips only. The laypersons performed the rate of each smile using a visual analog scale (VAS). Wilcoxon test, Student's t-test and Mann-Whitney test were applied, adopting a 5% level of significance. **Results:** Laypersons were able to perceive midline deviations starting at 1 mm. Statistically significant results ($p < 0.05$) were found for all multiple comparisons of the values in photographs of group LCN and for almost all comparisons in photographs of group L. Comparisons between the photographs of groups LCN and L showed statistically significant values ($p < 0.05$) when the deviation was 1 mm. **Conclusions:** Laypersons were able to perceive the upper dental midline deviations of 1 mm, and above when the adjacent structures of the smiles were included. Deviations of 2 mm and above when the lips only were included. The visualization of structures adjacent to the smile demonstrated influence on the perception of midline deviation.

Keywords: Esthetics, dental. Photography, dental. Perception. Orthodontics.

[1] Master's degree in Orthodontics, Universidade Federal Fluminense, Niterói/RJ, Brazil.

[2] Professor, Statistics Department, Universidade Federal Fluminense, Niterói/RJ, Brazil.

[3] Professor, Dental Clinics Department, Universidade Federal Fluminense, Niterói/RJ, Brazil.

[4] Full professor, Dental Clinics Department, Universidade Federal Fluminense, Niterói/RJ, Brazil.

» The authors report no commercial, proprietary or financial interest in the products or companies described in this article.

Andrea Fonseca Jardim da Motta
Rua Mário Santos Braga, 30, 2º andar, sala 214, Campus do Valonguinho, Centro, Niterói, RJ, Brazil, CEP: 24.020-140
E-mail: andreamotta@id.uff.br

INTRODUCTION

The dental literature available on the esthetics of the face and smile is very wide and always been discussed among dental professionals as well as has become interesting to people of different cultures, social classes and ages.[1-5] This interest is justified by the fact that persons with esthetically attractive smile have higher chances of acceptance by society, ensuring better interpersonal relations because they are considered friendly, popular, sociable and intelligent.[1,3,6-8]

However, esthetic perception of dental professionals do not always match the opinion of the patients and this different view implies that more research involving laypersons would help to better understand the perception and the esthetic effects of certain smile characteristics.[9-11]

Moreover, the importance of midline asymmetries on orthodontic diagnosis and treatment planning, is justified by the large number of cases with this malocclusion treated by orthodontists. Therefore, many studies have been done on the diagnosis and treatment of facial and dental asymmetry.[1,2,11-14] An individual's facial midline was defined by the soft tissue symmetry — base of the nose, nasal apex, center of the philtrum and central point of the chin[15] —, and the upper dental midline is evaluated by locating the tip of the gingival papilla between the maxillary central incisors. The gingival papilla should be located below the center of the philtrum of the upper lip.[16]

Although a subtle asymmetry between the facial and dental midlines may exist within acceptable limits, significant discrepancies can alter the level of dental attractiveness and may be detrimental to facial esthetics.[17] However, standards for evaluating midline discrepancy are difficult to established given the subjective nature of such assessment.[17,18]

Results from many studies that tried to determine the acceptability deviation of dental midline by dentists, orthodontists, patients, and laypersons are still conflicting.[17-19] Some studies found that the laypersons had considered the midline deviations as acceptable only under 2 mm deviation,[18,20-22] meanwhile other researches had found values around 3 mm to acceptability threshold.[15,22-24] Other controversial studies have found that 4 mm or less in midline deviations could not be perceived by layperson.[12,15,25]

A few studies used digitally modified images to determine the laypersons perception of the details that influence on the attractiveness of the smile. Disagreements between the values for acceptability may be related to differences in images manipulation among studies, the presence or not of anatomical structures surrounding to smile, the chosen model for handling as well as the size of images.[18,22,24-26]

Different methodologies were applied to evaluate the esthetic perception of the midline deviation, such as the kind of evaluators selection,[12,15,22,25] sample size,[4,12,15,18,20-23,25,27] evaluators calibrated or not,[12,15,18,20-25] different times for judgment,[12,15,20,21,23,24] number of smiling subjects to be evaluated,[4,15,18,22,24,25] photographs displayed size,[4,12,18,20-24,27] with and without anatomical structures adjacent to the smile,[4,12,15,18,20-25,27] amount of deviation in each studies,[12,18,20-25,27] different ways to define what would be assessed: perception, attractiveness, more or less esthetic, among other expressions.[4,12,15,18,20-25,27]

The acceptable deviation determination in midline is essential for decision making by the orthodontist. The solution for existing deviations from the midline may involve tooth movement, with or without dental extractions, orthopedic treatment or the need for orthognathic surgery. In some cases, the correction of the dental and facial midline is not simple and may increase the complexity and duration of orthodontic treatment.[2,4,20] Differential diagnosis makes it possible to discern the cause of the problem, enabling the use of proper mechanotherapy.[28]

Regardless of the orthodontists' desire to achieve all the orthodontic treatment goals, is their commitment to get the patient satisfaction, and the esthetic factor is prioritized by patients in orthodontic treatment.[8]

Based on this premise, we proposed in this research to evaluate the esthetic perception of the upper dental midline deviation by a group of laypersons, and to determine the influence of viewing the structures adjacent to the smile, such as lips, chin and nose, on the diagnosis of the midline deviation.

MATERIAL AND METHODS

This comparative and observational cross-sectional study was approved by the Ethics in Research Committee of the School of Medicine, *Universidade Federal Fluminense*, Niterói, Rio de Janeiro, Brazil, under control number 422.820.

One female subject with normal occlusion was selected among the residents at the postgraduate orthodontic residency program at *Universidade Federal Fluminense*, Niterói, Rio de Janeiro (Brazil), and agreed to participate in the study.

The frontal smiling photograph of the subject was obtained with a digital camera (EOS 60D; Canon, Tokyo, Japan). The photograph was altered using Adobe Photoshop software (Adobe Systems Inc, San Jose, USA) and progressive changes were applied to the upper dental midline relative to the facial midline at every 1 mm, from 0 to 5 mm. By altering the dental midline the entire adjacent tissue was held in position while the whole upper arch was gradually shifted only to the left.

The photographs were cropped in two different configurations and divided into two groups: Group LCN, including the lips, chin, and two thirds of the nose, and Group L, including the lips only. This resulted in twelve photographs for evaluation, two without midline shift and ten digitally altered that were standardized to replicate the subject's smile in its original size (real scale).

The twelve digital photographs (six from group LCN and six from group L) were printed and randomly arranged in an album. The photographs were coded to avoid identification discrepancies. The first part of the album contained group LCN photographs, and the second part, group L (Figs 1 and 2). Photograph evaluation was performed by 95 laypersons with a mean age of 21 years and 3 months. The type of sampling was based on cluster randomization and the evaluators were directly recruited by the researcher in the order they get in the university campus, and they had complete freedom to participate or not of the research. None had undergone orthodontic treatment prior to starting the evaluations and had no experience in Dentistry.

Before evaluating the photographs, a calibration was performed with the judges using two photographs, one without midline deviation (original) and one having a deviation of 6 mm to the left side. Visual Analog Scale (VAS) numbered from zero to 100 was used to mark the scores assigned to the photographs, with the lowest value assigned to the least esthetic smile and the highest value to the most esthetic. The mean value of 50 mm on the VAS was considered the cutoff between attractive and unattractive smile. The time limit for observing each photograph was 20 seconds with a maximum interval of ten seconds between photographs in order to enable the evaluators to assign a score to the smile on the VAS. The evaluators were instructed not to turn back to the previous page of the album to see a particular image again.

After marking the values assigned to the esthetics of the smile on their respective scales, measurements were performed by an operator with the aid of a digital caliper (Starret Indústria e Comércio Ltda., Itu, São Paulo) properly calibrated to the VAS, positioned at zero point, and extended as far as the marking made by the evaluator.

A sample size calculation was performed using the formula recommended by Pandis,[29] based on statistical power of 90% with a confidence interval of 95% ($\alpha = 0.05$) and standard deviation (SD = 20.88 mm) described by Motta[14] to detect a mean difference of 10 in VAS scores, which resulted in 92 evaluators.

To verify the method error, 21 evaluators randomly selected (representing 22% of the total) were asked to repeat the assessment after a 2-weeks interval. Student's *t*-test for paired samples was used for intrarater systematic error analysis, while intraclass correlation coefficient was applied to determine the calibration of the laypersons for photographs evaluation.

The data were tabulated and analyzed using the Statistical Package for the Social Sciences© software (SPSS Inc. Chicago, USA). Data normality was evaluated by the Kolmogorov-Smirnov statistical test.

To assess the influence of changes in the upper dental midline on the perception of smile esthetics, the Friedman test, followed by the Wilcoxon test considering the level of significance as corrected by the Bonferroni criterion ($\alpha = 0.0033$) were applied for multiple comparisons. Paired Student's *t*-test was used whenever data were considered normal, and Friedman test when the data were not considered normal, followed by Mann-Whitney test to assess the impact of structures adjacent to the smile on the perception of deviation in the upper dental midline. The level of significance adopted was 5% ($p < 0.05$).

Pearson's correlation coefficient and regression equation were formulated to determine the association between deviations in groups LCN and L, and the mean values assigned by the evaluators. The coefficient of determination was calculated to predict the accuracy of the regression equation.

Figure 1 - Group LCN photographs: the numbers on the photographs indicate the amount of deviation in millimeters.

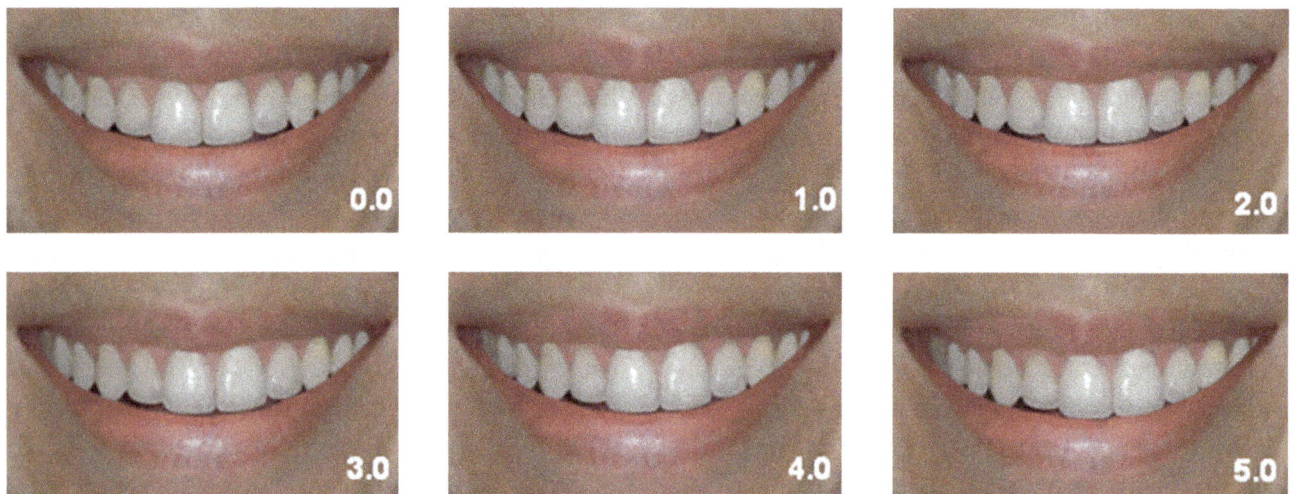

Figure 2 - Group L photographs: the numbers on the photographs indicate the amount of deviation in millimeters.

RESULTS

The paired Student t-test used to evaluate the systematic error, showed no significant difference ($p > 0.05$) and the ICC (0.953) showed an excellent calibration of the laypersons who performed the photographs evaluations.

Statistically significant values were found for all multiple comparisons of the attractiveness scores assigned to each midline shift in photographs of group LCN (Table 1). In group L there were statistical significant differences for almost all comparisons (Table 1). The only exceptions occurred in group L when the photograph that had no deviation was compared with the photograph with a 1 mm shift, and between photographs with 2 mm and 3 mm shifts.

Results of the tests performed to verify the impact of structures adjacent to the smile on the perception of upper dental midline deviations showed statistically significant difference ($p < 0.05$) for comparisons between the photographs of groups LCN and L only when the deviation was 1 mm (Table 1, Fig 3). For other situations of the midline deviation, the mean scores did not differ ($p > 0.05$).

The result of the Pearson's correlation coefficient showed strong negative correlation among deviations in groups LCN and L, and the mean values assigned by the evaluators (r = -0.9963). The value of the coefficient of determination ($r^2 = 0.9926$) and the linear regression equation (y = -7.366x + 80.741) were derived from the data collected for this study.

DISCUSSION

Although common sense tends to base the concept of facial esthetics on subjective opinions, the qualitative and quantitative processing of scientific orthodontic data regarding what is considered beautiful and pleasing is an element that can improve communication with the patient in order to meet their expectations. As the concept of beauty is personal, hence subjective, it requires a fast, straightforward and reliable evaluation method. Therefore, a VAS was used as research tool by the evaluators in this study.[12-15,20,25]

The methodology employed in the present study used photographs with alterations in the upper dental midline only to the left.[14] However, some authors who set out to evaluate the perception of the upper dental midline deviation also included the investigation of other potentially significant discrepancies in the smile attractiveness.[8,12,19,22-25,27] This methodology may produce questionable results given that the inclusion of numerous distinct features could confuse the evaluator.

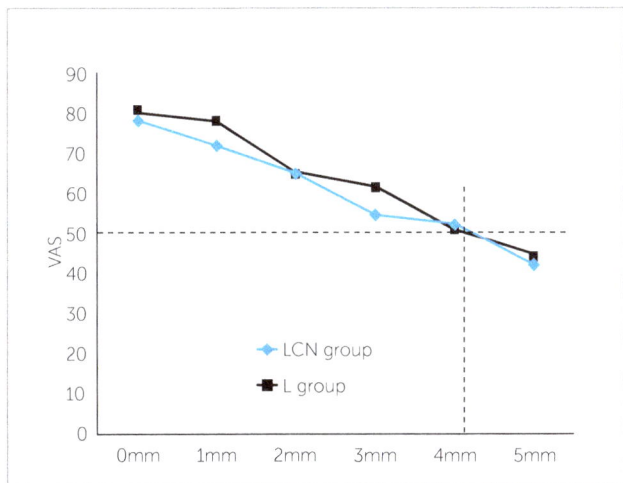

Figure 3 - Comparison between the overall scores assigned to the photographs in LCN and L groups.

Table 1 - Descriptive statistics (mm) and results for attractiveness scores and for comparisons between LCN group (including the lips, chin and nose) and L group (including the lips only).

Deviation (mm)	LCN group					L group					LCN x L
	Median	Mean	IQ	SD	Results*	Median	Mean	IQ	SD	Results*	
0	82.70	-	24.34	-	A	84.60	-	20.36	-	A	
1	75.66	-	22.51	-	B	80.26	-	18.55	-	A	†
2	70.31	-	23.91	-	C	70.54	-	28.43	-	B	
3	63.42	-	27.82	-	D	66.21	-	33.12	-	B	
4	51.68	-	35.28	-	E	53.68	-	36.93	-	C	
5	-	42.13	-	25.19	F	-	44.15	-	23.23	D	

*Variables with the same letter does not differ statistically ($p < 0.05$); † Statistical differences between groups of facial structures ($p < 0.05$).

Facial features, such as hair color, face pattern, skin color and gender, are factors that potentially affect the level of visual attention on the smile esthetic perception by laypersons.[5,25] Therefore, to gauge the interference of these structures of the face and evaluate the influence of structures that define the facial midline, two settings were applied to the photographs used in this study, which were divided into groups LCN and L. However, full face photographs were not employed.

The fact that they have assessed the photographs randomly and separately probably decreases the incorporation of bias. The evaluators could not compare the photographs at the same time like in previous studies,[22,23,26] which might have contributed to the results found in this study, since the variation from the least esthetic value to the most esthetic were limited between 42.13 mm and 84.60 mm (Table 1).

According to the findings of our study, laypersons were more critical in the perception of changes of the upper dental midline in the photographs of LCN group. There were statistically significant differences for all multiple comparisons between each midline shift in photographs of LCN group. These results evidence the capacity of laypersons to perceive each millimeter of deviation in photographs of LCN group. However, there were statistically significant differences for some multiple comparisons between each midline shift on photographs of L group. These results show the perception of laypersons to note midline deviations only from 2 mm, when anatomical details are suppressed in photographs arranged for evaluation. Likewise the evaluators failed to differentiate shifts between 2 and 3 mm or may not have detected significant difference between these midline variations (Table 1).

This result probably stemmed from the fact that LCN group photographs contained anatomical landmarks of the face such as the lips, chin, and nose, which are natural contributors to the diagnosis of upper dental midline deviation. Some investigations, using photographs of the whole face for evaluation of upper dental midline deviation, found that laypersons were able to notice deviations starting at 2 mm.[4,18,20,21] This divergence possibly resulted from the influence of other facial structures, which might potentially disperse the evaluation of smile esthetics by laypersons.[4,24]

Other studies analyzed the perception of dental midline deviations by laypersons in photographs showing only the smile, but with different methodologies. In the works of Ker et al[23] and Mc Leod et al[22], the evaluators accepted deviations in the upper midline of up to 2.9 mm, but they had judged all the photographs at the same time. Nevertheless, some studies reported that laypersons could only identify deviations from the upper midline of up to 3 mm[15,17] and 4 mm.[15] Furthermore, studies conducted by Kokich et al,[25] with pictures showing just the smile, concluded that 4 mm deviations might not be detectable by laypersons. These divergent results may have been due to the different methodologies used in the investigations as well as the heterogeneity of the population being studied.

In spite of the results of our study showing that the laypersons were able to identify deviations from the midline starting at 1 mm in LCN group and 2 mm in L group, it seems that only from a deviation of approximately 4 mm that the smile was considered not esthetically pleasing by laypersons. This can be explained by applying the mean value of 50 mm in the linear regression equation ($y = -7.366x + 80.741$) that provides the resulting value of 4.17 mm (Fig 3). This result confirms that, in many cases, even with a deviated midline, one could still have a beautiful smile and it could also explain the divergence among the results found by the various authors in their respective studies.

The almost perfect negative linear correlation ($r = -0.9963$) between the means and the deviations, demonstrated that the higher the deviation, the lower was the score assessed by the evaluators, and vice-versa. The coefficient of determination ($r^2 = 0.9926$) indicates that 99.26% of the variation of the mean scores assigned to the photographs can be explained by the amount of deviation. The evaluators were able to perceive the increase of the deviation despite the randomization of photographs.

This study is clinically important to the extent that it provides scientific data that makes it easier for professionals to better understand the patient's esthetic expectations and desires. Thus, it helps to outline the treatment plan and define which procedures should be performed during the final stage of orthodontic treatment. One last caveat is necessary: professionals should be aware that in some cases dental midline correction can prove a daunting task, which can involve complicated mechanic and result in increased complexity and duration of orthodontic treatment.

CONCLUSIONS

1) The laypersons were able to perceive the upper dental midline deviations of 1 mm and above when the adjacent structures of the smiles were viewed; and of 2 mm and above when only the lips were viewed.

2) Visualization of structures adjacent to the smile, such as lips, chin and nose demonstrated influence on the perception of upper dental midline deviation.

Author contributions

Conception/design of the study: JBF, AFJM, JNM. Data acquisition, analysis or interpretation: JBF, LES, AFJM. Writing the article: JBF, MTOC, AFJM, AACS, JNM. Critical revision of the article: MTOC, AFJM, AACS, JNM. Final approval of the article: AFJM, AACS, JNM. Overall responsibility: AFJM.

REFERENCES

1. Tjan AH, Miller GD, The JG. Some esthetic factors in a smile. J Prosthet Dent. 1984 Jan;51(1):24-8.

2. Beyer JW, Lindauer SJ. Evaluation of dental midline position. Semin Orthod. 1998 Sept;4(3):146-52.

3. Flores-Mir C, Silva E, Barriga MI, Lagravere MO, Major PW. Lay person's perception of smile aesthetics in dental and facial views. J Orthod. 2004 Sept;31(3):204-9; discussion 201.

4. Williams RP, Rinchuse DJ, Zullo TG. Perceptions of midline deviations among different facial types. Am J Orthod Dentofacial Orthop. 2014 Feb;145(2):249-55.

5. Richards MR, Fields HW Jr, Beck FM, Firestone AR, Walther DB, Rosenstiel S, et al. Contribution of malocclusion and female facial attractiveness to smile esthetics evaluated by eye tracking. Am J Orthod Dentofacial Orthop. 2015 Apr;147(4):472-82.

6. Shaw WC, Rees G, Dawe M, Charles CR. The influence of dentofacial appearance on the social attractiveness of young adults. Am J Orthod. 1985 Jan;87(1):21-6.

7. Badran SA The effect of malocclusion and self-perceived aesthetics on the self-esteem of a sample of Jordanian adolescents. Eur J Orthod. 2010 Dec;32(6):638-44.

8. Chang CA, Fields HW Jr, Beck FM, Springer NC, Firestone AR, Rosenstiel S, Christensen JC. Smile esthetics from patients' perspectives for faces of varying attractiveness. Am J Orthod Dentofacial Orthop. 2011 Oct;140(4):e171-80.

9. Bernabé E, Kresevic VD, Cabrejos SC, Flores-Mir F, Flores-Mir C. Dental esthetic self-perception in young adults with and without previous orthodontic treatment. Angle Orthod. 2006 May;76(3):412-6.

10. Pithonmm, Santos AM, Couto FS, Silva Coqueiro R, Freitas LM, Souza RA, et al. Perception of the esthetic impact of mandibular incisor extraction treatment on laypersons, dental professionals, and dental students. Angle Orthod. 2012 July;82(4):732-8.

11. Machado AW, Moon W, Gandini LG Jr. Influence of maxillary incisor edge asymmetries on the perception of smile esthetics among orthodontists and laypersons. Am J Orthod Dentofacial Orthop. 2013 May;143(5):658-64.

12. Pinho S, Ciriaco C, Faber J, Lenza MA. Impact of dental asymmetries on the perception of smile esthetics. Am J Orthod Dentofacial Orthop. 2007 Dec;132(6):748-53.

13. Pithonmm, Bastos GW, Miranda NS, Sampaio T, Ribeiro TP, Nascimento LE, et al. Esthetic perception of black spaces between maxillary central incisors by different age groups. Am J Orthod Dentofacial Orthop. 2013 Mar;143(3):371-5.

14. Motta AFJ. A influência de diferentes componentes dentários na estética do sorriso [tese]. Rio de Janeiro (RJ): Universidade do Brasil - UFRJ; 2009 [Acesso em: 10 maio 2015]. Disponível em: http://www.odontologia.ufrj.br/ortodontia/teses/doutorado/Andrea-Fonseca-Jardim-da-Motta-2009.pdf.

15. Normando ADC, Azevedo LA, Paixão PN. Quanto de desvio da linha média dentária superior ortodontistas e leigos conseguem perceber? Rev Dental Press Ortod Ortop Facial. 2009;14(2):73-80.

16. Kokich V. Esthetics and anterior tooth position: an orthodontic perspective. Part III: Mediolateral relationships. J Esthet Dent. 1993;5(5):200-7.

17. Janson G, Branco NC, Fernandes TM, Sathler R, Garib D, Lauris JR. Influence of orthodontic treatment, midline position, buccal corridor and smile arc on smile attractiveness. Angle Orthod. 2011 Jan;81(1):153-61.

18. Zhang YF, Xiao L, Li J, Peng YR, Zhao Z. Young people's esthetic perception of dental midline deviation. Angle Orthod. 2010 May;80(3):515-20.

19. España P, Tarazona B, Paredes V. Smile esthetics from odontology students' perspectives. Angle Orthod. 2014 Mar;84(2):214-24.

20. Johnston CD, Burden DJ, Stevenson MR. The influence of dental to facial midline discrepancies on dental attractiveness ratings. Eur J Orthod. 1999 Oct;21(5):517-22.

21. Shyagali TR, Chandralekha B, Bhayya DP, Kumar S, Balasubramanyam G. Are ratings of dentofacial attractiveness influenced by dentofacial midline discrepancies? Aust Orthod J. 2008 Nov;24(2):91-5.

22. McLeod C, Fields HW, Hechter F, Wiltshire W, Rody W Jr, Christensen J. Esthetics and smile characteristics evaluated by laypersons. Angle Orthod. 2011 Mar;81(2):198-205.

23. Ker AJ, Chan R, Fields HW, Beck M, Rosenstiel S. Esthetics and smile characteristics from the layperson's perspective: a computer-based survey study. J Am Dent Assoc. 2008 Oct;139(10):1318-27.

24. Springer NC, Chang C, Fields HW, Beck FM, Firestone AR, Rosenstiel S, et al. Smile esthetics from the layperson's perspective. Am J Orthod Dentofacial Orthop. 2011 Jan;139(1):e91-101.

25. Kokich VO Jr, Kiyak HA, Shapiro PA. Comparing the perception of dentists and lay people to altered dental esthetics. J Esthet Dent. 1999;11(6):311-24.

26. Pithonmm, Nascimento CC, Barbosa GC, Coqueiro Rda S. Do dental esthetics have any influence on finding a job? Am J Orthod Dentofacial Orthop. 2014 Oct;146(4):423-9

27. Talic N, AlOmar S, AlMaidhan A. Perception of Saudi dentists and lay people to altered smile esthetics. Saudi Dent J. 2013 Jan;25(1):13-21.

28. Jerrold L, Lowenstein LJ. The midline: diagnosis and treatment. Am J Orthod Dentofacial Orthop. 1990 June;97(6):453-62.

29. Pandis N. Sample calculations for comparison of 2 means. Am J Orthod Dentofacial Orthop. 2012 Apr;141(4):519-21.

3

Color changes of esthetic orthodontic ligatures evaluated by orthodontists and patients: a clinical study

Edilene Kawabata[1], Vera Lucia Dantas[1], Carlos Brito Kato[2], David Normando[3]

Objective: To evaluate *in vivo* changes in the color of esthetic elastomeric ligatures from different manufacturers. **Methods:** Four widely used commercial brands of elastomeric ligatures were selected and used in 20 adult patients in a split-mouth design. The ligatures were evaluated by orthodontists and patients in a double-blind manner on the day the ligatures were placed (T_0) and 30 days after intraoral exposure (T_1) by means of a system of staining scores. Groups were compared by Friedman test with $p < 0.05$. **Results:** Orthodontists and patients reported similar staining scores ($p > 0.05$). Results showed that all brands underwent significant staining when exposed to the intraoral environment. Modular-crystal Morelli™ (Sorocaba, SP, Brazil) showed the highest degree of staining with the median reaching the maximum value (3); while the other brands (3M Unitek™, American Orthodontics™ and GAC Dentsply™) showed the median equal to 1 ($p < 0.001$). A large individual variability in the degree of staining was also found for all brands. **Conclusions:** All four brands of esthetic ligatures showed significant staining, which appeared to be more pronounced for the Morelli™ brand. Changes in color of the elastomeric ligatures were perceived similarly by patients and orthodontists. The industry needs to improve the color stability of esthetic ligatures.

Keywords: Esthetic orthodontic ligatures. Esthetic elastomers. Pigmentation Orthodontic treatment.

[1] Specialist in Orthodontics, Associação Brasileira de Ortodontia, Belém, Pará, Brazil.

[2] Professor in Orthodontics, Associação Brasileira de Ortodontia, Belém, Pará, Brazil.

[3] Adjunct professor, Universidade Federal do Pará (UFPA), School of Dentistry, Belém, Pará, Brazil.

» The authors report no commercial, proprietary or financial interest in the products or companies described in this article.

David Normando
Universidade Federal do Pará, Belém, Brazil. Rua Augusto Corrêa, no 1, CEP: 66.075-110 – E-mail: davidnormando@hotmail.com

INTRODUCTION

Due to good color stability and improved adhesion, esthetic brackets have become very popular in Orthodontics in recent decades. Moreover, the demand of adult patients for orthodontic treatment performed with esthetic orthodontic brackets has increased substantially. Furthermore, as regards elastomeric ligatures used to tie the bracket/wire combination, clinical orthodontists are concerned and would like to make sure the ligatures' characteristics remain unchanged. Color changes caused by staining resulting from food ingestion or contact with intraoral fluids are particularly undesirable. These changes are due to swelling and discoloration when elastomers are exposed to the intraoral environment, and it is caused by buccal fluids and bacteria that fill up the spaces in the rubber matrix.[1,2,3] In order to minimize the influence of some types of food affecting the color of elastomeric ligatures, metallic pigments have been added during the manufacturing process; however, they reduce the level of force released, impairing their elastomeric properties.[1]

Many *in vitro* studies have evaluated the effects of the intraoral environment on the elastomeric properties of elastomers, such as force decay, friction and dimensional changes.[1-7] However, only a few *in vivo* studies have analyzed the behavior of orthodontic material after exposure to the intraoral environment,[8-11] particularly the changes in esthetics of the elastomeric ligatures used.

In vitro studies have shown that esthetic elastomers become stained after being immersed in liquids with high susceptibility to pigmentation.[12-18] However, these studies were conducted *in vitro*, which may not reflect the numerous factors present in the intraoral environment contributing to color change, such as the oral flora, temperature variation, the mechanical effect of brushing and solid and semi-solid food that cause pigmentation. Thus, clinical studies can yield a more realistic analysis of actual color changes taking place in orthodontic material after clinical use.[19]

Besides the need for clinical evaluation, patients' real perception of color changes undergone by elastomers is not yet known. Thus, this study aimed to investigate clinical changes in the color of esthetic elastomeric ligatures by means of direct visual analysis performed by both orthodontists and patients.

MATERIAL AND METHODS

This study was approved by the Ethics Committee of the Institute of Health Sciences, under protocol #15958513.7.0000.0018.

Four commercial brands of esthetic ligatures were selected based on a survey conducted on a social network of orthodontists. The following question was posted: "Which esthetic orthodontic ligature do you use in your practice?"

Relying on the collaboration of 94 orthodontists after ten days, the search resulted in the following brands: Obscure (3M Unitek™, Monrovia, CA, USA) with 22 indications (30.13%); followed by American Orthodontics™, pearl color (Sheboygan, Wisconsin, USA) with 21 indications (28.76%); Dentsply GAC™, clear (New York, NY, USA) with 20 (27.39%) and Modular-crystal Morelli™ (Sorocaba, SP, Brazil) with ten indications (13.69%).

A split-mouth, double-blind, prospective study was designed. A convenience sample included 20 adult volunteer patients (14 females and 6 males), aged between 20 and 57 years old (mean age of 38.5 years). All patients were treated with esthetic ceramic orthodontic appliances from six different orthodontic practices. In each patient, the four brands were randomly distributed by hemiarch and remained in the oral environment for 30 days (Fig 1). Randomization was performed by means of BioEstat 5.3 software (Mamirauá Institute, Belém, Pará, Brazil).

The scoring process was performed while patients were using the ligatures. The ligatures were scored on the same day they were placed (T_0), and after 30 days of exposure in the intraoral environment (T_1). Evaluation was carried out visually and under cold light, both by patients using a mirror (n = 20) and orthodontists (n = 6), by the same examiner in T_0 and T_1, under the same light conditions. No patient received any guidance regarding food restrictions in their diet. Analysis involved the use of scores according to the degree of staining,[19] in which: 0 = nonpigmented ligatures; 1 = slightly pigmented; 2 = moderately pigmented; and 3 = heavily pigmented.

Groups were statistically compared by Friedman test and ANOVA at 95% confidence level by means of BioEstat 5.3 software (Mamirauá Institute, Belém, Pará, Brazil).

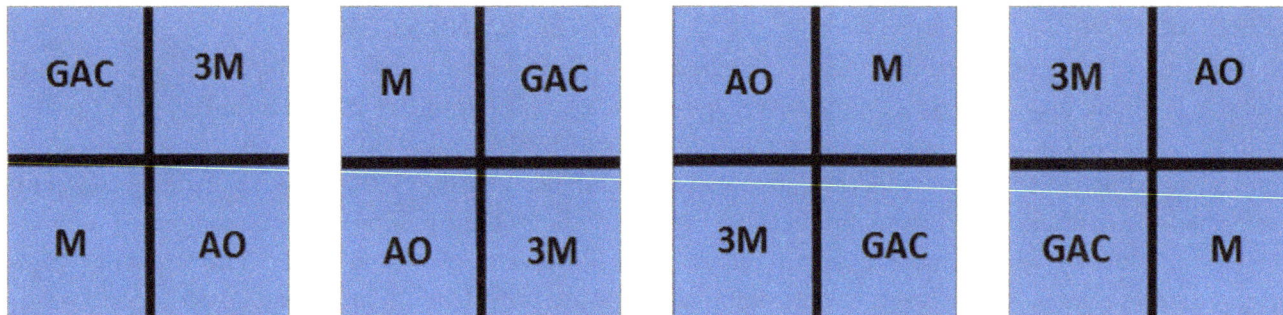

Figure 1 - Random distribution by quadrant: **M** = Morelli™, **GAC** = GAC™, **AO** = American Orthodontics™, **3M** = 3M Unitek™.

Table 1 - Median, interquartile range (IQR) and p-value of four commercial brands evaluated at T_0 by patients and orthodontists.

	GAC (n = 20)	3M (n = 20)	AO (n = 20)	Morelli (n = 20)	p value
Patients					
Median	0	0	0	0	0.96
IQR	0.25	1	0	0	
Orthodontist					
Median	0	0	0	0	0.14
IQR	0.25	1	1	0	

RESULTS

Evaluation performed by orthodontists and patients was not statistically different. The median score for the four as-received elastomer was zero ($p > 0.05$). Patients and orthodontists evaluated similarly the staining of all brands at T_0 (Table 1, Fig 2).

After a 30-day period of intraoral exposure (T_1), the four brands of elastomeric ligatures showed significant staining (Table 2). Differences were statistically significant in all groups ($p < 0.001$). The median observed at T_1 was equal to 1.0 (slightly pigmented) for the three brands manufactured in the United States (GAC™, 3M™ and American Orthodontics™), while the Brazilian brand (Morelli™) had a score of 3.0 (heavily pigmented) assigned. The American products manufactured by GAC™, 3M Unitek™ and American Orthodontics™ exhibited no significant differences when compared to one another (Table 2, Fig 2). However, a large variation in the degree of staining was observed in all brands. In patients' evaluation, GAC™ and 3M™ showed the greatest variation in staining, with scores ranging

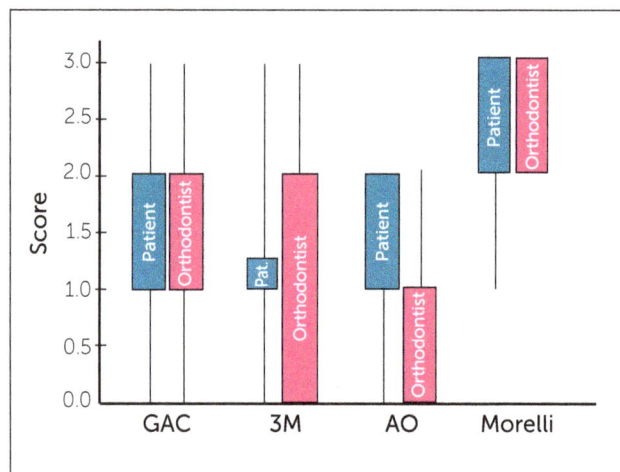

Figure 2 - Box-plot of medians and IQR of the scores assigned to the four brands according to orthodontists' and patients' assessment (T_1-T_0).

from 0 to 3, while American Orthodontics™ had scores between 0 and 2 assigned. The Brazilian ligatures (Morelli™) received scores ranging from 1 to 3 (Fig 2). This variation observed by orthodontists was similarly reported by patients (Fig 2).

Table 2 - Median, interquartile range (IQR) and p-value of four commercial brands evaluated at T_1-T_0 by patients and orthodontists.

	GAC (n = 20)	3M (n = 20)	AO (n = 20)	Morelli (n = 20)	p value (Friedman)
Patient					
Median	1(a)	1(a)	1(a)	3(b)	< 0.0001
IQR	1	0.25	1	1	
Orthodontist					
Median	1(a)	1(a)	1(a)	3(b)	< 0.0001
IQR	1	2	1	1	
p value					
Ortho x patient	0.823	1	0.263	0.823	

Different letters indicate $p < 0.05$.

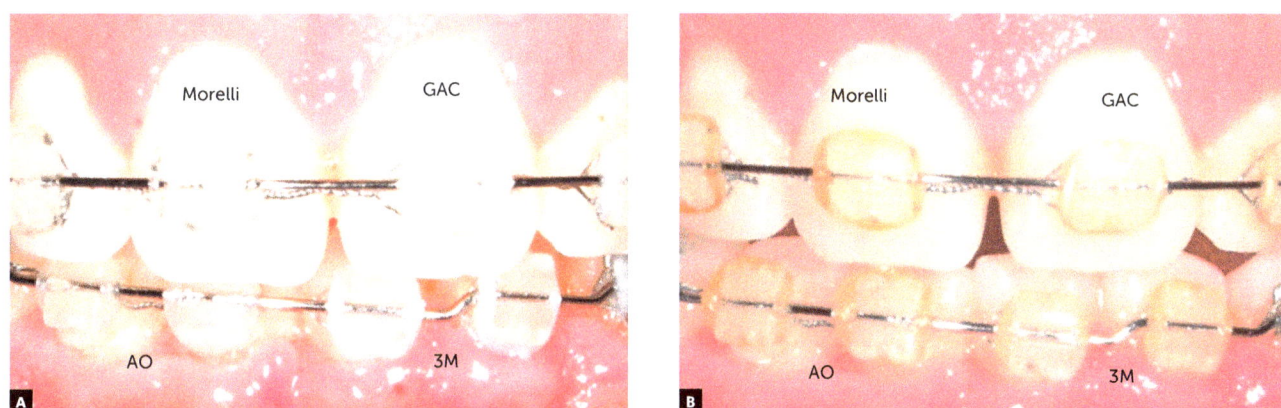

Figure 3 - Change in color of the ligatures before (**A**) and after exposure to the intraoral environment for 30 days (**B**): note that whereas the ligatures manufactured by GAC™, 3M™ and American Orthodontics™ show a pattern of less staining and are similar to each other, the ligature manufactured by Morelli™ exhibits a more pronounced pigmentation.

DISCUSSION

Patients' concerns about facial esthetics and properly aligned teeth have been combined with increased life expectancy and quality of life to boost the demand for orthodontic treatment in adult patients; and with it, the demand for esthetic orthodontic appliances. Despite great improvement in the quality and stability of bracket color, esthetic appliances are faced with the challenge of changes that occur in the color of esthetic orthodontic ligatures when exposed to the intraoral environment. Thus, patients' complaints are frequent, given that the whole bracket/ligature combination becomes less esthetic, as elastomers undergo undesirable staining.

Analyses of color changes in orthodontic ligatures are usually performed *in vitro*,[12-18] which does not reflect reality. In this study design, clear elastomers are dipped into high-pigmentation fluids and analyzed after a given period of time. Unlike the clinical design used in the present study, laboratory studies are not affected by oral fluids, oral microflora, diet and oral hygiene.

The *in vivo* model used in this study showed no significant difference between orthodontists and patients for all brands at the time the ligatures were placed (T_0). The median was the same for all brands, i.e., all values were equal to zero; thus, the metal pigments added during the manufacturing process of some of the esthetic orthodontic ligatures had no significant impact on the assessment of patients and orthodontists alike. Thirty days after exposure to the intraoral environment, all ligatures exhibited some degree of staining, but no significant differences were found between GAC™, 3M Unitek™ and American Orthodontics™. Morelli™ ligatures obtained a median of 3, showing greater susceptibility to pigmentation.

Moreover, it was observed that the pigmentation of elastomers made by the same manufacturer varied from patient to patient, which may have been related to diet and oral hygiene among the different experimental subjects. These results contradict the low pigmentation variability found in *in vitro* studies and further confirm the fact that individual factors can influence pigmentation intensity.

This clinical study differs from a previous *ex vivo* investigation[19] whereby analysis of elastomer pigmentation was carried outside the intraoral environment. The ligatures were removed, photographed and then analyzed, which could lead to interference in the results, depending on the calibration when capturing the images. *In vivo* analyses of staining in esthetic orthodontic ligatures could provide more accurate results, since different brands are examined through a direct visual analysis in the intraoral cavity by orthodontists and especially by patients themselves. However, even when evaluating American Orthodontics™ and Morelli™ ligatures, results do not seem to differ.

Dental material science has focused on the properties of as-received material rather than on changes produced after intraoral exposure.[20] The results of this study warrant the need for greater investment in research and technology to improve color stability of esthetic orthodontic ligatures. For now, a viable clinical option would be esthetic self-ligating brackets, which forestall the use of elastomeric ligatures. However, despite the elimination of undesirable staining in ligatures, metal clips, typically used in these attachments, contribute to substantial loss in appliance esthetics. Another option for the clinician, which happens to be more affordable than esthetic brackets, is the use of esthetic steel ligatures to tie the wire/bracket combination. The main drawback inherent to this method, however, is an increase in chair time compared to self-ligating brackets.[21]

CONCLUSIONS

After examining four brands of esthetic elastomeric ligatures, all of them showed significant staining, which appeared to be more pronounced in Morelli™ ligatures.[1] Changes in color of elastomeric ligatures were perceived similarly by patients and orthodontists.

REFERENCES

1. Wong A K. Orthodontic elastic materials. Angle Orthod. 1976 Apr; 46(2):196-205.
2. Ferriter JP, Meyers CE Jr, Lorton L. The effect of hydrogen ion concentration on the force-degradation rate of orthodontic polyurethane chain elastics. Am J Orthod Dentofacial Orthop. 1990 Nov;98(5):404-10.
3. von Fraunhofer JA, Coffelt MT, Orbell GM. The effects of artificial saliva and topical fluoride treatments on the degradation of the elastic properties of orthodontic chains. Angle Orthod. 1992 Winter;62(4):265-74.
4. Baccetti T, Franchi L. Friction produced by types of elastomeric ligatures in treatment mechanics with the preadjusted appliance. Angle Orthod. 2006 Mar;76(2):211-6.
5. Taloumis LJ, Smith TM, Hondrum SO, Lorton L. Force decay and deformation of orthodontic elastomeric ligatures. Am J Orthod Dentofacial Orthop. 1997 Jan;111(1):1-11.
6. De Genova DC, McInnes-Ledoux P, Weinberg R, Shaye R. Force degradation of orthodontic elastomeric chains—a product comparison study. Am J Orthod. 1985 May;87(5):377-84.
7. Baty DL, Volz JE, von Fraunhofer JA. Force delivery properties of colored elastomeric modules. Am J Orthod Dentofacial Orthop. 1994 July;106(1):40-6.
8. Eliades T, Bourauel C. Intraoral aging of orthodontic materials: the picture we miss and its clinical relevance. Am J Orthod Dentofacial Orthop. 2005 Apr;127(4):403-12.
9. Marques IS, Araújo AM, Gurgel JA, Normando D. Debris, roughness and friction of stainless steel archwires following clinical use. Angle Orthod. 2010 May;80(3):521-7.
10. Araújo RC, Bichara LM, Araujo AM, Normando D. Debris and friction of self-ligating and conventional orthodontic brackets after clinical use. Angle Orthod. 2015 July;85(4):673-7.
11. Normando D, Araújo AM, Marques I da S, Barroso Tavares Dias CG, Miguel JA. Archwire cleaning after intraoral ageing: the effects on debris, roughness, and friction. Eur J Orthod. 2013 Apr;35(2):223-9.
12. Ardeshna AP, Vaidyanathan TK. Colour changes of orthodontic elastomeric module materials exposed to in vitro dietary media. J Orthod. 2009 Sept;36(3):177-85.
13. Kim SH, Lee YK. Measurement of discolouration of orthodontic elastomeric modules with a digital camera. Eur J Orthod. 2009 Oct;31(5):556-62.
14. Lew KK. Staining of clear elastomeric modules from certain foods. J Clin Orthod. 1990 Aug;24(8):472-4.
15. Cavalcante JS, Barbosa MC, Sobral MC. Evaluation of the susceptibility to pigmentation of orthodontic esthetic elastomeric ligatures. Dental Press J Orthod. 2013 Mar 15;18(2):20.e1-8.
16. Soldati DC, Silva RC, Oliveira AS, Kaizer MR, Moraes RR. Color stability of five orthodontic clear elastic ligatures. Orthodontics (Chic.). 2013;14(1):e60-5.
17. Fernandes AB, Ribeiro AA, Araujo MV, Ruellas AC. Influence of exogenous pigmentation on the optical properties of orthodontic elastic ligatures. J Appl Oral Sci. 2012 July-Aug;20(4):462-6.
18. Fernandes AB, Ruellas AC, Araújo MV, Sant'Anna EF, Elias CN. Assessment of exogenous pigmentation in colourless elastic ligatures. J Orthod. 2014 Jun;41(2):147-51.
19. Silva AM, Mattos GV, Kato CM, Normando D. In vivo color changes of esthetic orthodontic ligatures. Dental Press J Orthod. 2012;17(5):76-8.
20. Eliades T, Bourauel C. Intraoral aging of orthodontic materials: the picture we miss and its clinical relevance. Am J Orthod Dentofacial Orthop. 2005 Apr;127(4):403-12.
21. Chen SS, Greenlee GM, Kim JE, Smith CL, Huang GJ. Systematic review of self-ligating brackets. Am J Orthod Dentofacial Orthop. 2010 Jun;137(6): 726.e1-726.e18; discussion 726-7.

4

Efficiency of two protocols for maxillary molar intrusion with mini-implants

Juliana Volpato Curi Paccini[1], Flávio Augusto Cotrim-Ferreira[2], Flávio Vellini Ferreira[2],
Karina Maria Salvatore de Freitas[3], Rodrigo Hermont Cançado[3], Fabrício Pinelli Valarelli[3]

Objective: The aim of this study was to compare the efficiency of two protocols for maxillary molar intrusion with two or three mini-implants. **Methods:** Twenty five maxillary first molars extruded for loss of their antagonists in adult subjects were selected. The sample was divided into two groups, according to the intrusion protocol with two or three mini-implants. Group 1 consisted of 15 molars that were intruded by two mini-implants. Group 2 consisted of 10 molars intruded by three mini-implants. Changes with treatment were analyzed in lateral cephalograms at the beginning and at the end of intrusion of maxillary molars. **Results:** Results showed that there was no difference in efficiency for the two intrusion protocols. It was concluded that extruded maxillary molars can be intruded with two or three mini-implants with similar efficiency.

Keywords: Corrective Orthodontics. Tooth intrusion. Bone screws.

» The authors report no commercial, proprietary or financial interest in the products or companies described in this article.

[1] MSc, Universidade Cidade de São Paulo (UNICID), Department of Orthodontics, São Paulo, São Paulo, Brazil.
[2] Professor, Universidade Cidade de São Paulo (UNICID), Department of Orthodontics, São Paulo, São Paulo, Brazil.
[3] Professor, Faculdade Ingá, Department of Orthodontics, Maringá, Paraná, Brazil.

Karina Maria Salvatore de Freitas
Av. Colombo, 9.727 Km 130 - Maringá, PR, Brazil. CEP: 87070-810
E-mail: kmsf@uol.com.br

INTRODUCTION AND STATEMENT OF THE PROBLEM

One of the most difficult movements in orthodontic mechanics requiring efficient anchorage to achieve success is tooth intrusion. This movement is usually necessary when a tooth has extruded, especially due to absence of the antagonist tooth. Extrusion can cause several problems, such as occlusal interferences and consequent functional problems.[1-4] It is, therefore, necessary to correct this condition to further promote prosthetic rehabilitation of the antagonist tooth.

There are several intra- and extraoral areas to be used as anchorage. Conventional methods present some inconvenience, including esthetic implications, anchorage loss and the need for patient's compliance, greatly compromising the success of intrusion mechanics.[2,5,6] It is extremely necessary to differentiate the intrusion of maxillary first molars from the extrusion of adjacent teeth, which can occur when proper anchorage is not used, representing a relative intrusion and not a true one.[3,6]

The use of miniscrews and the possibility to obtain absolute anchorage has provided new perspectives for Orthodontics. It created a stable point within the oral cavity, so that movements are performed in a more controlled and predictable way, with minimal need for patient's compliance.[3,4] Currently, there are mini-implants available in a wide variety of sizes, allowing their insertion in several locations of the maxilla and mandible.[7] Mini-implants remained in the dental market due to several advantages, such as the absence of complex surgical procedures, low cost and great patient acceptance.[8]

Currently, intrusive mechanics of maxillary molars anchored in mini-implants uses several protocols.[3,9-12] However, there is a concern regarding the best protocol to perform molar intrusion with maximum efficiency and the ideal number of mini-implants to be used during this mechanics.

The aim of this study was to compare the dental and skeletal changes produced by intrusion of maxillary first molars anchored in mini-implants, using two different protocols, and to evaluate the efficiency of these protocols based on the ratio between the amount and duration of intrusion.

MATERIAL AND METHODS

This study was approved by the Ethics Research Committee of Universidade Cidade de São Paulo (UNICID) (protocol 13599774).

Sample size calculation was based on an alpha significance level of 5% (0.05) and a beta of 20% (0.20) to achieve 80% power test to detect a mean difference of 0.78 mm with standard deviation of 0.6 for maxillary molar intrusion.[24] Thus, sample size calculation revealed the need for 10 individuals in each group.

This study was retrospective, and sample selection followed the following criteria: presence of at least an extruded maxillary first molar due to loss of the antagonist tooth, patients with no growth potential, absence of chronic systemic problems, presence of lateral cephalograms from the beginning of orthodontic treatment and from the end of intrusion, presence of completed files with information concerning the procedure for intrusion of maxillary first molars and absence of endodontic treatment in the intruded molar. None of the individuals in the sample had previous orthodontic treatment or periodontal disease in the beginning of treatment.

According to these criteria for selecting the sample, 19 patients (four males, 15 females) were selected, 13 with unilateral and six with bilateral extrusion, thereby totalling 25 first molars which had undergone mechanical intrusion, anchored in mini-implants and associated with fixed appliances. All patients were treated by graduate students supervised by the same professor at FACSETE, Porto Velho, Rondônia, Brazil. Thus, the sample was divided into two groups, according to the protocol of two or three mini-implants used for molar intrusion.

» Group 1 (G1): Composed of 15 maxillary first molars which were intruded by two mini-implants, one on the buccal side and one on the palatal side (Fig 1).

» Group 2 (G2): Composed of 10 maxillary first molars which were intruded by three mini-implants, two on the buccal side and one on the palatal side (Fig 2).

In patients of G1, elastomeric chains (Dental Morelli Ltda, Sorocaba, São Paulo, Brazil) were anchored in the mini-implants, passing through the occlusal surface of first molar crown (Fig 1). In patients of G2, elastomeric chains (Dental Morelli Ltda, Sorocaba, São Paulo, Brazil) were placed as follows: from the two mini-implants placed buccally to the tube of the first molar band, and from the mini-implant placed palatally to the button soldered on the first molar band, on the palatal side (Fig 2). Intrusion mechanics

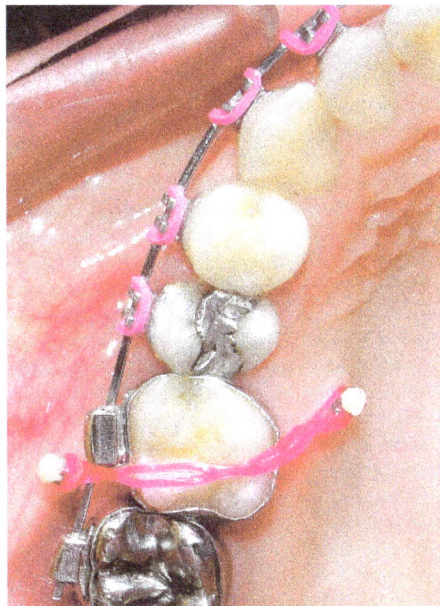

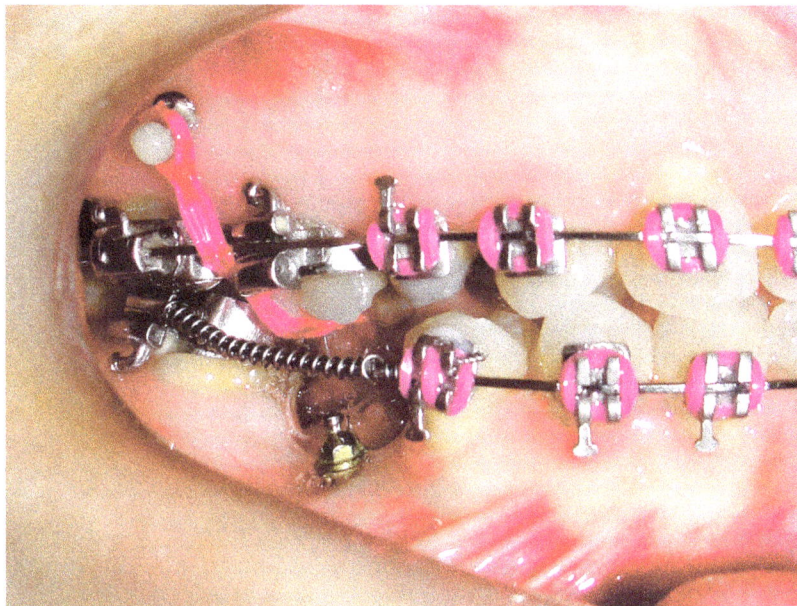

Figure 1 - First molar intrusion in Group 1.

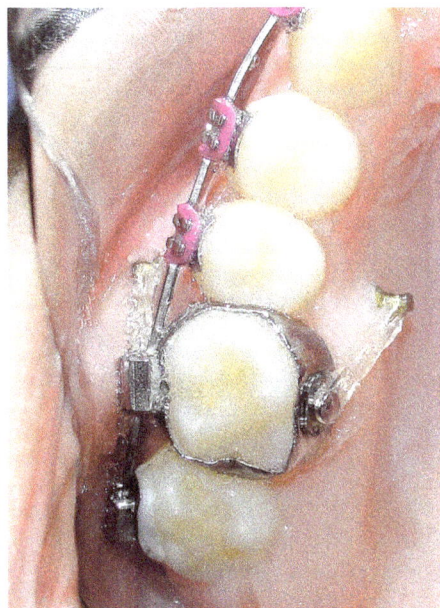

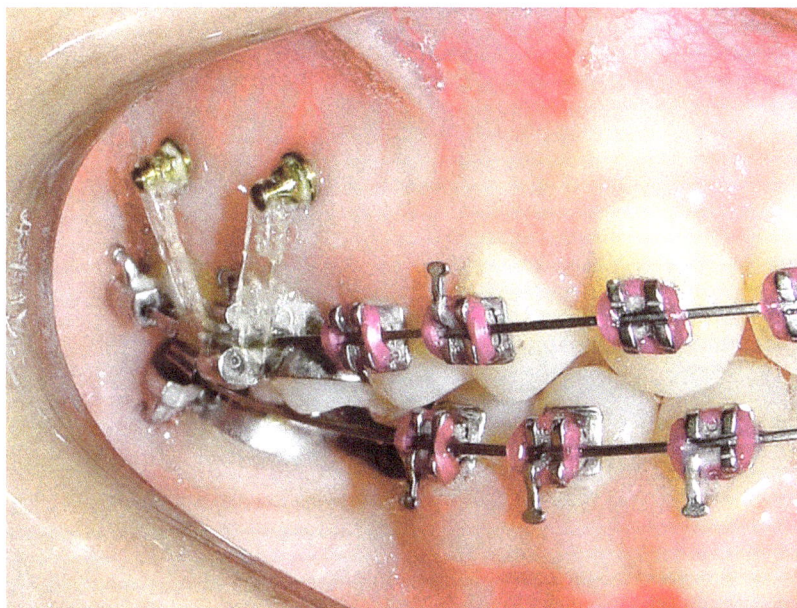

Figure 2 - First molar intrusion in Group 2.

was applied immediately after mini-implant placement, with approximately 150 g of force being applied to each mini-implant.[13,14,15] This force was measured by a tensiometer (50-500 g, Dental Morelli Ltda, Sorocaba, São Paulo, Brazil). The elastomeric chains were changed every four weeks and intrusion force was checked at each appointment. Retention of the intruded molars was performed with ligature wires (0.010-in).

Simultaneously to intrusion of maxillary first molars, the cases were treated with preadjusted appliances (Roth prescription, slot 0.022 x 0.028-in, Dental Morelli Ltda. Sorocaba, SP, Brazil). Patients received self-drilling mini-implants (S.I.N. Implant System, São Paulo, São Paulo, Brazil), with dimensions of 1.4 x 6 x 1 mm for the buccally installed and 1.4 x 8 x 3 mm for the palatally installed mini-implants.[16]

The mean initial age of patients was 34.25 years (SD = 8.22, minimum 22.66, maximum 46.99) for Group 1 and 39.47 years (SD = 8.12, minimum 21.07, maximum 47.44) for Group 2. Mean intrusion duration was 0.81 years (SD = 0.35, minimum 0.41, maximum 1.64) for Group 1 and 1.17 years (SD = 0.48, minimum 0.75, maximum 2.14) for Group 2.

METHODS

Initial and final lateral cephalograms were not taken by the same equipment. Therefore, in order to increase reliability of results, correction of the magnification factor of each cephalogram was performed.[17]

Cephalograms were scanned in Microtek ScanMaker i800 (9600 x 4800 dpi, Microtek International, Inc., Carson, CA, USA) connected to a microcomputer Compaq Pavilion B6000BR board Intel Dual Core E5300 2.6 GHz, 2 GB memory RAM. Images were transferred to Dolphin Imaging Premium 5.10 software (Dolphin Imaging &Management Solutions, Chatsworth, CA, USA), through which points were marked by the same examiner and measurements were processed. The examiner was blinded regarding the group of each patient.

For better identification of maxillary first molars in the lateral cephalograms, clinical and cephalometric characteristics were associated: presence of restorations, level of extrusion, crown angulation and general characteristics of maxillary first molars as well as adjacent and antagonist teeth. Patients who had bilateral extrusions were measured twice separately.

Skeletal, dental and soft tissue variables were used, as shown in Figure 3. In initial and final cephalograms, the centroid point was built in the crown of the intruded first molar, and a vertical line was drawn perpendicular to the palatal plane, touching the centroid point. This way, the amount of intrusion of the maxillary first molar was measured. The centroid point is less influenced by potential side effects because it is a point on the longitudinal axis. Moreover, the palatal plane was used as a reference to measure intrusion of maxillary teeth[6] (Fig 4).

To evaluate the efficiency of the two studied intrusion protocols, the following formula was used:

$$Efficiency = \frac{Amount\ of\ intrusion}{Intrusion\ time}$$

With this formula, an efficiency value for molar intrusion was determined for each group separately.

Statistical analysis

To evaluate intraexaminer error, 15 randomly selected radiographs were remeasured after a month interval. Dependent t-test was applied to estimate systematic error. For evaluation of the random error, Dahlberg's formula was used.

In order to check for comparability between Groups 1 and 2 regarding the initial age, independent t-test was applied. Fisher exact test was used to evaluate intergroup comparability in relation to sex and type of malocclusion at the beginning of the study.

Independent t-test was used to compare variables between Groups 1 and 2 at the initial stage and during the intrusion period. The independent t-test was also used to compare intrusion duration between groups as well as intrusion efficiency. All statistical analyses were performed with Statistica for Windows software (Statsoft, Tulsa, Oklahoma, USA). Results were considered significant for $p < 0.05$.

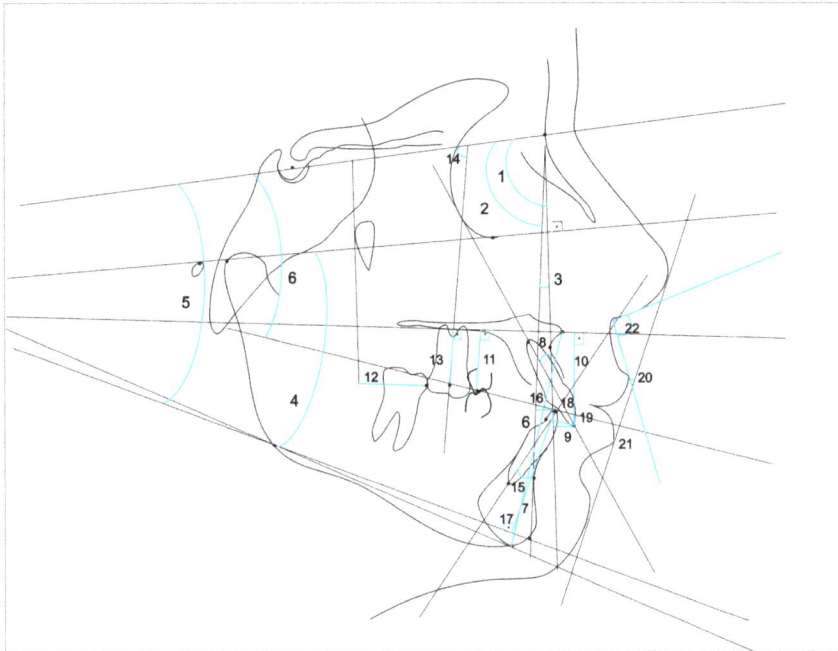

Figure 3 - Cephalometric variables: **1)** SNA, **2)** SNB, **3)** ANB, **4)** FMA, **5)** SN.GoGn, **6)** SN.Ocl, **7)** LAFH, **8)** U1.NA, **9)** U1-NA, **10)** U1-PP, **11)** U5-PP, **12)** U6-PTV, **13)** U6-PP, **14)** U6.SN, **15)** L1.NB, **16)** L1-NB, **17)** L1-GoGn, **18)** Overjet, **19)** Overbite, **20)** UL-E, **21)** LL-E, **22)** Nasolabial Angle.

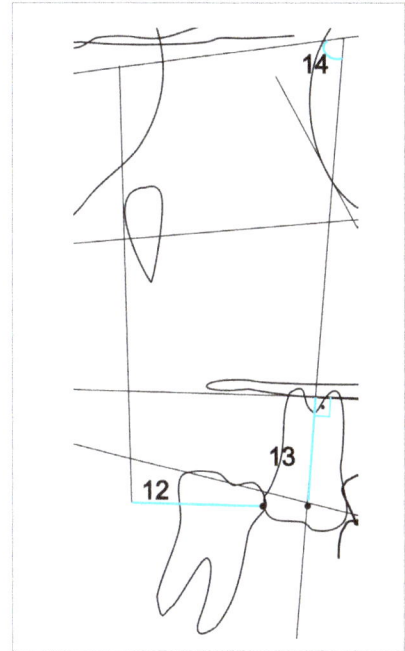

Figure 4 - Cephalometric variables relative to the maxillary first molar: **12)** U6-PTV, **13)** U6-PP, **14)** U6.SN.

RESULTS

No systematic error was detected and random errors varied from 0.18 mm (UL-E) to 0.47 mm (U6-PTV) in linear measurements and from 0.21° (FMA) to 0.95° (ANB). The groups were compatible regarding age, sex and type of malocclusion (Tables 1, 2 and 3). Table 4 showed that groups were also cephalometrically compatible at the beginning of treatment. During treatment/intrusion phase, only the variable LL-E showed statistically significant difference between groups (Table 5).

There was statistically significant difference for the time of intrusion, but there was no significant difference regarding the efficiency of intrusion between the two groups (Table 6).

Table 1 - Intergroup comparability of initial age (independent t-test).

| Variable (Years) | Group 1 | | Group 2 | | P Value |
	Mean	SD	Mean	SD	
Initial age	34.25	8.22	39.47	8.12	0.131

Table 2 - Intergroup comparability of sex distribution (Fisher exact test).

Sex / Group	Female	Male	Total
Group 1	12	3	15
Group 2	8	2	10
Total	20	5	25
Fisher Exact Test		DF=1	p = 1.000

Table 3 - Intergroup comparability of type of malocclusion (Fisher exact test).

Type of malocclusion	Group 1 (n = 15)	Group 2 (n = 10)
Class I	8	3
Class II	7	7
Fisher Exact Test	DF=1	p = 0.413

Table 4 - Intergroup comparison of cephalometric variables at the initial stage (T₁) (independent t-tests).

Variables	Group 1		Group 2		ρ value
	Mean	SD	Mean	SD	
Maxillary Component					
SNA (degrees)	85.18	3.20	85.56	3.81	0.7897
Mandibular Component					
SNB (degrees)	81.43	3.75	81.48	2.20	0.9681
Maxillomandibular Relationship					
ANB (degrees)	3.77	2.41	4.08	4.75	0.8328
Vertical Component					
FMA (degrees)	27.51	4.96	27.76	6.03	0.9119
SN.GoGn (degrees)	29.98	5.63	30.60	4.55	0.7744
SN.Ocl (degrees)	6.08	7.05	7.96	3.67	0.4477
LAFH (mm)	63.24	5.32	60.12	6.98	0.2174
Maxillary Dentoalveolar Component					
U1.NA (degrees)	26.01	8.00	23.61	8.19	0.4747
U1-NA (mm)	4.80	2.77	3.15	2.76	0.1572
U1-PP (mm)	26.98	3.26	24.88	3.06	0.1196
U5-PP (mm)	23.82	2.68	22.11	4.10	0.2177
U6-PTV (mm)	19.65	2.75	19.47	3.53	0.8853
U6-PP (mm)	21.58	2.83	19.79	3.17	0.1530
U6.SN (degrees)	80.81	5.30	81.00	6.92	0.9376
Mandibular Dentoalveolar Component					
L1.NB (degrees)	27.33	5.94	22.34	5.94	0.0514
L1-NB (mm)	5.83	2.22	3.98	2.26	0.0548
L1-GoGn (mm)	37.45	2.47	37.11	3.94	0.7944
Dental Relationships					
Overjet (mm)	3.84	1.11	4.32	2.71	0.5437
Overbite (mm)	2.99	0.94	3.49	2.38	0.4717
Soft Tissue Component					
UL-E (mm)	-3.75	2.43	-4.24	3.84	0.6965
LL-E (mm)	-1.21	2.40	-1.65	2.96	0.6835
Nasolabial angle (degrees)	100.56	7.45	103.48	11.60	0.4495

Table 5 - Intergroup comparison of cephalometric changes during treatment/intrusion (T_2-T_1) (independent t -ests).

Variables	Group 1		Group 2		p value
	Mean	SD	Mean	SD	
Maxillary Component					
SNA (degrees)	0.06	1.42	0.36	1.43	0.6104
Mandibular Component					
SNB (degrees)	-0.09	1.27	0.48	0.90	0.2295
Maxillomandibular Relationship					
ANB (degrees)	0.13	0.99	-0.11	1.33	0.6134
Vertical Component					
FMA (degrees)	-0.47	1.60	-1.24	0.98	0.1863
SN.GoGn (degrees)	0.34	1.27	-0.57	1.20	0.0864
SN.Ocl (degrees)	4.81	3.66	3.44	3.39	0.3539
LAFH (mm)	-0.16	2.11	0.16	1.80	0.6978
Maxillary Dentoalveolar Component					
U1.NA (degrees)	2.33	4.98	2.13	7.76	0.9368
U1-NA (mm)	0.52	1.88	-0.12	1.97	0.4215
U1-PP (mm)	-0.59	3.23	1.73	9.32	0.3808
U5-PP (mm)	-1.39	1.90	-1.31	1.67	0.9183
U6-PTV (mm)	-0.08	2.66	0.50	2.62	0.5963
U6-PP (mm)	-1.79	1.28	-2.12	1.25	0.5253
U6.SN (degrees)	1.17	3.29	-0.42	5.02	0.3458
Mandibular Dentoalveolar Component					
L1.NB (degrees)	2.51	2.80	0.21	4.07	0.1059
L1-NB (mm)	0.33	0.95	0.15	1.13	0.6761
L1-GoGn (mm)	-0.75	1.18	-0.37	1.42	0.4780
Dental Relationships					
Overjet (mm)	0.55	1.32	-0.51	2.23	0.1484
Overbite(mm)	-1.49	1.24	-1.57	2.46	0.9117
Soft Tissue Component					
UL-E (mm)	0.30	1.98	-0.13	2.24	0.6188
LL-E (mm)	1.11	1.02	-0.65	2.65	0.0275*
Nasolabial angle (degrees)	-1.07	8.92	-4.44	8.73	0.3601

* Statistically significant for $p < 0.05$.

Table 6 - Intergroup comparison of intrusion duration and efficiency (independent t-tests).

Variables	Group 1		Group 2		P Value
	Mean	SD	Mean	SD	
Intrusion duration (years)	0.81	0.35	1.17	0.48	0.045*
Intrusion efficiency	-2.18	1.14	-1.86	1.07	0.489

* Statistically significant for $p < 0.05$

DISCUSSION

An important criterion for sample selection was to include only patients with no growth potential. In a growing patient, vertical maxillary growth and development could possibly result in a relative molar intrusion, i.e., it would be questionable whether an actual intrusion occurred or presented as a result of alveolar process growth.[6]

Patients with systemic diseases, such as diabetes, osteoporosis, heart disease, clotting disorders and metabolic bone disorders, were excluded from the sample, as these factors could influence root resorption and stability of mini-implant and consequently in treatment/intrusion time.[18] Endodonticaly treated teeth were also excluded from the sample, since they could present an injury in healing process or root resorption, and these factors could influence the amount of intrusion.[18,19]

The study sample consisted of two lateral cephalograms of each patient. Lateral cephalograms for evaluation of skeletal and dental changes produced by intrusion mechanics are widely used in the literature, including assessment of maxillary molar intrusion.[4,20,21] Dolphin Imaging software computerized method also minimized errors in the determination of cephalometric values.[22] Several authors have used this software in other studies, thus ensuring its reliability.[22]

Groups were compatible regarding initial age (Table 1), sex distribution (Table 2), type of malocclusion (Table 3) and cephalometry at the beginning of treatment (Table 4). This allows comparability of groups, excluding factors influencing the results.

The sample was retrospectively selected, and there was probably some influence of the amount of intrusion required regarding the choice of protocols with two or three mini-implants. This possibly generated a difference between groups regarding the amount of intrusion achieved, being higher in the group in which the three mini-implant protocol was used (Table 5). This fact also explains the longer intrusion duration of this group (Table 6). However, to minimize this difference, intrusion efficiency was compared, which is the amount of intrusion achieved divided by intrusion duration, thus allowing intergroup comparison.

Cephalometric changes

During treatment/intrusion phase, there was no difference in skeletal and dental changes, except for the variable LL-E that showed a statistically significant difference between groups (Table 5).

According to specific first molar variables, i.e. U6-PTV, U6-PP and U6.SN, it was observed that both G1 and G2 showed a significant reduction in U6-PP during treatment, demonstrating effectiveness of the intrusion mechanics. In G1, mean intrusion of the maxillary first molar of 1.79 mm was obtained; while for G2, the mean intrusion of the first molar was of 2.12 mm. Mean molar intrusion was similar between groups (Table 5, Figs 5 and 6). Molar intrusion was finished when the tooth was leveled with adjacent teeth. Therefore, the amount of intrusion ranged from 0.6 to 5 mm, which was reasonable considering the different amount of overeruption of the tooth in each patient. The amount of intrusion varied in the literature according to the clinical needs. Carrillo et al[23] achieved 1.2 to 2.3 mm, Heravi et al[24] ranged from 1.5 to 4.5 mm and Al-Fraidiand Zawawi[25] achieved 4 mm in their studies.

There was also intrusion of second maxillary premolars in both groups (mean of 1.39 and 1.31 mm for Groups 1 and 2, respectively); however, without significant diffcrence between them (Table 5). Intrusion of premolars and molars was caused by intrusion mechanics with mini-implant anchorage. Since a leveling arch was used in fixed appliances in maxillary premolars and molars, this result was already expected. If the orthodontic mechanics of leveling and alignment was being held without intrusive force in the maxillary first molar region, premolars would probably extrude.[26] In the work by Yao et al,[3] there was a mean intrusion of first molars and second premolars of 3 mm and 2 mm, respectively.[3] These results corroborate the present study, since they show that the intrusion mechanics of the first molar also provides intrusion of the second premolar.

Both protocols in this study used forces from buccally and palatally placed mini-implants to prevent the overerupted molar from tipping either labio-palatally or mesio-distally as it was intruded. There was a small variation, in both groups, in mesiodistal angulation and anteroposterior movement of maxillary molars (U6.SN and U6-PTV, respectively, Table 5). This evinced a purely intrusive mechanics, without molar angulation that could camouflage the vertical positioning of these teeth.[27]

The method used in this study for molar intrusion produced an excellent control of labio-palatal maxillary molar position during intrusion with elastomeric chains attached to the mini-implants.

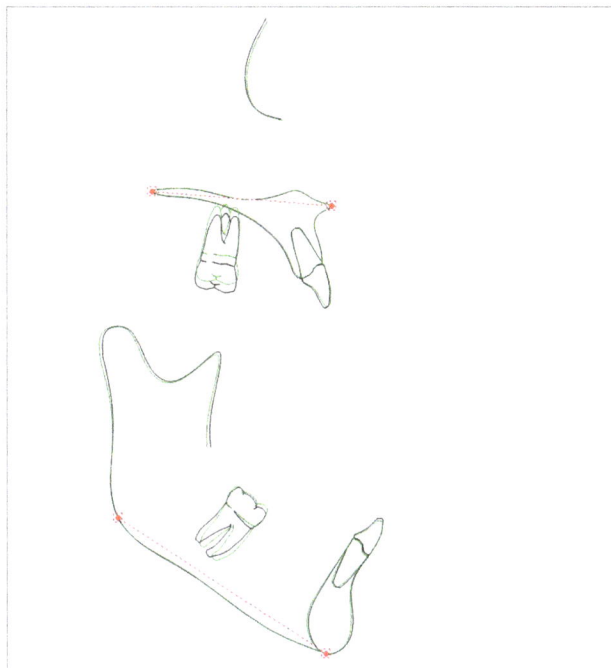

Figure 5 - Initial and final average tracings superimposition of Group 1.

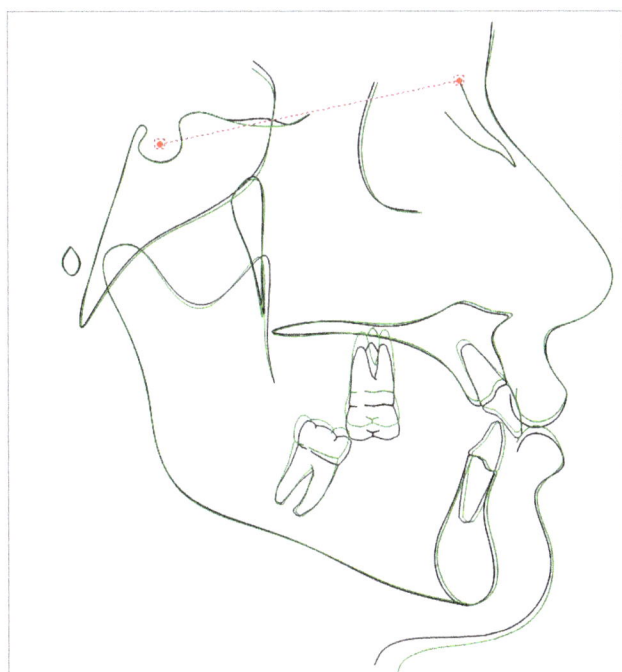

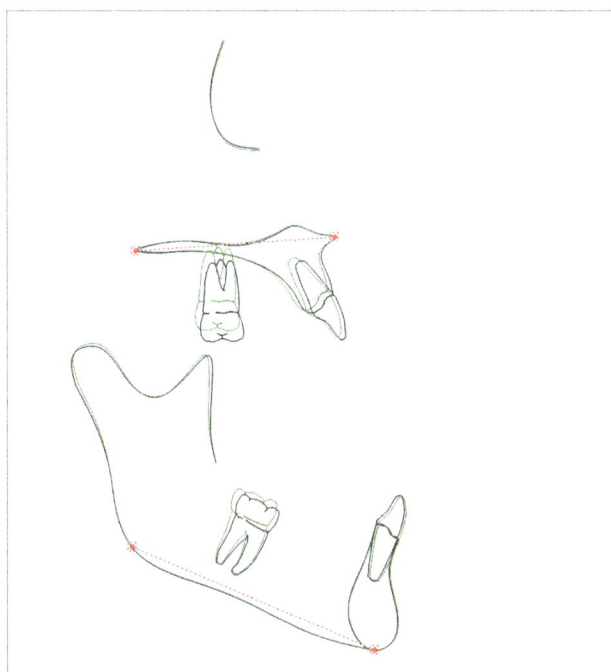

Figure 6 - Initial and final average tracings superimposition of Group 2.

There is no agreement in the literature on the optimum force to be used for molar intrusion. Some authors suggest forces ranging from 30 to 100 g,[24,28] whereas others have recommended using greater force for intrusion (150 to 500 g).[29,30] In this study, approximately 150 g of force was delivered from a short length of elastomeric chain. Force was carefully measured to ensure that it did not exceed the desired force level.

Regarding intrusion duration, there was statistically significant difference between groups, indicating that Group 2, the protocol with three mini-implants, showed longer intrusion duration, when compared to Group 1, the protocol with two mini-implants. However, these results are influenced by the greater or lesser need for intrusion in each case, as described above.

Maybe it is interesting that the tooth with the greatest need for intrusion has three mini-implants

placed, so as to increase reinforcement of anchorage.

There was no significant difference regarding intrusion efficiency between the two groups (Table 6).

CONCLUSION

Protocols of maxillary molar intrusion with two or three mini-implants presented the same efficiency of skeletal anchorage.

Authors contribution

Conception or design of the study: JVCP, FACF, FVF. Data acquisition, analysis or interpretation: JVCP, KMSF, RHC, FPV. Writing of the article: JVCP, KMSF, RHC. Critical revision of the article: KMSF, FACF, FVF, FPV. Final approval of the article: KMSF, FACF, RHC, FVF, FPV. Obtained funding: JVCP, FACF, FVF. Overall responsibility: JVCP.

REFERENCES

1. Cheng SJ, Tseng IY, Lee JJ, Kok SH. A prospective study of the risk factors associated with failure of mini-implants used for orthodontic anchorage. Int J Oral Maxillofac Implants. 2004 Jan-Feb;19(1):100-6.

2. Melsen B. Limitation in adults Orthodontics. In: Melsen B, editor. Current controversies in Orthodontics. Chicago: Quintessence; 1991. p. 147-80.

3. Yao CC, Lee JJ, Chen HY, Chang ZC, Chang HF, Chen YJ. Maxillary molar intrusion with fixed appliances and mini-implant anchorage studied in three dimensions. Angle Orthod. 2005 Sept;75(5):754-60.

4. Yao CC, Wu CB, Wu HY, Kok SH, Chang HF, Chen YJ. Intrusion of the overerupted upper left first and second molars by mini-implants with partial-fixed orthodontic appliances: a case report. Angle Orthod. 2004 Aug;74(4):550-7.

5. Chun YS, Lim WH. Bone density at interradicular sites: implications for orthodontic mini-implant placement. Orthod Craniofac Res. 2009 Feb;12(1):25-32.

6. Ng J, Major PW, Flores-Mir C. True molar intrusion attained during orthodontic treatment: a systematic review. Am J Orthod Dentofacial Orthop. 2006 Dec;130(6):709-14.

7. Chen CH, Chang CS, Hsieh CH, Tseng YC, Shen YS, Huang IY, et al. The use of microimplants in orthodontic anchorage. J Oral Maxillofac Surg. 2006 Aug;64(8):1209-13.

8. Brandão LBC, Mucha JN. Rate of mini-implant acceptance by patients undergoing orthodontic treatment - A preliminary study with questionnaires. Dental Press J Orthod. 2008 Sept-Oct;13(5):118-27.

9. Lee SJ, Jang SY, Chun YS, Lim WH. Three-dimensional analysis of tooth movement after intrusion of a supraerupted molar using a mini-implant with partial-fixed orthodontic appliances. Angle Orthod. 2013 Mar;83(2):274-9.

10. Grenga V, Bovi M. Corticotomy-enhanced intrusion of an overerupted molar using skeletal anchorage and ultrasonic surgery. J Clin Orthod. 2013 Jan;47(1):50-5; quiz 64.

11. Sawhney C, Kumar S. Technique tips--modified transpalatal appliance: a simple non-invasive technique for maxillary molar intrusion. Dent Update. 2012 Apr;39(3):228.

12. Lee M, Shuman J. Maxillary molar intrusion with a single miniscrew and a transpalatal arch. J Clin Orthod. 2012 Jan;46(1):48-51.

13. Bae SM, Park HS, Kyung HM, Kwon OW, Sung JH. Clinical application of micro-implant anchorage. J Clin Orthod. 2002 May;36(5):298-302.

14. Park HS, Bae SM, Kyung HM, Sung JH. Micro-implant anchorage for treatment of skeletal Class I bialveolar protrusion. J Clin Orthod. 2001 July;35(7):417-22.

15. Lin JC, Liou EJ. A new bone screw for orthodontic anchorage. J Clin Orthod. 2003 Dec;37(12):676-81.

16. Crismani AG, Bertl MH, Celar AG, Bantleon HP, Burstone CJ. Miniscrews in orthodontic treatment: review and analysis of published clinical trials. Am J Orthod Dentofacial Orthop. 2010 Jan;137(1):108-13.

17. Janson G, Valarelli FP, Henriques JF, de Freitas MR, Cançado RH. Stability of anterior open bite nonextraction treatment in the permanent dentition. Am J Orthod Dentofacial Orthop. 2003 Sept;124(3):265-76; quiz 340.

18. Abuabara A. Biomechanical aspects of external root resorption in orthodontic therapy. Med Oral Patol Oral Cir Bucal. 2007 Dec 1;12(8):E610-3.

19. Chung KR, Kim SH, Kang YG, Nelson G. Orthodontic miniplate with tube as an efficient tool for borderline cases. Am J Orthod Dentofacial Orthop. 2011 Apr;139(4):551-62.

20. Erverdi N, Keles A, Nanda R. The use of skeletal anchorage in open bite treatment: a cephalometric evaluation. Angle Orthod. 2004 Jun;74(3):381-90.

21. Moon CH, Wee JU, Lee HS. Intrusion of overerupted molars by corticotomy and orthodontic skeletal anchorage. Angle Orthod. 2007 Nov;77(6):1119-25.

22. Thurzo A, Javorka V, Stanko P, Lysy J, Suchancova B, Lehotska V, et al. Digital and manual cephalometric analysis. Bratisl Lek Listy. 2010;111(2):97-100.

23. Carrillo R, Rossouw PE, Franco PF, Opperman LA, Buschang PH. Intrusion of multiradicular teeth and related root resorption with mini-screw implant anchorage: a radiographic evaluation. Am J Orthod Dentofacial Orthop. 2007 Nov;132(5):647-55.

24. Heravi F, Bayani S, Madani AS, Radvar M, Anbiaee N. Intrusion of supra-erupted molars using miniscrews: clinical success and root resorption. Am J Orthod Dentofacial Orthop. 2011 Apr;139(4 Suppl):S170-5.

25. Al-Fraidi AA, Zawawi KH. Clinical showcase. Selective intrusion of overerupted upper first molars using a temporary anchorage device: case report. J Can Dent Assoc. 2010;76:a9.

26. Armbruster P, Sheridan JJ, Nguyen P. An Essix intrusion appliance. J Clin Orthod. 2003 Aug;37(8):412-6.

27. Romeo A, Esteves M, García V, Bermúdez J. Movement evaluation of overerupted upper molars with absolute anchorage: an in-vitro study. Med Oral Patol Oral Cir Bucal. 2010 Nov 1;15(6):e930-5.

28. Melo AC, Jawonski ME, Largura LZ, Thomé G, Souza JR, Silva MA. Upper molar intrusion in rehabilitation patients with the aid of microscrews. Aust Orthod J. 2008 May;24(1):50-3.

29. Umemori M, Sugawara J, Mitani H, Nagasaka H, Kawamura H. Skeletal anchorage system for open-bite correction. Am J Orthod Dentofacial Orthop. 1999 Feb;115(2):166-74.

30. Park YC, Lee SY, Kim DH, Jee SH. Intrusion of posterior teeth using mini-screw implants. Am J Orthod Dentofacial Orthop. 2003 Jun;123(6):690-4.

5

Orthodontic intrusion of maxillary incisors: a 3D finite element method study

Armando Yukio Saga[1], Hiroshi Maruo[2], Marco André Argenta[3], Ivan Toshio Maruo[4], Orlando Motohiro Tanaka[5]

Objective: In orthodontic treatment, intrusion movement of maxillary incisors is often necessary. Therefore, the objective of this investigation is to evaluate the initial distribution patterns and magnitude of compressive stress in the periodontal ligament (PDL) in a simulation of orthodontic intrusion of maxillary incisors, considering the points of force application. **Methods:** Anatomic 3D models reconstructed from cone-beam computed tomography scans were used to simulate maxillary incisors intrusion loading. The points of force application selected were: centered between central incisors brackets (LOAD 1); bilaterally between the brackets of central and lateral incisors (LOAD 2); bilaterally distal to the brackets of lateral incisors (LOAD 3); bilaterally 7 mm distal to the center of brackets of lateral incisors (LOAD 4). **Results and Conclusions:** Stress concentrated at the PDL apex region, irrespective of the point of orthodontic force application. The four load models showed distinct contour plots and compressive stress values over the midsagittal reference line. The contour plots of central and lateral incisors were not similar in the same load model. LOAD 3 resulted in more balanced compressive stress distribution.

Keywords: Orthodontics. Tooth intrusion. Finite element analysis.

[1] Professor, Pontifícia Universidade Católica do Paraná (PUC-PR), School of Health and Biosciences, Residency in Orthodontics, Curitiba, Paraná, Brazil.

[2] Professor, Associação Brasileira de Odontologia (ABO-PG), Ponta Grossa, Paraná, Brazil.

[3] Adjunct professor, Universidade Federal do Paraná (UFPR), Department of Civil Engineering, Graduate Program in Numerical Methods, Curitiba, Paraná, Brazil.

[4] Professor, Pontifícia Universidade Católica do Paraná (PUC-PR), Residency in Orthodontics, and Associação Brasileira de Odontologia (ABO-PR), Curitiba, Paraná, Brazil.

[5] Professor, Pontifícia Universidade Católica do Paraná (PUC-PR), School of Health and Biosciences, Graduate Dentistry Program in Orthodontics, Curitiba, Paraná, Brazil.

» The authors report no commercial, proprietary or financial interest in the products or companies described in this article.

Orlando Tanaka
Rua Imaculada Conceição, 1155 – CEP: 80.215-901 – Curitiba/PR, Brazil
E-mail: tanakaom@gmail.com

INTRODUCTION

Regardless of genetic or treatment-related factors, maxillary incisors consistently feature more external apical root resorption (EARR) than any other tooth.[1,2] With respect to the type of movement, intrusion movement appeared to be the most predictive for EARR.[3,4,5] However, frequently, in orthodontic treatment, intrusion movement of an entire segment consisting of four maxillary incisors is necessary, as in cases of deep overbite correction.

With tridimensional (3D) numeric computer analysis, such as the finite element analysis (FEA), valuable information can be obtained, since various orthodontic clinical conditions can be simulated, and stress distribution in the individual constituents of the periodontium can be evaluated qualitatively and quantitatively.[6,7]

Studies relating the distribution of compression stress in the periodontal ligament (PDL) to the intrusion of maxillary incisors are scarce and approached in nonclinical conditions, since an intrusive force coincident with the long axes of four maxillary incisors is impossible to obtain clinically.[8,9]

Therefore, the objective of this investigation is to evaluate the initial distribution patterns and magnitude of compressive stress in the PDL in a simulation of orthodontic intrusion of maxillary incisors, considering the points of force application.

MATERIAL AND METHODS

A maxilla from a dry adult human skull was reconstructed based on cone-beam computed tomography scans (i-CAT™, Imaging Sciences, Hatfield, PA, USA), yielding a stack of 256 slices with 0.25 mm thickness, converted into exportable DICOM files.

The limits of the compact and trabecular layers of bone, enamel and dentin were determined by using digital edge detection technology. The edges were then used to generate the 3D geometry with commercial computer-aided design software (Simpleware™, Innovation Centre, Exeter, United Kingdom). The generated solid was exported as STL file (Stereolithography CAD) extension to Solidworks™ (Dessault Systèmes Solidworks Corp., Concord, MA, USA) in order to convert into bilinear nonuniform rational B-spline (NURBS). The 0.022-in standard nontorqued, nonangulated edgewise orthodontic brackets and a cross section of 0.021 x 0.025-in arch wire were also 3D modeled. A 0.25-mm gap between roots and alveolar bone socket surfaces was considered as the space of the PDL.

This file was exported to ANSYS™ v12.1 (Swanson Analysis System Inc., Canonsburg, PA, USA), the FEA solver software. The model was meshed by using tetrahedral elements of which quadratic shape allowed capturing the complex, curved surfaces in the modeling accuracy. The final model consisted of 322450 elements with edge length ranging from 0.25 mm to 1.50 mm and 603380 nodes.

Dental and bone material were assumed to be homogeneous, isotropic, and linearly elastic with specific Young's modulus and Poisson's ratios (Table 1).[10,11] To represent the nonlinear mechanical behavior of the PDL, parameters of the hyperelastic instantaneous response were used (Table 2).[12]

The points of force application were selected based on simulated clinical situations and considering points which the clinician usually would choose to intrude maxillary incisors. Thus, the points of force application were:

- LOAD 1: centered between central incisors brackets (Fig 1A).
- LOAD 2: bilaterally between central and lateral incisors brackets (Fig 1B).
- LOAD 3: bilaterally distal to lateral incisors brackets (Fig 1C).
- LOAD 4: bilaterally 7 mm distal to the center of lateral incisors brackets (Fig 1D).

To LOADs 2, 3 and 4, the points were selected also considering the approximate location of the center of resistance (CRes) of maxillary incisors. As a reference, it could lie apical of a point between the distal root side of the lateral incisor and the distal root side of the canine.[13-16] No consensus has been reached in the literature in terms of the exact localization of CRes of maxillary incisors. Therefore, the points of force application varied in the 3D model in an attempt to approach, as close as possible, the center of resistance, which would result in more balanced stress distribution.

An intrusive force of 15 gf per tooth was applied to the model vertically, upwards and direct to the cross section of the 0.021 x 0.025-in archwire, since previous studies recommended a force magnitude varying from 10 to 20 gf per tooth, depending on the amount of periodontal support.[17,18] It was imposed zero-displacement and zero-rotation boundary conditions on the nodes along the sliced maxilla in supra-apical horizontal plane.

Table 1 - Basic material properties of teeth and bone.

Material	Young's modulus (MPa)	Poisson's ratios
Enamel	84100[a]	0.20[a]
Dentin	18600[a]	0.31[a]
Compact bone	13800[a]	0.26[a]
Trabecular bone	345[a]	0.31[a]
Stainless steel	200000[b]	0.30[c]

a = Source: Jones et al.[10]; b = Source: Kojima and Fukui.[11]

Table 2 - Parameters of the hyperelastic instantaneous response of the PDL.[12]

C1 (MPa)	C2(MPa)	C3(MPa)	Kᵥ (MPa)	β
0.004	0.002	0.004	1000	3.5

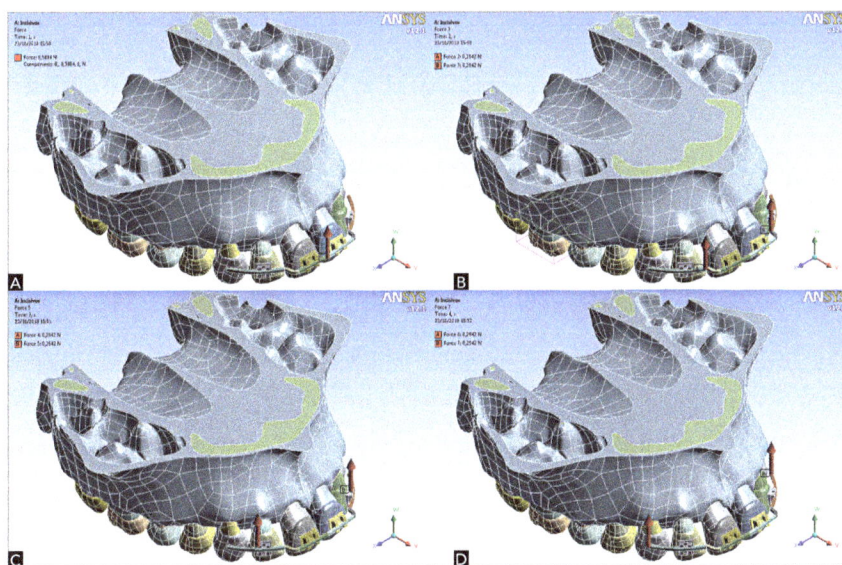

Figure 1 - Selected points of force application. A) LOAD 1; B) LOAD 2; C) LOAD 3; D) LOAD 4.

XY scatter charts of stress values in a representative sagittal labial-apex-palatal (LAP) line were also considered, since the latter is located in the main plane to visualize maxillary incisors intrusion movement. The LAP representative line was defined by a reference line from the labial side of the PDL alveolar crest, going up to the apex to the palatal side of the alveolar crest, and matching, as close as possible, the midsagittal plane of the tooth.[5,19,20] A total of 79 nodes were selected along this line for central incisors (relabeled from 1 to 79) and 88 for lateral incisors (relabeled from 1 to 88). Once the anatomical traits of the maxilla and teeth were clinically symmetrical, only teeth on the right side were considered for the XY scatter charts.

Figure 2 illustrates just the location of the odd numbered nodes for right maxillary central and lateral incisors in the LAP representative line.

RESULTS

The results are graphically demonstrated in two manners: contour plots and XY scatter charts representing nodal stress data in the PDL side of the PDL-socket bone interface, since stress in the PDL can be used to predict potential sites of bone remodeling.[21]

Records according to the minimum, mid and maximum principal stresses were obtained. In this study, minimum principal stress (MinPS) was equivalent to compressive stress. Hence, MinPS will be approached.

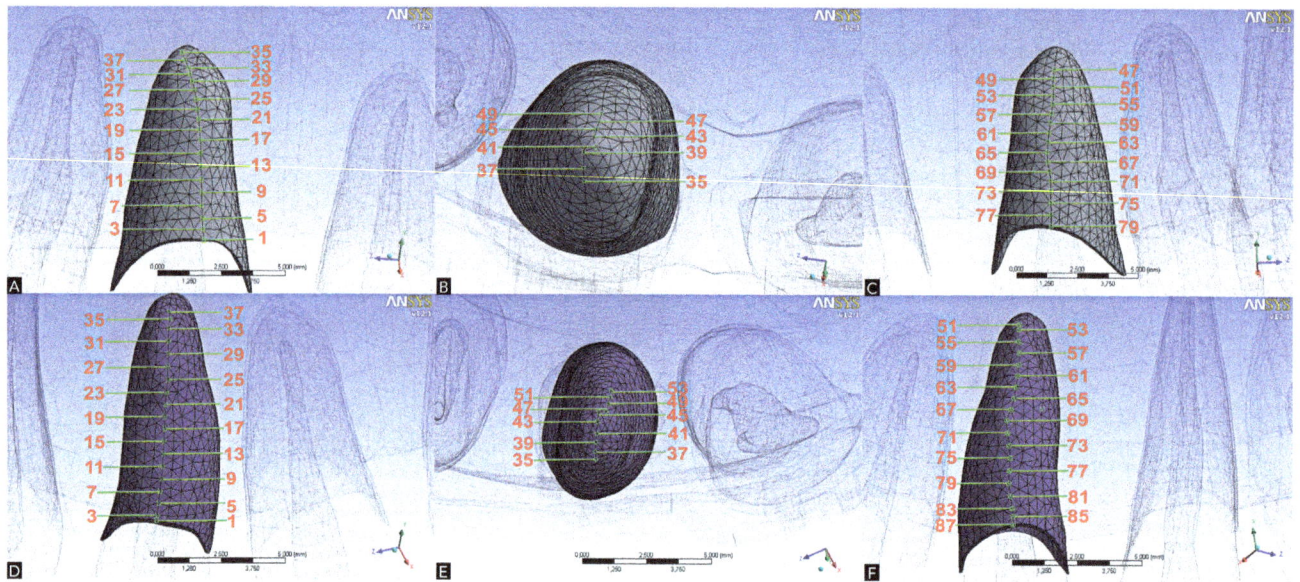

Figure 2 - Position of the odd numbered nodes in the LAP referential plane to right maxillary central incisor (**A** - labial view; **B** - apical view; **C** - palatal view) and to right maxillary lateral incisor (**D** - labial view; **E** - apical view; **F** - palatal view).

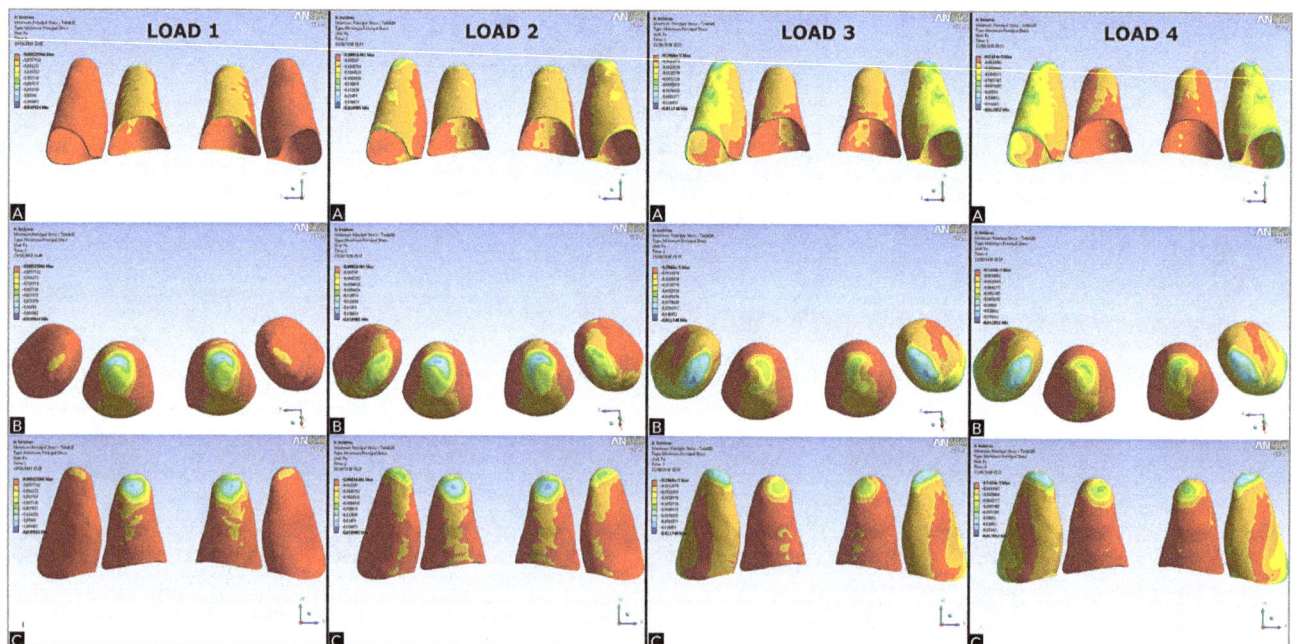

Figure 3 - MinPS (compression stress) distribution for maxillary incisors to LOADS 1, 2, 3 and 4: **A**) labial view; **B**) apical view; **C**) palatal view.

Contour plots

The contour plots for MinPS distribution are illustrated in Figure 3. Blue color shows areas of higher compression while red color refers to areas of lower compression. Throughout the simulation, the highest compressive areas were located at the apex.

In LOAD 1, the highest compression occurred mainly at the apex of central incisors. Overall, the labial side of the PDL presented a more extended compressive region than the palatal side.

In LOAD 2, the highest compressive areas were observed at the apex of central incisors as well, but these areas shifted to mesial. Areas of compression were observed in the lateral incisors apex. Both central and lateral incisors exhibited higher compressive areas on the labial side in comparison to the palatal side, especially at the PDL labial margin of lateral incisors.

In LOAD 3, the highest compressive areas shifted to lateral incisors apex. Compression areas in the PDL labial middle region and at the PDL labial margin were also present in these teeth. For central incisors, the palatal side of the apex exhibited higher compressive stress and almost the entire labial side of the PDL presented lower compression in comparison to the palatal side.

Similarly to LOAD 3, in LOAD 4, the highest compression was observed at the lateral incisors apex as well. In the labial middle region and at the labial and mesial margin of lateral incisors PDL, compression was also present. Comparatively to LOAD 3, central incisors PDL labial side was less compressive. MinPS magnitudes (milliPascal, or mPa) for the four loading models are given in Table 3.

MinPS XY scatter charts - Right maxillary central incisor (Fig 4)

In every loading model, node 45, located in the PDL apex, showed the highest compression; i.e., most negative values. In LOAD 1, on the labial side, higher compression in the PDL cervical third occurred comparatively to the palatal side. From node 25 (labial apical third) to node 35, a sharper compression increase occurred. Node 45, located at the PDL apex, presented the highest compression (-40.14 mPa). From node 45,

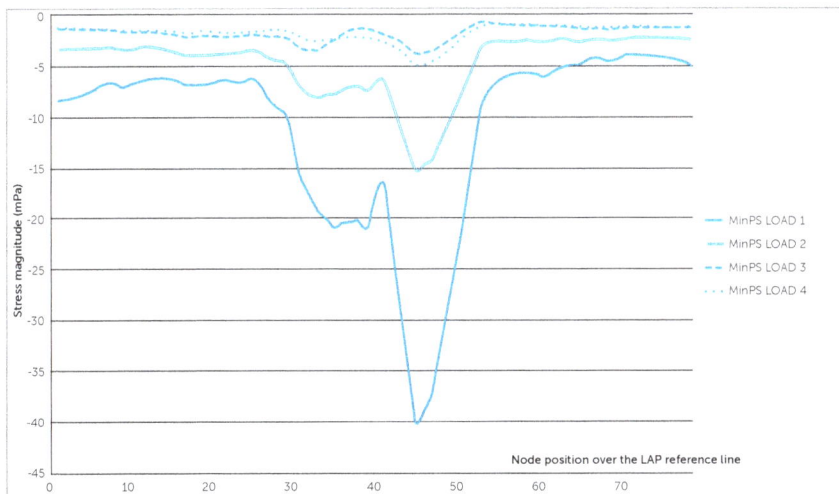

Figure 4 - MinPS (compression stress) scatter chart to the four loading simulations according to node position over the LAP reference line for the right maxillary central incisor.

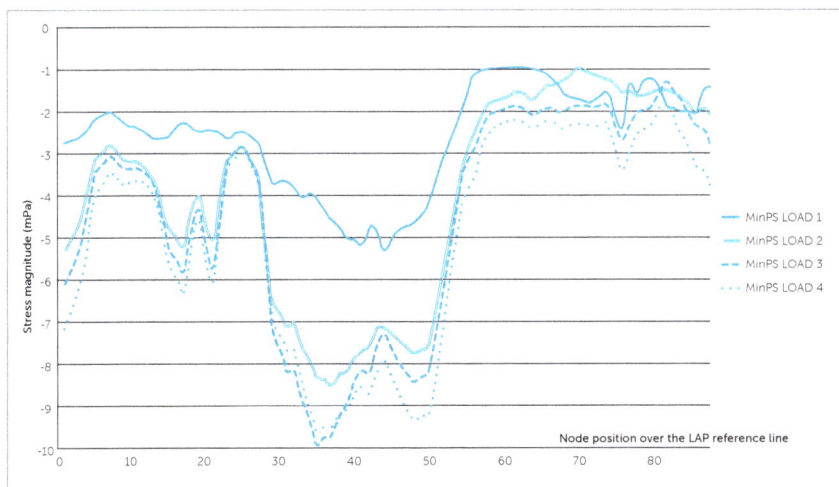

Figure 5 - MinPS (compression stress) scatter chart to the four loading simulations according to node position over the LAP reference line for the right maxillary lateral incisor.

Table 3 - MinPS values (mPa) of the four loading simulation to maxillary right central and lateral incisors.

MinPS	LOAD 1		LOAD 2		LOAD 3		LOAD 4	
	Max	Min	Max	Min	Max	Min	Max	Min
Central incisor	-7.72	-40.14	-2.20	-15.30	-0.69	-3.80	-0.90	-5.06
Lateral incisor	-0.94	-5.30	-0.99	-8.49	-1.29	-9.89	-1.74	-9.57

Note: the more negative the value, the higher the compressive stress.

compression descended steeply. The line between nodes 55 and 79 referred approximately to the cervical and middle thirds of the PDL palatal side.

LOAD 2 had a similar behavior to LOAD 1; however, in all nodes, less compression was observed; e.g., in node 45, MinPS was -15.30 mPa (2.62 less compression than in LOAD 1). Moreover, from node 1 to 25, on PDL labial side, compression was relatively constant.

LOADS 3 and 4 revealed the lowest compression (-3.80 mPa and -5.06 mPa, respectively) and variations of stress along the LAP reference line, showing the smallest differences between maximum and minimum values. Thus, they demonstrated a more balanced distribution of stress.

MinPS XY scatter charts - Right maxillary lateral incisor (Fig 5)

Comparatively to central incisors, stress distribution over the LAP reference line was more irregular for lateral incisors, with more up and down variations. For LOAD 1, there was a tendency from node 1 to 44 towards a moderate compression decrease. Node 44 had the highest compression stress (-5.30 mPa). From this node until node 56, the decrease in compression stress was followed by a tendency towards stabilization of compression. For LOADs 2, 3 e 4, the graphic line behavior was similar. The PDL labial side demonstrated great nodal stress variations along the LAP reference line. Compression stress was observed in the PDL labial margin in LOAD 4 (-7.11 mPa), followed by LOAD 3 (-6.08 mPa) and 2 (-5.29 mPa).

In the PDL apex, the highest compression stress was observed at the apical area at node 35 to LOAD 4 (-9.57 mPa) and LOAD 3 (-9.89 mPa), at node 36 to LOAD 2 (-8.33 mPa) and at node 44 (-5.30 mPa) to LOAD 1.

DISCUSSION

FEA is a computer engineering numeric method that has allowed solution of biomechanical problems not involving live organisms. The 3D model of the maxilla and teeth obtained from a real anatomic skull and the discretization of individual components of bone (trabecular and cortical bone) and tooth (enamel and dentin) in this study render the results as closer as possible to a real situation.

Clinically, intrusive forces have been traditional suspect in severe cases of root resorption.[4,5,22] The present finite element model study showed that there was stress concentration at the PDL of the root apex. Shaw, Sameshima and Vu,[7] as well as Parker and Harris,[5] reported that intrusive movement and increase in incisor proclination were the most powerful predictors of EARR. Comparatively, LOADs 1 and 2 were mechanical configurations with the highest compression in the apical region of the PDL, and also had the greatest tendency towards buccal proclination of central incisors. Thus, from a biological and mechanical standpoint, they could be the least desirable points of force application for intrusion of maxillary incisors. Even though this study has demonstrated stress concentration in the apical region of the PDL, clinical studies[20,23] showed no differences in the amount of root resorption between intrusion and other orthodontic movements, demonstrating that there are still other factors or variables to be explored.

In addition, factors that alter the position of the CRes of four maxillary incisors are the shape of surrounding bone, root morphology, position of each tooth, and structure of the periodontal attachment.[9,24] Since these factors will generally be different for each patient, the location of the CRes of anterior arch segments in these patients will also be different.

In vitro studies using different methods[13,15,25,26] showed that the CRes of the four incisors lies 8-10 mm apical and 5-7 mm distal to lateral incisors. A more anterior location of the point of force application causes flaring, whereas a more posterior location will cause uprighting of anterior teeth. When the axial inclination of incisors is different, so is the location of the axes of resistance in relation to the position of incisors crowns. More flared incisors should have a more distal point of force application than retroclined incisors.[16] However, it is important to report that the 3D model produced had just a slight maxillary incisor protrusion, and this fact might have influenced the results in relation to stress distribution. Even if there is no common center or axis of resistance to the four incisors, it is necessary to determine a line of action of force that promotes a more balanced stress distribution.

LOAD 1 and LOAD 2 mechanical configurations, especially LOAD 1, showed a strong tendency towards proclination of maxillary central incisors; whereas for LOAD 3 and LOAD 4, the orthodontic movement likely to occur would be intrusion with little or no protrusion, but with distal inclination of lateral incisors in LOAD 4.

Although LOAD 3 and LOAD 4 presented more balanced stress distribution, in agreement with Reimann et al,[25] it is important to note that the central incisors are loaded with smaller force systems than lateral incisors. This, in turn, means that lateral incisors are loaded higher by the applied force system, which could compromise periodontal support, since lateral incisors usually have a smaller root surface area than central incisors.

As in most computer simulations of biological situations, the limitations of the study are mainly regarding material parameters. It must be stated that values reported in the literature differ significantly from each other, especially in terms of the PDL. These differences are due to experimental designs, large variation in the complexity and geometry of numerical models.[27]

Evidently the applied parameters did not reproduce perfectly the complex structure and behavior of dental, bone and PDL tissues. Nevertheless, it was assumed that this behavior idealization was suitable to describe theoretically the initial stress distribution of maxillary incisors orthodontic intrusion and that the results could be considered in clinical treatment planning.

Computed tomography scans and 3D reconstructions have become common examinations in orthodontic diagnosis. They allow individual determination of the most suitable points/axes of force application by computer modeling and numerical simulation. Thus, in the treatment of patients with complex problems, in which risks are greater, they may assist the implementation of a more effective orthodontic mechanics in order to obtain greater predictability of orthodontic movement with minimal side effects.

CONCLUSIONS

Within the study methodology, it is possible to conclude the following:

1. Stress is concentrated at the PDL apex region, irrespective of the point of orthodontic force application;

2. The four load models showed distinct contour plots and compressive stress values over the LAP reference line;

3. The contour plots of central and lateral incisors were not similar in the same load model;

4. LOAD 3 resulted in more balanced compressive stress distribution.

Authors contribution

Conceived and designed the study: AYS, ITM. Drafted the study: AYS. Data acquisition, analysis or interpretation: AYS, MAA, ITM. Wrote the article: AYS. Critical revision of the article: OMT. Final approval of the article: HM. Overall responsibility: AYS

REFERENCES

1. Kennedy DB, Joondeph DR, Osterberg SK, Little RM. The effect of extraction and orthodontic treatment on dentoalveolar support. Am J Orthod. 1983 Sep;84(3):183-90.

2. Linge BO, Linge L. Apical root resorption in upper anterior teeth. Eur J Orthod. 1983 Aug;5(3):173-83.

3. Baumrind S, Korn EL, Boyd RL. Apical root resorption in orthodontically treated adults. Am J Orthod Dentofacial Orthop. 1996 Sep;110(3):311-20.

4. Han G, Huang S, Von den Hoff JW, Zeng X, Kuijpers-Jagtman AM. Root resorption after orthodontic intrusion and extrusion: an intraindividual study. Angle Orthod. 2005 Nov;75(6):912-8.

5. Parker RJ, Harris EF. Directions of orthodontic tooth movements associated with external apical root resorption of the maxillary central incisor. Am J Orthod Dentofacial Orthop. 1998 Dec;114(6):677-83.

6. Sung SJ, Jang GW, Chun YS, Moon YS. Effective en-masse retraction design with orthodontic mini-implant anchorage: a finite element analysis. Am J Orthod Dentofacial Orthop. 2010 May;137(5):648-57.

7. Shaw AM, Sameshima GT, Vu HV. Mechanical stress generated by orthodontic forces on apical root cementum: a finite element model. Orthod Craniofac Res. 2004 May;7(2):98-107.

8.   Rudolph DJ, Willes PMG, Sameshima GT. A finite element model of apical force distribution from orthodontic tooth movement. Angle Orthod. 2001 Apr;71(2):127-31.

9.   Kamble RH, Lohkare S, Hararey PV, Mundada RD. Stress distribution pattern in a root of maxillary central incisor having various root morphologies: a finite element study. Angle Orthod. 2012 Sep;82(5):799-805.

10. Jones ML, Hickman J, Middleton J, Knox J, Volp C. A validated finite element method study of orthodontic tooth movement in the human subject. J Orthod. 2001 Mar;28(1):29-38.

11. Kojima Y, Fukui H. A numerical simulation of tooth movement by wire bending. Am J Orthod Dentofacial Orthop. 2006 Oct;130(4):452-9.

12. Natali A, Pavan P, Carniel E, Dorow C. Viscoelastic response of the periodontal ligament: an experimental-numerical analysis. Connect Tissue Res. 2004;45(4-5):222-30.

13. Vanden Bulcke MM, Dermaut LR, Sachdeva RC, Burstone CJ. The center of resistance of anterior teeth during intrusion using the laser reflection technique and holographic interferometry. Am J Orthod Dentofacial Orthop. 1986 Sep;90(3):211-20.

14. Pedersen E, Isidor F, Gjessing P, Andersen K. Location of centres of resistance for maxillary anterior teeth measured on human autopsy material. Eur J Orthod. 1991 Dec;13(6):452-8.

15. Matsui S, Caputo AA, Chaconas SJ, Kiyomura H. Center of resistance of anterior arch segment. Am J Orthod Dentofacial Orthop. 2000 Aug;118(2):171-8.

16. van Steenbergen E, Burstone CJ, Prahl-Andersen B, Aartman IH. The relation between the point of force application and flaring of the anterior segment. Angle Orthod. 2005 Sep;75(5):730-5.

17. Melsen B, Agerbaek N, Markenstam G. Intrusion of incisors in adult patients with marginal bone loss. Am J Orthod Dentofacial Orthop. 1989 Sep;96(3):232-41.

18. Weiland FJ, Bantleon HP, Droschl H. Evaluation of continuous arch and segmented arch leveling techniques in adult patients--a clinical study. Am J Orthod Dentofacial Orthop. 1996 Dec;110(6):647-52.

19. Costopoulos G, Nanda R. An evaluation of root resorption incident to orthodontic intrusion. Am J Orthod Dentofacial Orthop. 1996 May;109(5):543-8.

20. Bellamy LJ, Kokich VG, Weissman JA. Using orthodontic intrusion of abraded incisors to facilitate restoration: the technique's effects on alveolar bone level and root length. J Am Dent Assoc. 2008 Jun;139(6):725-33.

21. Field C, Ichim I, Swain MV, Chan E, Darendeliler MA, Li W, et al. Mechanical responses to orthodontic loading: a 3-dimensional finite element multi-tooth model. Am J Orthod Dentofacial Orthop. 2009 Feb;135(2):174-81.

22. Harris DA, Jones AS, Darendeliler MA. Physical properties of root cementum: part 8. Volumetric analysis of root resorption craters after application of controlled intrusive light and heavy orthodontic forces: a microcomputed tomography scan study. Am J Orthod Dentofacial Orthop. 2006 Nov;130(5):639-47.

23. Polat-Ozsoy O, Arman-Ozcirpici A, Veziroglu F. Miniscrews for upper incisor intrusion. Eur J Orthod. 2009 Aug;31(4):412-6.

24. Heravi F, Salari S, Tanbakuchi B, Loh S, Amiri M. Effects of crown-root angle on stress distribution in the maxillary central incisors' PDL during application of intrusive and retraction forces: a three-dimensional finite element analysis. Prog Orthod. 2013 Sep 11;14:26.

25. Reimann S, Keilig L, Jäger A, Bourauel C. Biomechanical finite-element investigation of the position of the centre of resistance of the upper incisors. Eur J Orthod. 2007 Jun;29(3):219-24. Epub 2007 Feb 22.

26. Sia S, Koga Y, Yoshida N. Determining the center of resistance of maxillary anterior teeth subjected to retraction forces in sliding mechanics. An in vivo study. Angle Orthod. 2007 Nov;77(6):999-1003.

27. Poppe M, Bourauel C, Jäger A. Determination of the elasticity parameters of the human periodontal ligament and the location of the center of resistance of single-rooted teeth a study of autopsy specimens and their conversion into finite element models. J Orofac Orthop. 2002 Sep;63(5):358-70.

6

Force decay evaluation of latex and non-latex orthodontic intraoral elastics: *in vivo* study

Daniela Ferreira de Carvalho Notaroberto[1], Mariana Martins e Martins[2],
Maria Teresa de Andrade Goldner[3], Alvaro de Moraes Mendes[3], Cátia Cardoso Abdo Quintão[3]

Objective: This clinical study was conducted in order to evaluate force decay over time of latex and non-latex orthodontic intraoral elastics. **Methods:** Patients (n = 15) were evaluated using latex and non-latex elastics in the periods of : 0, 1, 3, 12 and 24 hours. The rubber bands were transferred to the testing machine (EMIC DL-500 MF), and force values were recorded after stretching the elastic to a length of 25mm. Paired *t* test was applied and analysis of variance (ANOVA) was used to evaluate the variation of force generated. LSD (Fisher's least significant difference) *post-hoc* test was thus employed. **Results:** As regards the initial forces (zero time), the values of force for non-latex elastic were slightly higher than for the latex elastic. In the subsequent times, the forces generated by the latex elastic showed higher values. Regarding the material degradation, at the end of 24 hours the highest percentage was observed for non-latex elastic. **Conclusions:** The latex elastics had a more stable behavior during the studied period, compared with non-latex.

Keywords: Elastomers. Tensile strength. Latex. Silicone elastomers.

[1] Universidade do Estado do Rio de Janeiro, Programa de Pós-graduação em Odontologia, Departamento de Odontologia Preventiva e Comunitária (Rio de Janeiro/RJ, Brazil).
[2] Universidade Federal Fluminense, Faculdade de Odontologia, Disciplina de Ortodontia (Niterói/RJ, Brazil).
[3] Universidade do Estado do Rio de Janeiro, Departamento de Odontologia Preventiva e Comunitária, Disciplina de Ortodontia (Rio de Janeiro/RJ, Brazil).

Daniela Ferreira de Carvalho Notaroberto
Rua Eduardo Guinle, 55/1001, bloco 02, Botafogo, Rio de Janeiro/RJ
CEP: 22.260-090 – Email: danielafcn@yahoo.com.br

» The authors report no commercial, proprietary or financial interest in the products or companies described in this article.

INTRODUCTION

Orthodontic elastics are still valuable devices, widely used in clinical practice, because they present many varieties of application regarding the direction of force applied to the teeth to be moved, thus helping in the correction of several malocclusions.[1]

Initially, these elastics were composed of natural rubber (latex), a raw material discovered and used for centuries by the ancient Inca and Mayan civilizations.[2] They are still widely used today,[3,4] mainly because of the high flexibility and low cost.[5] However, by the 1980s, allergic reactions to latex became more prevalent and better recognized.[6,7] With the aim of maintaining the mechanical properties of the elastics, without causing allergy in patients with hypersensitivity to latex, orthodontic rubber elastics based on synthetic rubber (non-latex) have been used more frequently.[8-10] So, it is imperative to evaluate and compare the mechanical properties of these two different materials.

Some laboratory studies were performed to analyze the behavior of non-latex elastics compared to latex elastics.[4,6,9,11-13] Most of these studies showed a marked reduction in the strength levels of these elastics within the first 24 hours, showing the non-latex elastics limitation in maintaining a constant force for an extended period.[4,6,11,12] Manufacturers have added chemical substances to retard these effects and extend the lifetime of these elastomers.[2]

However, in the oral cavity, the characteristics of elastics materials are affected by physical, chemical and biological factors, some of them related to functional activities, salivary changes and nutrition habits.[3,14] Non-latex elastics also must be tested in the oral environment and, at our knowledge, just one clinical study[15] was reported in the literature. The related article did not evaluate the first hours of use, which are described as being critical in relation to the greatest force loss of the intermaxillary elastics. Other few clinical studies evaluating intraoral elastics were performed evaluating only latex elastics.[3,16]

Thus, the purpose of the present study was to evaluate *in vivo* the force degradation of latex and non-latex elastics exchanged at different times, over a period of 24 hours.

MATERIAL AND METHODS

A prospective controlled clinical trial with split-mouth design was conducted to evaluate the behavior of latex and non-latex elastics over 24 hours.

This study was approved by the Research Ethics Committee of Hospital Universitário Pedro Ernesto/UERJ (Ethics Committee document #285.772). All participants received prior information about the research and signed an informed consent form.

Intraoral latex ($n = 75$) and non-latex elastics ($n = 75$) (American Orthodontics, Sheboygan, USA), at a 3/16-inch size were tested. They were within the expiration dates and stored in sealed plastic packages in a cool and dark environment.

Using a specific formula for split-mouth or crossover studies,[17] sample size calculation was performed based in a pilot study ($n = 5$), in which the values in gram-force (gf) generated by the elastics of the five patients were used. The sample size of the present study was then determined to be 13 patients, with 80% of test power, 5% of alpha level, 24.75 of standard deviation of difference, and 20 of average difference; however, to avoid missing data, 15 patients were selected for the study.

Systematic convenience sampling was used, in which participants were selected in a post-graduate orthodontic program of a public university, following dental appointment schedules between February 2016 and August 2016.

Patients ($n = 15$) with mean age of 20.16 years, who were undergoing orthodontic treatment were selected. As inclusion criteria they should be in final phase of the treatment, using rectangular or round arches of 0.020-inch of diameter, with no extractions and with a prescription for using Class II or Class III intermaxillary elastics, on both side of the mouth.

The side selection for the use of each elastic material (latex or non-latex) was randomized and sequential, using sealed brown envelopes, so that the patient #1 would use latex on the right side and non-latex on the left side (Fig 1), patient #2 would use non-latex on the right side and latex on the left side, and so on.

The elastics were attached to canine and first molars hooks (Fig 1). The mean value of the distance between the hooks for the placement of the elastic was 25 mm. The patients were instructed to use an intermaxillary elastic for 1, 3, 12 and 24 hours. They could only remove the elastic to eat or brush the teeth, replacing the same elastic then.

By the time of elastic removal, the patient was referred to the clinic next to the laboratory, allowing

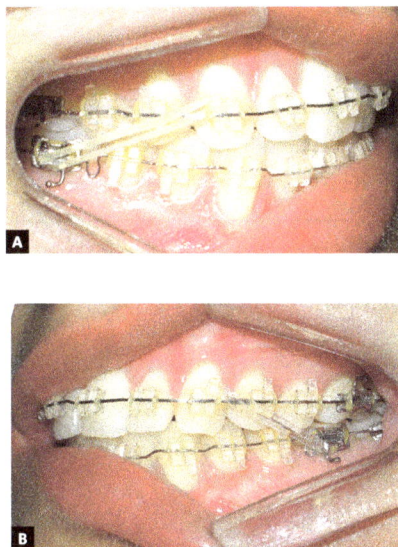

Figure 1 A) Latex elastic on the right side, B) non-latex elastic on the left side.

the elastics to be removed from the patient mouth and immediately adapted to the mechanical testing machine (EMIC DL-500 MF), for force measurement. Each elastic was carefully transferred with a pair of tweezers by the same operator from the patient's mouths to the test machine, and was then discarded after measurement.

The cross-head speed of the testing machine was 30 mm/min, as recommended by Fernandes et al[18] and Lopez et al,[12] and the calibrated load cell capacity was 2.0 Kgf. Extension force magnitudes of the elastics were immediately recorded after they were removed from the patient's mouth and stretched at a distance of 25 mm. All procedures were performed by the same operator.

Descriptive statistics were used as mean, median, standard deviation, maximum and minimum, relative to the elastic force values measured in grams/force and organized for the amounts of liberated force observed at different time intervals.

The collected data were analyzed by paired t test, in order to compare the different types of elastic at each time; and by analysis of variance (ANOVA), to evaluate the variation of the forces generated at all selected times. A *post-hoc* test (Fisher's least significant difference, LSD) was applied to identify which pairs of the force remained significantly different during the study (SPSS software version 20.0; IBM, Armonk, NY). A p value less than 0.05 was considered statistically significant.

RESULTS

Although in baseline (control group) non-latex elastics have generated higher values than latex elastics when stretched to 25mm, in all the other periods the latex strength force values were superior to non-latex elastics. Paired t test showed significant difference between latex and non-latex elastics in almost all observed times, except in baseline (control group) (Table 1).

Analysis of variance for paired data (ANOVA) detected significant differences when comparing the strength force values of latex and non-latex elastics between all times studied ($p < 0.001$). Then, LSD *post-hoc* test was performed and statistical differences were found (Table 1).

Force degradation percentages for latex and non-latex elastics, between all the times are shown in Figure 2. The highest percentage difference generated of force decay occurred between baseline and 1 hour (14.60% for latex elastics and 27.32% for non-latex elastics). Over the next intervals (1-3 hours; 3-12 hours and 12-24 hours), the percentage difference generated of force decay occurred more subtly. After 24 hours of the study, the biggest difference between the degradation percentage of the force was observed for non-latex elastics (39.23%) compared to latex elastics (19.92%).

All the participants had an excellent cooperation with the use of elastic, but of the 15 evaluated patients, 7 needed to repeat the use of the elastics during the 24-hour period, due to the rupture of the non-latex elastics.

Table 1 - Mean and standard deviation of the forces (gf) generated by intermaxillary orthodontic latex and non-latex elastics, according to time of experiment.

Type of elastic	Time				
	0h	1h	3h	12h	24h
Latex	224.49 ± 11.09[a]	191.70 ± 11.92[b]	186.18 ± 10.25[bc]	179.13 ± 10.41[c]	179.75 ± 16.45[c]
Non-latex	228.03 ± 13.33[a]	165.72 ± 10.19[b]	162.43 ± 13.68[b]	146.43 ± 13.27[c]	138.56 ± 14.14[d]
Paired t test	p = 0.470	p < 0.001	p < 0.001	p < 0.001	p < 0.001

Values with different superscript letters (a, b, c, d) indicate significant differences, over time (LSD post-hoc test).

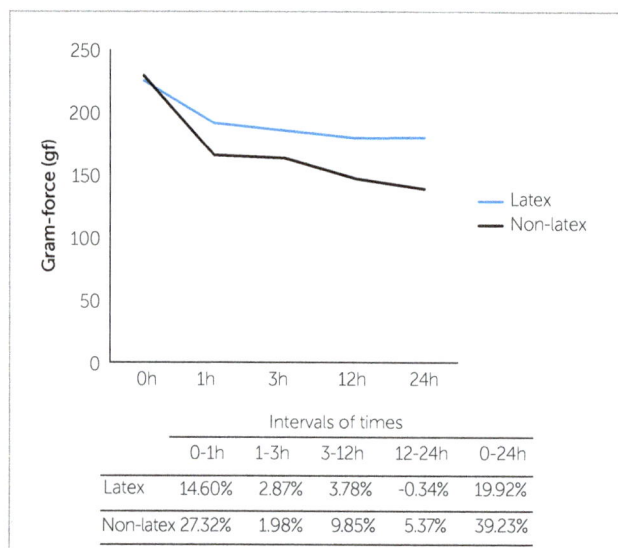

	0-1h	1-3h	3-12h	12-24h	0-24h
Latex	14.60%	2.87%	3.78%	-0.34%	19.92%
Non-latex	27.32%	1.98%	9.85%	5.37%	39.23%

Figure 2 - Latex and non-latex elastics behavior in the 24-hour period.

DISCUSSION

The literature has provided several studies evaluating the force released by the intermaxillary elastics conducted in laboratorial environment.[5,6,8-13,18-21] Some have evaluated the differences between the forces released by latex and non-latex elastics.[4,6,9,11-13] However, it is known that the oral medium is much more complex, with a great variety of interacting factors such as salivary pH, diet, oral hygiene conditions and oral habits.[3,14] *In situ* study, as conducted in this research, is the more precise method to test materials that will be held in the oral environment. A split-mouth study model was adopted, reducing variability and allowing a smaller sample.[17]

The elastic force was measured at 0 (baseline), 1, 3, 12 and 24 hours, considering the fact that laboratory studies indicate the greatest force drop occurring in the first hours.[5,18,19,22,23] The only clinical study found in our literature review that analyzed the differences between the forces released by the latex and non-latex elastics was conducted by Pithon et al[15] and evaluated only 0, 12 and 24 hours. The total time of 24 hours was chosen because this is the period in which routinely it is asked the patient to replace the elastics by new ones.

The results showed that both elastics (latex and non-latex) have progressive force reductions over time (24 hours period).

The biggest drop of the force unleashed by the latex elastics occurred in the first hour, with significant difference. On subsequent times, the decrease in strength was softer, without statistical significance (Table 1). These results are in agreement with the findings of laboratory studies affirming that the greatest fall in the values of the forces generated by the latex intermaxillary elastics occur in the first hours after their distension and as time progressed, the degradation became slower.[5,18,19,24] The few clinical studies conducted also reported this behavior. Wang et al[3] and Qodcieh et al[16] found that the large force loss occurred within the first hour.

The non-latex elastics also demonstrated a significant large decrease in the amount of force generated between 0 and 1 hour, but continued to show significant loss of force within 3 to 12 hours and within 12 to 24 hours (Table 1). Similarly, Kersey et al,[4] in a study involving the non-latex intermaxillary elastics of 1/4-in diameter, noticed a decrease in the values of forces generated between 20% and 30% in the first hour, and 40% to 60% after 24 hours. However, higher percentage values than those obtained in this study were reported by Araujo and Ursi,[23] who observed a reduction in the amount of force generated by the non-latex elastics from 20.31% to 38.47% in the first hour, and from 47.7% to 75.95% on 28 days of stretching. The only clinical study with non-latex elastics did not evaluate the first hours, but showed a progressive and significant reduction of the force generated by these elastics from 0 to 12 hours and also from 12 to 24 hours.[15]

When the forces generated by the intermaxillary elastics of the two types (latex and non-latex) were compared, significant differences were found in all the times studied, except for the baseline (Table 1). These data are in agreement with the study by Pithon et al,[15] who found that latex intermaxillary elastics with 1/8-in diameter lose less force over time compared to non-latex elastics. However, in the study of Pithon et al,[15] latex and non-latex elastics 1/4-in and 5/16-in in diameter demonstrated no significant differences after 24 hours.

The most significant decrease in force values occurred in the first hour, for both latex and non-latex elastics, with the difference percentage higher for non-latex elastic, of 27.32%, compared to the difference for latex, 14.60%. After 24 hours, the percentage difference for non-latex elastics was 39.23% and for latex was 19.92% (Fig 2). The laboratory studies[9,12] found similar results, detecting greater loss of strength for the non-latex elastics, when compared to the latex ones. Kersey et al[4], when comparing latex and non-latex elastics from a single manufacturer (American Orthodontics, the same manufacturer used in this study), found that latex elastics maintain higher strength levels over 24 hours, retaining 83% of initial strength, compared to 69% retained by non-latex elastics. The clinical study showed the same results, a greater loss of the initial force in 24 hours for the non-latex elastics.[15]

Of the 15 patients evaluated, 7 needed to repeat the use of the elastics during the 24-hour period, due to the rupture of the non-latex elastics. This limitation of non-latex elastics was also observed in the studies of Russell et al[6] and Hwang and Cha.[13] No fracture was observed in latex elastic throughout the clinical study.

These findings are important because non-latex elastics are an alternative for patients with latex sensitivity. It is necessary to understand the clinical behavior of these elastics in order to establish the best way to use them. As the clinical behavior was different at all times tested in the oral cavity (1, 3, 12, 24 hours) and having these non-latex elastics released smaller forces and losing greater amount of force over time, it is suggested that the non-latex elastics must be changed more frequently in order to obtain a better action during their use in orthodontic treatment.

It is important to emphasize that this study evaluated the difference in composition between elastics. Thus, only one trademark and one size were evaluated, for a better interpretation of the results. Other brands and diameters may perform differently and must be tested.

CONCLUSIONS

Latex elastics showed a more stable behavior within 24 hours, when compared to non-latex elastics.

During the oral experimental time (3, 12 and 24 hours), the latex elastics had higher force released values, when compared to non-latex elastics.

Author's contribution (ORCID ⓘ)

Daniela F. C. N. (DFCN): 0000-0002-3834-1797 ⓘ
Mariana M. Martins (MMM): 0000-0002-1237-1947 ⓘ
Maria T. A. Goldner (MTAG): 0000-0003-4690-9562 ⓘ
Cátia C. A. Quintão (CCAQ): 0000-0003-4627-8190 ⓘ
Álvaro de M. Mendes (AMM): 0000-0002-3428-0296 ⓘ

Conception or design of the study: DFCN, AMM. Data acquisition, analysis or interpretation: DFCN, MMM, MTAG, CCAQ, AMM. Writing the article: DFCN, MTAG. Critical revision of the article: DFCN, MMM, MTAG, CCAQ, AMM. Final approval of the article: DFCN, MMM, MTAG, CCAQ, AMM. Obtained funding: DFCN. Overall responsibility: DFCN.

REFERENCES

1. Singh VP, Pokhrael PR, Pariekh K, Roy DK, Singla A, Biswas KP. Elastics in orthodontics: a review. Health Renaissance. 2012;10(1):49-56.

2. Baty DL, Storie DJ, Von Fraunhofer JA. Synthetic elastomeric chains: a literature review. Am J Orthod Dentofacial Orthop. 1994 June;105(6):536-42.

3. Wang T, Zhou G, Tan X, Dong Y. Evaluation of force degradation characteristics of orthodontic latex elastics in vitro and in vivo. Angle Orthod. 2007;77(4):688-93.

4. Kersey ML, Glover KE, Heo G, Major PW. A comparison of dynamic and static testing of latex and nonlatex orthodontic elastics. Angle Orthod. 2003 Apr;73(2):181-6.

5. Kanchana P, Godfrey K. Calibration of force extension and force degradation characteristics of orthodontic latex elastics. Am J Orthod Dentofacial Orthop. 2000 Sept;118(3):280-7.

6.   Russel KA, Milne AD, Khanna RA, Lee JM. In vitro assessment of the
      mechanical properties of latex and non-latex orthodontic elastics. Am J
      Orthod Dentofacial Orthop. 2001 July;120(1):36-44.

7.   Hain MA, Longman LP, Field EA, Harrison JE. Natural rubber latex allergy:
      implications for the orthodontist. J Orthod. 2007 Mar;34(1):6-11.

8.   Hanson M, Lobner D. In vitro neuronal cytotoxity of latex and
      nonlatex orthodontic elastics. Am J Orthod Dentofacial Orthop. 2004
      July;126(1):65-70.

9.   Aljhani AS, Aldrees AM. The effect of static and dynamics testing on
      orthodontic latex and non-latex elastics. Orthod Waves. 2010;69(3):117-
      22.

10.   Alavi S, Tabatabaie AR, Hajizadeh F, Ardekani AH. An In-vitro comparison
      of force loss of orthodontic non-latex elastics. J Dent (Tehran). 2014
      Jan;11(1):10-6.

11.   Kamisetty SK, Nimagadda C, Begam MP, Nalamotu R, Srivastav T,
      Shwetha GS. Elasticity in Elastics-An in-vitro study. J Int Oral Health. 2014
      Apr;6(2):96-105.

12.   López N, Vicente A, Bravo LA, Calvo JL, Canteras M. In vitro study of
      force decay of latex and non-latex orthodontic elastics. Eur J Orthod.
      2012 Apr;34(2):202-7.

13.   Hwang CJ, Cha JY. Mechanical and biological comparison of latex
      and silicone rubber bands. Am J Orthod Dentofacial Orthop. 2003
      Oct;124(4):379-86.

14.   De Genova DC, McInnes-Ledoux P, Weinberg R, Shaye R. Force
      degradation of orthodontic elastomeric chains-a product comparison
      study. Am J Orthod. 1985 May;87(5):377-84.

15.   Pithon MM, Mendes JL, Silva CA, Santos RL, Coqueiro RD. Force decay of
      latex and non-látex intermaxillary elastics: a clinical study. Eur J Orthod.
      2016 Feb;38(1):39-43.

16.   Qodcieh SMA, Al-Khateeb SN, Jaradat ZW, Abu Alhaija ESJ. Force
      degradation of orthodontic latex elastics: An in-vivo study. Am J Orthod
      Dentofacial Orthop. 2017 Mar;151(3):507-12.

17.   Pandis N. Sample calculation for split-mouth designs. Am J Orthod
      Dentofacial Orthop. 2012 June;141(6):818-9.

18.   Fernandes DJ, Fernandes GMA, Artese F, Elias CN, Mendes AM. Force
      extension relaxation of medium force orthodontic latex elastics. Angle
      Orthod. 2011 Sept;81(5):812-9.

19.   Bishara SE, Andreasen GF. A comparison of time related forces between
      plastics alastiks and latex elastics. Angle Orthod. 1970 Oct;4(4):319-28.

20.   Sauget PS, Stewart KT, Katona TR. The effect of pH levels on non-latex
      latex interarch elastics. Angle Orthod. 2011;81(6):1070-4.

21.   Santos RL, Pithon MM, Romanos MTV. The influence of pH levels on
      mechanical and biological properties of nonlatex and latex elastics. Angle
      Orthod. 2012 July;82(4):709-14.

22.   Oesterle LJ, Owens JM, Newman SM, Shellhart WC. Perceived vs
      measured forces of interarch elastics. Am J Orthod Dentofacial Orthop.
      2012 Mar;141(3):298-306.

23.   Araújo FBC, Ursi WJS. Study of the degradation of the force generated
      by synthetic orthodontic elastics. Rev Dental Press Ortod Ortop Facial.
      2006;11(6):52-61.

24.   Moris A, Sato K, Facholli AFL, Nascimento JE, Sato FRL. In vitro study of
      the strength degradation of latex orthodontic elastics under dynamic
      conditions. Rev Dental Press Ortod Ortop Facial. 2009;14(2):95-108.

7

Influence of occlusal plane inclination and mandibular deviation on esthetics

Cristiane Cherobini Dalla Corte[1], Bruno Lopes da Silveira[2], Mariana Marquezan[3]

Objective: The aim of this study was to assess the degree of perception of occlusal plane inclination and mandibular deviation in facial esthetics, assessed by laypeople, dentists and orthodontists. **Methods:** A woman with 5.88° of inclination and 5.54 mm of mandibular deviation was selected and, based on her original photograph, four new images were created correcting the deviations and creating more symmetric faces and smiles. Examiners assessed the images by means of a questionnaire. Their opinions were compared by qualitative and quantitative analyses. **Results:** A total of 45 laypeople, 27 dentists and 31 orthodontists filled out the questionnaires. All groups were able to perceive the asymmetry; however, orthodontists were more sensitive, identifying asymmetries as from 4.32° of occlusal plane inclination and 4.155 mm of mandibular deviation ($p < 0.05$). The other categories of evaluators identified asymmetries and assigned significantly lower grades, starting from 5.88° of occlusal plane inclination and 5.54 mm of mandibular deviation ($p < 0.05$). **Conclusion:** Occlusal plane inclination and mandibular deviation were perceived by all groups, but orthodontists presented higher perception of deviations.

Keywords: Smiling. Face. Esthetics. Facial asymmetry. Photography.

[1] Specialist in Orthodontics, Centro Universitário Franciscano (UNIFRA), Santa Maria, Rio Grande do Sul, Brazil.
[2] Professor, Universidade Federal de Santa Maria (UFSM), Department of Restorative Dentistry, Santa Maria, Rio Grande do Sul, Brazil.
[3] Postdoc resident, Universidade Federal do Rio de Janeiro (UFRJ), Department of Pediatric Dentistry and Orthodontics, Rio de Janeiro, Rio de Janeiro, Brazil.
Dentist, Universidade Federal de Santa Maria (UFSM), Department of Restorative Dentistry, Santa Maria, Rio Grande do Sul, Brazil.

» The authors report no commercial, proprietary or financial interest in the products or companies described in this article.

Mariana Marquezan
Rua Dr Alberto Pasqualini, 70/809, Santa Maria/RS – Brazil – CEP 97015-010
E-mail: marianamarquezan@gmail.com

INTRODUCTION

Perfect facial symmetry is a theoretical concept. There is no perfectly symmetrical human face, even the most beautiful face exhibits some degree of asymmetry.[1,2] Asymmetry in craniofacial areas can be recognized as differences in size or relationship between the two sides of the face. This may be the result of discrepancies either in shape of individual bones, or a malposition of one or more bones in the craniofacial complex.[3] From the point of view of esthetics, it is challenging to establish the threshold level of mild facial asymmetry. It is difficult to find a cutoff point that distinguishes a pleasing asymmetrical face, an acceptable asymmetrical face and an asymmetrical face that requires intervention. Despite the subjectivity of beauty, it becomes necessary to acknowledge and study facial esthetics, bearing in mind the concept of normality which serves as a guide during orthodontic treatment planning.[4]

Craniomandibular structural asymmetry can be congenital or hereditary, or can be acquired as a result of trauma or infection. During growth, quantitative and qualitative alterations of functional loads applied to the bones might modify their developmental pattern and lead to asymmetry.[5] Facial asymmetry may be present in the upper, middle and lower thirds of the face. The majority of asymmetries are usually concentrated in the lower third of the face due to being involved in the masticatory structures[6,7,8] and subject to masticatory and occlusal problems.[9]

Many patients with facial asymmetry present occlusal plane inclination caused by unilaterally extruded maxillary molars or asymmetrical mandibular vertical development.[10] Because the occlusal plane is an important element in the position and adaptation of the mandible,[11] inclination is usually associated with mandibular deviation and vice-versa.[12,13] The degree of inclination of the maxilla is proportional to the degree of mandibular deviation in both hard and soft tissues.[13] The prevalence of inclination is about 41%, but many cases are not perceptible due to being of minor severity.[14]

Facial asymmetries in soft tissues influence patient's expectations regarding orthodontic treatment.[8] In order to prevent disagreements between patient's and orthodontist's treatment objectives, the normal range of facial asymmetry needs to be determined in a given population.[1] Therefore, the aim of this research was to assess the influence of occlusal plane inclination and consequent mandibular deviation on esthetics in the opinion of laypeople, dentists and orthodontists.

METHODS

This study was characterized as an observational, descriptive, transverse study with quantitative and qualitative analysis of data. It was submitted to and approved by the Human Research Ethics Committee of Centro Universitário Franciscano (UNIFRA) (CAAE: 11097113.5.0000.5306, #265.831, issued on 21st of May, 2013). A model with an esthetically pleasant face, but with severe occlusal plane inclination (5.88°) and mandibular deviation (5.54 mm), both of which led her to seek orthodontic treatment, was selected for the study.

Based on patient's original photograph, a professional designer created four smiles by means of Adobe Photoshop CS5 (Adobe Systems, San Jose, California) software. Firstly, the pupillary plane was traced and positioned parallel to the ground. A new line was traced starting from the center of the left pupil up to the tip of the maxillary left canine cusp.[23] The distance between these points was transferred to the right side, and, thus, it was possible to trace the ideal occlusal plane. The difference between the angle formed by the patient's real inclination and the digital manipulation at an angle equal to zero resulted in 5.88°. The four manipulated smiles had occlusal plane inclination progressively corrected by 1.47° in each photo, until the smile became symmetrical. As the occlusal plane was being altered, mandibular deviation was also manipulated until it was completely corrected (1.385 mm for each photograph, totaling 5.54 mm), rendering the face more symmetrical and making the facial midline match with the center of the mentum (Fig 1). It is emphasized that the model agreed with the use of her image in the research by signing a term of authorization for image use.

The five images were identified with colored labels (Fig 1) and randomly disposed in a photograph album. There was only one photograph on each page of the album, so that the images were not compared side by side. The evaluators were not allowed to return to the previous photo or move on without attributing a score to the photograph. No set time was established for the evaluations. The albums were made available to three categories of evaluators: laypeople, dentists and orthodontists; together with a questionnaire in which the evaluators could express their esthetic preference by attributing

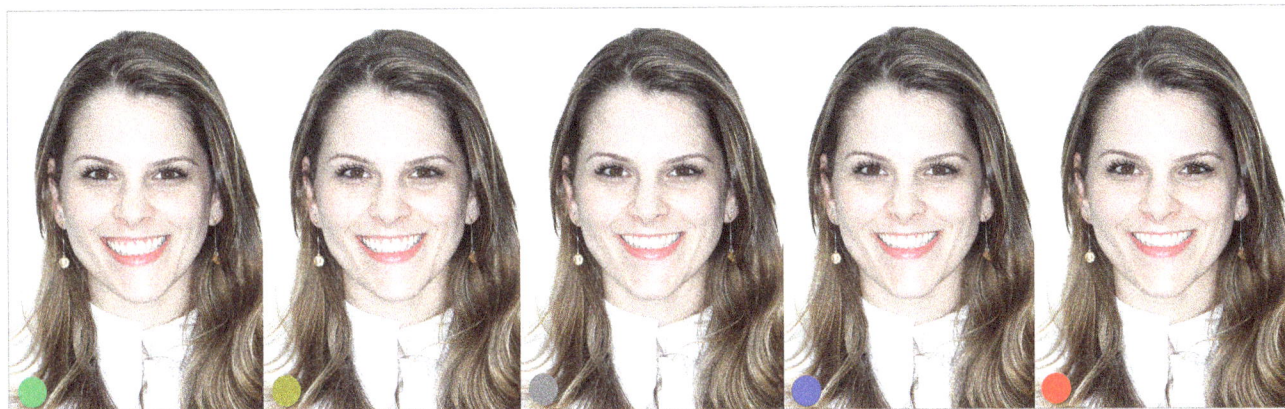

Figure 1 - Original smile (green label), with 5.88° of inclination and 5.54 mm of mandibular deviation, and their corrections (1.47° and 1.385 mm in each photo).

scores from 0 to 10 (zero to ten) to each image. In the questionnaire, the evaluators were also asked whether they perceived anything that called their attention in each one of the photographs, so as to justify the score attributed to them.

A total of 150 questionnaires were distributed in Dental Schools and Dental Clinics of Santa Maria (Rio Grande do Sul, Brazil). These are the places where dentists and orthodontists work, and laypeople can also be found (employees, patients' relatives and friends).

Quantitative data were tabulated in SPSS Statistics version 20 for statistical analysis. The scores attributed to each smile in the categories of evaluators were compared by ANOVA/Tukey tests.

RESULTS

Of the 150 questionnaires, 103 were returned duly filled out: 45 by laypeople, 27 by dentists and 31 by orthodontists. All groups were able to perceive asymmetry; however, orthodontists were more sensitive, identifying asymmetries as from 4.32° of inclination and 4.155 mm of mandibular deviation ($p \leq 0.05$). The other categories of evaluators identified asymmetries and assigned significantly lower grades, starting from 5.88° of inclination and 5.54 mm of mandibular deviation ($p \leq 0.05$). All three groups of evaluators considered the original photograph (green) as the least attractive one, followed by gold and silver photographs. Laypeople and orthodontists considered the most symmetrical face and smile (red photograph) to be the most attractive. Dentists, on the other hand, preferred the blue photograph. The results of the qualitative and quantitative analyses (means, standard

deviation and results of ANOVA/Tukey tests) as regards the esthetic preference of laypeople are shown in Table 1, whereas the preference of dentists is shown in Table 2 and orthodontists' preference is shown in Table 3.

DISCUSSION

Although no face is perfectly symmetrical, a face is only considered asymmetrical when there is perceptible disharmony between homologous parts. It is known that a certain degree of asymmetry is beautiful, but the border line between normal asymmetry and asymmetry that requires treatment is subjective[15] and varies among professionals and laypeople.[16] In order to assess the threshold of esthetic tolerance for occlusal plane inclination and mandibular lateral deviation, the photographs of a model with an asymmetrical face were gradually edited until these parameters became symmetrical. In the qualitative analysis, it was perceived that the largest number of evaluators detected the asymmetry of the smile (inclination) rather than that of the face itself (mandibular shift). In the three categories, a lower number of evaluators reported deviation of the mandible or chin. According to a previous study, frontal photographs of the face allow facial symmetry, and numerous other factors such as eyes, size and shape of the face, to be assessed. These aspects can divert attention from potential skeletal-facial changes.[17]

Laypeople, dentists and orthodontists were capable of perceiving occlusal plane inclination associated with mandibular lateral deviation. The original photograph (green), with an inclination of 5.88° and 5.54 mm of lateral deviation of the mandible, was the one that received the lowest

Table 1 - Perception of laypeople.

Preferably sequence	Smile	Qualitative analysis	Quantitative analysis mean (SD)	ANOVA/ Tukey*
1st	Red	» White teeth (3 people) » Perfect teeth, aligned (3 people) » Thin upper lip (3 people) » Gingival exposure (2 people) » Harmony (2 people) » Deviated chin » Narrow mouth » Narrow smile » Aligned chin » Different earrings » Happiness	8.68 (1.39)	a
2nd	Blue	» Good gingival exposure (5 people) » White teeth (4 people) » Bent smile (3 people) » Beautiful teeth, perfect (3 people) » Problem in the height of the teeth » The right side of the patient is higher » Thin upper lip » Problems in the teeth, gingiva and lip » Great alignment » The smile expresses pleasure, happiness, sympathy	8.60 (1.13)	a
3rd	Silver	» Asymmetry (6 people) » Yellow teeth (2 people) » Lighten teeth (2) » Perfect teeth (2) » Deviated chin » Difference in posterior teeth » Thin upper lip » Beautiful smile » Mouth and face in harmony » Happiness, sympathy	8.31 (1.25)	a,b
4th	Gold	» Asymmetric smile (13 people) » White teeth (3 people) » Symmetric teeth (3 people) » Happy person (2 people) » Beautiful smile (2 people) » Asymmetric face » Deviated chin » One side of the mouth is more open » Aligned teeth » Happiness, sympathy in the look and smile	8.04 (1.52)	a,b
5th	Green	» Asymmetric smile (20 people) » One side of the mouth is more open » Bent upper lip » Deviated chin » Posterior teeth are different » Lighten teeth, perfect » Smile revels teeth well » Happiness, sympathy	7.75 (1.54)	b

* ANOVA showed statistical difference among groups ($p = 0.016$). Different letters indicate statistical difference for post hoc Tukey.

Table 2 - Perception of dentists.

Preferably sequence	Smile	Qualitative analysis	Quantitative analysis mean (SD)	ANOVA/ Tukey*
1st	Blue	» Lower midline deviation (7 people) » Inclination (4 people) » Smile line (2 people) » Chin deviation (2 people) » Increased buccal corridor » Small left eye » Bent nose » Thin upper lip	8.42 (1.11)	a
2nd	Red	» Lower midline deviation (8 people) » Low smile line (8 people) » Chin deviation (2 people) » Narrow buccal corridor (2 people) » Thin upper lip » Seems to have many teeth » Tooth 23 bucally positioned	8.13 (1.50)	a
3rd	Silver	» Inclination (11 people) » Lower midline deviation (8 people) » Chin deviation (5 people) » Low smile line » Acute zenith on the right side » Buccal corridor » Color of the teeth » Tooth 23 bucally positioned	7.85 (1.26)	a,b
4th	Gold	» Inclination (20 people) » Lower midline deviation (11 people) » Chin deviation » Small left eye » Increased buccal corridor	7.50 (1.13)	a,b
5th	Green	» Inclination (23 people) » Lower midline deviation (7 people) » Chin deviation (2 people) » Buccal corridor (2 people) » Tooth 23 bucally positioned	6.87 (1.51)	b

* ANOVA showed statistical difference among groups (p = 0.000). Different letters indicate statistical difference for post hoc Tukey.

score in the three categories, followed by photographs with gold (4.32° and 4.155 mm of deviation) and silver (2.88° and 2.77 mm of deviation) labels. The photographs with blue and red labels received the highest scores, being red (symmetrical) preferred by laypeople and orthodontists. Nevertheless, the photograph with a blue label was preferred by dentists who probably did not identify the small degree of inclination (1.47°) and small mandible deviation (1.385 mm) and perceived the more harmonious smile line (Table 2). It has been shown that a smile with the upper lip resting on the gingival margin of maxillary incisors (as found in the blue photograph) is considered the most esthetic for a female subject.[18]

Orthodontists were more sensitive to perceiving inclination and chin deviation. When verifying the scores attributed to the photographs, orthodontists assigned significantly lower grades ($p \le 0.05$) to the smile in the gold label photograph ($p \le 0.05$) (Table 3). This means they identified asymmetries as from 4.32° of inclination and 4.155 mm of mandibular deviation. Unlikewise, dentists and laypeople assigned significantly lower grades ($p \le 0.05$) only to green label photographs (Tables 1 and 2). This means that they identified asymmetries as from 5.88° of inclination and 5.54 mm of mandibular deviation. Previous studies have shown lower cutoff values for inclination and mandibular deviation. Padwa et al[19] considered an inclination of 4° as the threshold for recognition by laypeople and trained evaluators. For mandibular deviation, Da Silva et al[20] found that orthodontists and laypeople only perceived shifts greater than or equal

Table 3 - Perception of orthodontists.

Preferably sequence	Smile	Qualitative analysis	Quantitative analysis mean (SD)	ANOVA/Tukey*
1st	Red	» Lower midline deviation (15 people) » Chin deviation (6 people) » Little gingival exposure (4 people) » Artificial smile (3 people) » Larger buccal corridor on left side » Greater exposure of left teeth » Decreased vertical dimension	8.48 (1.37)	a
2nd	Blue	» Lower midline deviation (17 people) » Mandibular asymmetry (8 people) » Inclination (3 people) » Thin upper lip (2 people) » Nose (2 people) » Little exposure of lower incisors » Mild crowding of tooth #21 » Low smile line	8.15 (0.74)	a,b
3rd	Silver	» Inclination (15 people) » Mandibular asymmetry (11 people) » Lower midline deviation (11 people) » Upper lip (3 people) » Buccal corridor » Nose	7.58 (1.10)	a,b
4th	Gold	» Inclination (22 people) » Mandibular asymmetry (10 people) » Lower midline deviation (9 people) » Buccal corridor » Little exposure of lower incisors » Nose	7.25 (1.05)	b
5th	Green	» Inclination (24 people) » Mandibular asymmetry (11 people) » Lower midline deviation (8 people) » Buccal corridor (2 people) » Upper central incisor inclined to the left » Nose	6.20 (1.58)	c

* ANOVA showed statistical difference among groups (p = 0.000). Different letters indicate statistical difference for post hoc Tukey.

to 4 mm when analyzing a woman's photographs (rest position). When examining a man's photographs, orthodontists perceived shifts greater than or equal to 4 mm, but laypeople did not perceive any changes (up to 6 mm). On the other hand, in a classification proposed by Kim et al,[13] used to assess facial asymmetry in diagnosis for orthognathic surgeries, mandibular and occlusal plane deviations greater than 2 mm were considered as asymmetries.

Although some laypeople perceived inclination and mandibular deviation, these deviations were mentioned by a larger number of orthodontists. While dentists and orthodontists analyzed the smile more carefully, detailing problems such as buccal corridor and midline deviation, the attention of laypeople did not focus so much on the oral region, as they reported details of the face other than the teeth, such as earrings and eyes, in addition to subjective characteristics such as sympathy and happiness. According to Jackson et al,[21] orthodontists have a clear advantage in assessing facial symmetry when compared with laypeople, and an advantage over general clinical dentists in the most difficult cases.

The more symmetrical the smile, the more details, such as color and anatomy of teeth, were perceived and described by the interviewees; however, with increasing inclination and mandibular deviation, the negative influence of these features was perceived and described by the three groups of evaluators.

Although laypeople perceived the asymmetries, the mean scores attributed to the photograph with green label (the most asymmetric one) was still high (7.75). This fact makes one wonder if this amount of asymmetry is clinically significant for patients as far as esthetics is concerned.

Some limitations were detected and need to be addressed by future studies, such as the number of questionnaires. Sample size should be increased to reduce the possibility of type II error (failure to reject a false null hypothesis; in other words, failure to detect difference between photographs). It would also be interesting to use different models, varying the sex, ethnicity, color of the hair, skin, and eyes. It would also be interesting to register more detailed data about the evaluators, such as the time elapsed since their graduation (experience time).

CONCLUSION

The three groups of evaluators perceived inclination and mandibular deviation; however, orthodontists were those with the greatest perception.

REFERENCES

1. Alqattan M, Djordjevic J, Zhurov AI, Richmond S. Comparison between landmark and surface-based three-dimensional analyses of facial asymmetry in adults. Eur J Orthod. 2015;37(1):1-12.
2. Primozic J, Perinetti G, Zhurov A, Richmond S, Ovsenik M. Assessment of facial asymmetry in growing subjects with a three-dimensional laser scanning system. Orthod Craniofac Res. 2012;15(4):237-44.
3. Bishara SE, Burkey PS, Kharouf JG. Dental and facial asymmetries: a review. Angle Orthod. 1994;64(2):89-98.
4. Peron APLM, Morosini IC, Correia KR, Moresca R, Petrelli E. Photometric study of divine proportion and its correlation with facial attractiveness. Dental Press J Orthod. 2012;17(2):8-11.
5. Schmid W, Mongini F. [Factors in craniomandibular asymmetry: diagnostic principles and therapy]. Mondo Ortod. 1990;15(1):91-104.
6. Vig PS, Hewitt AB. Asymmetry of the human facial skeleton. Angle Orthod. 1975;45(2):125-9.
7. Shah SM, Joshi MR. An assessment of asymmetry in the normal craniofacial complex. Angle Orthod. 1978;48(2):141-8.
8. Masuoka N, Momoi Y, Ariji Y, Nawa H, Muramatsu A, Goto S, et al. Can cephalometric indices and subjective evaluation be consistent for facial asymmetry? Angle Orthod. 2005;75(4):651-5.
9. Lundstrom A. Some asymmetries of the dental arches, jaws, and skull, and their etiological significance. Am J Orthod. 1961;47(2):81-106.
10. Jeon YJ, Kim YH, Son WS, Hans MG. Correction of a canted occlusal plane with miniscrews in a patient with facial asymmetry. Am J Orthod Dentofacial Orthop. 2006;130(2):244-52.
11. Ishizaki K, Suzuki K, Mito T, Tanaka EM, Sato S. Morphologic, functional, and occlusal characterization of mandibular lateral displacement malocclusion. Am J Orthod Dentofacial Orthop. 2010;137(4):454.e1-e9; discussion 54-5.

12. Hashimoto T, Fukunaga T, Kuroda S, Sakai Y, Yamashiro T, Takano-Yamamoto T. Mandibular deviation and canted maxillary occlusal plane treated with miniscrews and intraoral vertical ramus osteotomy: functional and morphologic changes. Am J Orthod Dentofacial Orthop. 2009;136(6):868-77.
13. Kim JY, Jung HD, Jung YS, Hwang CJ, Park HS. A simple classification of facial asymmetry by TML system. J Craniomaxillofac Surg. 2014;42(4):313-20.
14. Severt TR, Proffit WR. The prevalence of facial asymmetry in the dentofacial deformities population at the University of North Carolina. Int J Adult Orthodon Orthognath Surg. 1997;12(3):171-6.
15. Lee MS, Chung DH, Lee JW, Cha KS. Assessing soft-tissue characteristics of facial asymmetry with photographs. Am J Orthod Dentofacial Orthop. 2010;138(1):23-31.
16. Edler R, Wertheim D, Greenhill D. Clinical and computerized assessment of mandibular asymmetry. Eur J Orthod. 2001;23(5):485-94.
17. Morihisa O, Maltagliati LA. Avaliação comparativa entre agradabilidade facial e análise subjetiva do Padrão Facial. Rev Dental Press Ortod Ortop Facial. 2009;14(6):46.e1-e9.
18. Dutra MB, Ritter DE, Borgatto A, Derech CD, Rocha R. Influence of gingival exposure on the smile esthetics. Dental Press J Orthod. 2011;16(5):111-8.
19. Padwa BL, Kaiser MO, Kaban LB. Occlusal cant in the frontal plane as a reflection of facial asymmetry. J Oral Maxillofac Surg. 1997;55(8):811-6; discussion 17.
20. Silva NCF, Aquino ERB, Mello KCFR, Mattos JNR. Orthodontists' and laypersons' perception of mandibular asymmetries. Dental Press J Orthod. 2011;16(4):38.e1-e8.

8

The influence of sagittal position of the mandible in facial attractiveness and social perception

Lorena Marques Ferreira de Sena[1], Lislley Anne Lacerda Damasceno e Araújo[2],
Arthur Costa Rodrigues Farias[1], Hallissa Simplício Gomes Pereira[3]

Objective: This study aims at comparing the perception of orthodontists, maxillofacial surgeons, visual artists and lay-persons when evaluating the influence of sagittal position of the mandible — in lateral view — in facial attractiveness; at a job hiring; and in the perception of socioeconomic profile. **Methods:** A black male, a white male, a black female and a white female with harmonic faces served as models to obtain a facial profile photograph. Each photograph was digitally manipulated to obtain seven facial profiles: an ideal, three simulating mandibular advancement and three simulating mandibular retrusion, producing 28 photographs. These photographs were evaluated through a questionnaire by orthodontists, maxillofacial surgeons, visual artists and laypersons. **Results:** The anteroposterior positioning of the mandible exerted strong influence on the level of facial attractiveness, but few significant differences between the different groups of evaluators were observed ($p < 0.05$). **Conclusions:** The profiles pointed as the most attractive were also pointed as more favorable to be hired to a job position and pointed also as having the best socioeconomic condition.

Keywords: Mandible. Social values. Esthetics.

[1] Post-graduation program, Department of Dentistry, Universidade Federal do Rio Grande do Norte, Natal, RN, Brazil.
[2] Federal University of Rio Grande do Norte, Department of Dentistry, Natal, RN, Brazil.
[3] Adjunct professor in Orthodontics, Department of Dentistry, Universidade Federal do Rio Grande do Norte, Natal, RN, Brazil.

» The authors report no commercial, proprietary or financial interest in the products or companies described in this article.

Lorena Marques Ferreira de Sena
Av. Senador Salgado Filho, nº 1787. Natal/RN – Brazil - CEP: 59.056-000
E-mail: lorena.mf@hotmail.com.

INTRODUCTION

Facial esthetics has been researched for a long time. Some studies show that people with attractive dentition are considered more intelligent, more popular and more easily employed than other people with less attractive teeth.[1,2,3] In addition, the desire to improve facial esthetics is one of the main reasons why people seek orthodontic treatment.[4,5,6]

Some authors believe that reaching the esthetic standard desired by the patient is a challenging task for dentists due to the subjective nature of the evaluation and perception of facial esthetics.[7] According to Kumar et al.[8] and Cochrane et al.[9], professionals and laypersons perceive facial esthetics differently, with laypersons demonstrating a larger variation on what is considered to be attractive. However, there is not a consensus on the matter. Other authors[7,10-11] have concluded that there is not any difference between professionals and laypersons when it comes to the perception of facial esthetics.

Among the facial structures capable of influencing the level of facial attractiveness, mandible position is highlighted. According to some authors[12,13], the sagittal prominence of the mandible is an important determinant in the attractiveness of facial profile. For Naini et al,[14] it is one of the facial characteristics that society tends to associate with the personality of the individual.

Considering the importance of the sagittal prominence of the mandible in facial attractiveness and the contradictory results in regard to the perception of facial esthetics by different evaluators, this study has as objective to compare the perception of orthodontists, maxillofacial surgeons, visual artists and laypersons when evaluating the influence of the sagittal positioning of the mandible, in lateral view, in facial attractiveness; in hiring the individual for a job; and in perception of the socioeconomic profile.

MATERIAL AND METHODS
Ethical considerations

All the criteria prescribed by Resolution 466/12 of the National Health Council (NHC), which deals with ethics in research with human beings were obeyed in implementing this study. The research project was approved by a Research Ethics Committee (REC) under number 012-04.

Model selection

Four adult individuals, being two white individuals (one male and one female) and two black individuals (one male and one female), at the average age of 25, were selected as models. All individuals had faces considered harmonic in the vertical plane[15] and in the horizontal plane.[16] The individuals authorized the use of their images for scientific purposes through an Informed Consent Form.

Photographs acquisition

All photographs were taken with the individuals seated, with the Frankfurt plane and the interpupillary line parallel to the ground, using the auricular positioners of a cephalostat. The individuals were oriented to maintain their teeth in the maximum intercuspation position. The facial profile was obtained by turning the positioner to the zero degree point, where the two positioners were in the same distance to the camera, up to 85°, with the aim of obtaining a real outline of the profile. This position was determined through the coincidence of two previously marked points in the cephalostat, one at the base and another at the swivel mount, with the aid of a protractor. This provided the photograph of the right side facial profile, including the visualization of part of the left eyebrow. All individuals were instructed to remove makeup or facial accessories. The individuals with long hair were instructed to put the hair backwards. During the photography session, semiprofessional photographic equipment was used.

Manipulation of the photographs

The four photos with the original profiles, considered harmonic, were manipulated on a computer, using the Photoshop CS2 9® software (Adobe Inc., San Jose, CA, USA), in order to generate four ideal profiles. Details that could distort the perception of the evaluator, such as skin spots and excessive adipose tissue in the region of the cervical mandibular angle, were corrected. The following points were marked in the photographs to standardize the alterations:

» Glabella (G): most prominent point of the forehead.
» Subnasal (Sn): limit point between the nasal septum and the cutaneous part of the superior lip.
» Pogonion (Pg): most anterior point of the soft tissue of the chin.
» Menton (Me): most inferior point of the soft tissue of the chin.
» Superior Lip (SL): most prominent point of the superior lip.

» Inferior Lip (IL): most prominent point of the inferior lip.

The vertical proportions of the faces of the individuals were standardized in a manner that the proportion between middle and inferior thirds was close to 1:1. The middle third was measured in a line perpendicular to the Frankfurt plane, from G point to Sn point, and the inferior third from the Sn point to Me point.[15] The profiles were analyzed and altered, in the horizontal direction, according to angle of facial convexity. This angle, formed by a line that connects G point to Sn point and by another that connects Sn point to Pg, should be 12° in adult individuals, with a standard deviation of 4°.[16] For this purpose, 12° was the measure established for convexity angles of the four ideal profiles.

The degree of lip protrusion considered as ideal was different for white and black individuals. For white individuals, it was considered the standard lip protrusion established by Steiner.[17] This author suggests that the inferior and superior lips touch the line that connects the half of the nose base to the Pogonion. For black individuals, it was considered the standard lip protrusion degree proposed by Farrow et al,[18] in which the inferior and superior lips must be between 3 and 6 mm in front of a line perpendicular to the Frankfurt plane, passing by the G point. These measures were set, in each profile, to produce friendly changes according to each ethnicity.

From each profile considered ideal, the Pg was advanced, by decreasing the G.Sn.Pg angle, at a rate of 4°, sequentially, down to 0°. In addition, the Pg was retracted, by increasing the G.Sn.Pg angle, at a rate of 4°, up to 24°. There were obtained , in this manner, seven profiles of each individual, one ideal, three simulating mandibular advancement and three simulating mandibular retrusion. The menton, the inferior lip and the mentolabial sulcus were advanced or retracted in a similar magnitude to Pg movement. All the modifications in the profile were made in a way that the manipulations were imperceptible. At the end, the 28 photographs of the different facial profiles were printed (9x13cm size, 1200 dpi) and used to create an album with four pages of 29.5 x 40.5 cm dimensions. In each page, seven photographs of the same individual were organized, three photos in the superior part, one in the middle, and three in the inferior part of the page, according to Figure 1. All photographs were identified with letters, to make easier for evaluators to answer the questionnaire.

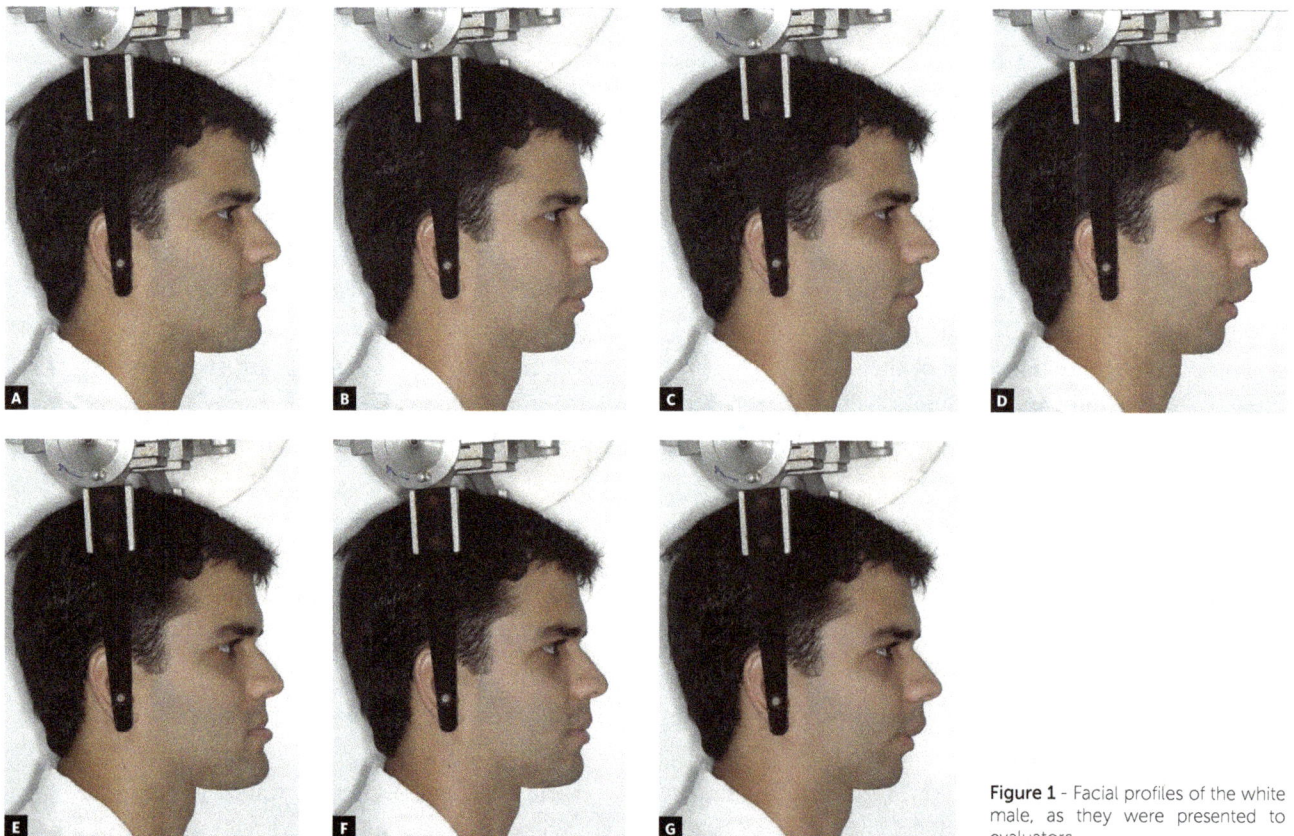

Figure 1 - Facial profiles of the white male, as they were presented to evaluators.

Selection of evaluators

For the evaluation of the 28 facial profiles, 20 orthodontists, associated to the *Associação Brasileira de Ortodontia* (Brazilian Orthodontics Association); 20 maxillofacial surgeons, members of the *Colégio Brasileiro de Cirurgia e Traumatologia Buco-Maxilo-Facial* (Brazilian College of Oral and Maxillofacial Surgery); 20 Visual Arts students at the *Universidade Federal do Rio Grande do Norte* (Rio Grande do Norte Federal University); and 22 laypersons (people without academic or professional qualifications in the areas of Dentistry or Visual Arts) were selected.

Evaluation of the photographs

Together with the photo album, each evaluator received four questionnaires, one for each page of the photo album. In the first item of each questionnaire, there was a ruler (analog visual scale), so the evaluators would mark the level of attractiveness that each photo exerted on them. The marks were identified with the letter corresponding to the photograph. Each evaluator was told that it was possible to mark the ruler at any point, and it was also possible to mark two or more letters at the same point. The analog visual scale had 116 mm, and it was written on the extreme left VERY BAD and, on the extreme right, VERY GOOD. In the center of the ruler, the word REGULAR was written. The distance (mm) between the point marked by the evaluator and the extreme left point was measured, originating the level of attractiveness of each face. In the second item, the evaluators were asked about the relation between facial attractiveness and the feeling of trust, and had to point which of the individuals they would hire for a job position. In the third item, the evaluators were asked which one of the individuals presented a better social condition.

All the evaluators examined the album and answered the questions individually, in the same room and under the same lighting conditions. The presence of other individuals in the room was not permitted as to not influence the judgment of the evaluator. The evaluator could view the album as much as needed, until all questions were answered. All evaluators were told they could refuse to answer any question.

Data analysis

The data were treated statistically at the SPSS® (Statistical Package for Social Sciences) software.

In order to analyze the first question (Facial attractiveness), a descriptive analysis was obtained from the average and the standard deviation of each group. The Kolmogorov-Smirnov test was used to verify the distribution of data.

The variance analysis (ANOVA One-Way) was performed to verify if there were any differences among the groups and the Tukey testing to identify between which groups the differences happened. In all cases, the significance level considered was 5%.

For the following questions, Employability and Socioeconomic condition, only descriptive analysis was performed by percentage data.

RESULTS

Table 1 shows the average and the standard deviation of the level of attractiveness that the different profiles exerted on the evaluators, regardless of the group that they belonged. Tables 2, 3, 4 and 5 show the level of attractiveness that the facial profiles of the black male, white male, black female and white female, respectively exerted on the different groups of evaluators.

Table 1 -Mean (M) and Standard Deviation (SD) of the level of attractiveness that the different facial profiles exerted on the evaluators.

Facial convexity angle	Black male M/SD	White male M/SD	Black female M/SD	White woman M/SD
0°	1.07/0.86	1.80/1.53	0.84/0.66	0.86/0.86
4°	3.55/2.27	6.24/2.41	2.36/1.49	2.31/1.5
8°	8.21/2.34	9.36/2.17	6.33/2.62	6.34/2.19
12°	9.41/2.16	8.43/2.65	9.01/2.11	9.25/1.91
16°	5.66/2.18	4.99/2.06	6.64/2.39	7.03/2.12
20°	2.32/1.72	2.11/1.64	3.56/2.20	4.87/2.08
24°	1.12/1.07	1.07/1.24	1.57/1.22	2.07/2.09

Confidence interval = 95%.

Table 2 -Mean and standard deviation of the level of facial attractiveness of the black male, according to each group of evaluators.

Facial convexity angle	Orthodontists		Surgeons		Visual artists		Laypersons	
	Mean	SD	Mean	SD	Mean	SD	Mean	SD
0°	0.74*	0.60	0.75**	0.57	1.30	0.94	1.50 *, **	1.01
4°	3.85	2.17	3.73	2.08	3.29	2.42	3.33	2.51
8°	7.77*	2.45	8.37	1.89	9.68 *, **	1.46	7.04 **	2.66
12°	10.83*	0.80	10.60**	0.95	8.93 *, **, ***	1.86	7.30 *, **, ***	2.42
16°	6.24	2.06	5.87	1.46	5.78	2.39	4.76	2.52
20°	2.31	1.95	2.30	1.85	2.36	1.61	2.33	1.59
24°	0.77*	0.91	0.68**	0.52	1.27	0.77	1.78 *, **	1.51

*, **, *** Statistically significant difference among the groups of evaluators ($p<0,05$).

Table 3 -Mean and standard deviation of the level of facial attractiveness of the white male, according to each group of evaluators.

Facial convexity angle	Orthodontists		Surgeons		Visual artists		Laypersons	
	Mean	SD	Mean	SD	Mean	SD	Mean	SD
0°	1.69	1.79	1.54	0.93	2.41	1.66	2.37	1.49
4°	6.75	1.76	6.74	2.12	6.17	2.79	6.11	2.91
8°	11.30*	0.58	10.91**	0.74	8.21 *, **	2.04	7.83 *, **	2.10
12°	10.23*	1.74	10.38**	1.37	7.18 *, **	2.27	6.75 *, **	2.69
16°	5.05	1.79	5.44	1.85	4.73	2.30	5.56	2.29
20°	1.71*	1.21	1.54**	0.99	3.09 *, **	1.95	2.89	1.71
24°	0.62*	0.36	1.20	1.73	1.73*	1.27	1.54	0.97

*, ** Statistically significant difference among the groups of evaluators ($p<0,05$).

Table 4 - Mean and standard deviation of the level of face attractiveness of the black female, according to each group of evaluators.

Facial convexity angle	Orthodontists		Surgeons		Visual artists		Laypersons	
	Mean	SD	Mean	SD	Mean	SD	Mean	SD
0°	0.57*	0.46	0.57**	0.43	1.10 *, **	0.77	1.12 *, **	0.71
4°	2.59	1.80	2.60	1.59	2.15	1.27	2.10	1.26
8°	6.47	2.59	6.26	2.49	6.32	2.76	6.28	2.82
12°	10.98*	0.70	10.68**	1.02	7.47 *, **	1.30	6.92 *, **	1.06
16°	7.69*	2.34	8.07**	2.15	5.44 *, **	1.88	5.38 *, **	1.89
20°	3.93	2.39	3.70	2.05	3.01	2.14	3.60	2.29
24°	1.14	1.19	1.20	0.98	1.93	1.19	2.01	1.29

*, **, *** Statistically significant difference among the groups of evaluators ($p < 0,05$).

Table 5 - Mean and standard deviation of the level of face attractiveness of the white female, according to each group of evaluators.

Facial convexity angle	Orthodontists		Surgeons		Visual artists		Laypersons	
	Mean	SD	Mean	SD	Mean	SD	Mean	SD
0°	0.37*	0.25	0.37**	0.35	1.38 *, **	0.88	1.34 *, **	1.03
4°	1.84	0.95	2.20	1.39	2.65	1.75	2.57	1.74
8°	6.25	2.11	6.41	2.09	6.39	2.40	6.34	2.29
12°	10.75*	1.16	10.65**	0.98	7.96 *, **	1.45	7.66 *, **	1.37
16°	6.81	1.82	7.02	1.77	7.15	2.53	7.17	2.38
20°	4.84	1.50	4.93	1.42	4.91	2.66	4.80	2.57
24°	1.07 *, **	1.09	1.04	0.83	3.09 *, **	2.48	3.08 *, **	2.42

*, ** Statistically significant difference among the groups of evaluators ($p < 0,05$).

Table 6 - Percentage of evaluators per group that chose each facial profile as the most trustworthy to hire for a job position.

	0°	4°	8°	12°	16°	20°	24°
Black male							
Orthodontists	0%	0%	10%	90%	0%	0%	0%
Surgeons	0%	0%	0%	100%	0%	0%	0%
Visual artists	0%	0%	25%	50%	25%	0%	0%
Laypersons	0%	0%	20%	60%	15%	0%	5%
White male							
Orthodontists	0%	0%	60%	40%	0%	0%	0%
Surgeons	0%	0%	50%	50%	0%	0%	0%
Visual artists	0%	35%	50%	15%	0%	0%	0%
Laypersons	0%	14%	54%	14%	14%	0%	4%
Black female							
Orthodontists	0%	0%	10%	90%	0%	0%	0%
Surgeons	0%	0%	10%	90%	0%	0%	0%
Visual artists	0%	0%	10%	75%	15%	0%	0%
Laypersons	0%	0%	9%	73%	14%	0%	4%
White female							
Orthodontists	0%	0%	0%	80%	20%	0%	0%
Surgeons	0%	0%	0%	70%	30%	0%	0%
Visual artists	0%	0%	0%	50%	50%	0%	0%
Laypersons	0%	4%	10%	41%	37%	4%	4%

Table 7 - Percentage of evaluators that chose each profile as the one presenting better social-economic condition.

	0°	4°	8°	12°	16°	20°	24°
Black male							
Orthodontists	0%	0%	10%	90%	0%	0%	0%
Surgeons	0%	0%	30%	70%	0%	0%	0%
Visual artists	0%	0%	45%	55%	0%	0%	0%
Laypersons	0%	0%	50%	41%	9%	0%	0%
White male							
Orthodontists	0%	0%	50%	50%	0%	0%	0%
Surgeons	0%	0%	40%	60%	0%	0%	0%
Visual artists	0%	30%	45%	25%	0%	0%	0%
Laypersons	0%	14%	59%	23%	4%	0%	0%
Black female							
Orthodontists	0%	0%	0%	100%	0%	0%	0%
Surgeons	0%	0%	0%	100%	0%	0%	0%
Visual artists	0%	0%	20%	70%	10%	0%	0%
Laypersons	0%	0%	18%	64%	18%	0%	0%
White female							
Orthodontists	0%	0%	0%	90%	10%	0%	0%
Surgeons	0%	0%	0%	80%	20%	0%	0%
Visual artists	0%	0%	0%	55%	45%	0%	0%
Laypersons	0%	4%	14%	50%	28%	4%	0%

According to these results, the anteroposterior positioning of the mandible exerts strong influence on the level of facial attractiveness, but there are few significant differences among the different groups of evaluators.

Table 6 shows the percentage of evaluators per group that chose each facial profile as the most trusted profile for a job position. In general, orthodontists and surgeons follow a similar line of thinking, agreeing, in most cases, on which profile they would hire for a job position.

Table 7 shows the percentage of evaluators per group that chose each facial profile as the profile that presented a better socioeconomic condition. In general, those profiles chosen as the most attractive were also indicated as the ones deserving the job positions.

DISCUSSION

Contemporary orthodontics has been suffering a great influence of the appeal for attractive facial esthetics. In order to ensure that the esthetic goals of an orthodontic treatment will be achieved, orthodontists must make a treatment plan substantiated by a thorough evaluation of the patient's face. By using the clinical examination of the frontal and profile views of the face, it's possible to evaluate the harmony of the structures that compose it.[19]

The soft tissue profile should be taken into consideration for the evaluation of underlying skeletal discrepancy itself, due to differences in the soft tissue thickness.[20,21] Soft tissue outline largely determines the esthetics of the face. For this reason, the facial profile has been extensively studied in Orthodontics.[7,22-26]

In addition, many studies[11,24,25,27] have discussed whether there is any difference in esthetic perception between professionals and laypersons, with the objective to allow the construction of treatment plans that contemplate not only the technical requirements desired by professionals, but also the needs of the patients.

The present study evaluated the influence of sagittal positioning of the mandible in facial attractiveness, from the perception of different groups of evaluators, including professionals and laypersons. Some authors have carried out similar studies.[11,23-25] However, none of them had evaluated the influence of sagittal positioning of the mandible and the perception of socioeconomic profile. Another interesting aspect of the present study is the inclusion of a group of visual artists. These pro-

fessionals do not have the same technical formation as orthodontists and surgeons, but they can also base their judgement on esthetics principles.

During data collection, it was opted for the use of colored photos of patients' profiles, since photographs give more realism to facial esthetics when compared to drawings of profile silhouettes.[7] However, facial characteristics of the patient, such as eye color, nose size, hair, and others, may influence the judgement of the evaluator.[23] For this reason, these characteristics were preserved in the different profiles with the help of Adobe Photoshop CS2® software.

Facial attractiveness

In the first item of the questionnaire, the answers were obtained with the aid of an analog visual scale. To Maple et al,[7] this scale permits a quick measurement, easy reading and greater freedom in data analysis. According to Orsini et al,[28] the use of words with contrasting meanings is ideal to measure the reactions of people to specific stimuli.

As to the results, it was observed that the anteroposterior positioning of the mandible exerts strong influence on the level of facial attractiveness, but there were few significant differences among the different groups of evaluators (Tables 1 to 5). Some authors[7,23,25] performed similar studies and did not observe significant differences between the groups of evaluators. McKeta et al,[27] when comparing the perception of the results of orthodontic treatment between patients —considered as laypersons— and dentists, observed that patients have a less significantly favorable perception of their own esthetics when compared to orthodontists. In the cited study, the laypersons evaluated their own cases, while in the present study, laypersons evaluated photographs of other patients, tending, thus, to be less critical. It is important to highlight that orthodontists and surgeons did not show results with statically significant differences for any of the facial profiles analyzed, which may be attributed to the fact that only these two groups could make a judgement based on technical criteria.

When observing Table 1, it can be noticed that the extreme angulations of Class II (0°) and Class III (24°) received the lower scores, regardless of ethnicity, being that, for male individuals, the most pronounced Class II was the profile that received the lowest scores, while for the female faces, the lowest scores were attributed to the most pronounced Class III. Fabré et al.[11] also found distinct results according to the gender of facial profiles, but the authors did not believe that the gender may influence the esthetic analysis by the evaluators. Almeida et al.[23] believe that both gender and race of the facial profile may have influence on esthetic evaluation. According to Cochrane et al.[9], regardless of gender, Class II is less attractive than Class III.

In regard to the faces considered ideal, the straight profile showed higher acceptance, in agreement to the majority of the studies in the literature.[11,22-23] For the black male and the black female, the straight profile with an angulation of 12° obtained the higher acceptance. This straight profile is characterized by low protruded lips. According to the literature[18,29], black faces, when compared to white faces, are considered more attractive when presenting a slighter lip protrusion. For the white woman, the straight profile with angulation of 12° also obtained higher acceptance. In the case of the white male, the straight profile with slight mandibular protrusion (8°) was the most accepted one, in agreement to the results of Almeida et al.[23], that used a similar methodology, working with colored photographs and with an analog visual scale during data collection. Czarnecki et al.[30], when evaluating the role of the nose, lips and chin in obtaining a balanced facial profile, also found similar results and concluded that straight profiles, with the menton slightly prominent, are more accepted to white male faces than to white female faces.

As for the evaluators, for the black male, there was a statically significant difference among the groups. According to the visual artists, the profile considered as the most harmonic was the straight one with slight mandibular protrusion (8°) and not the profile of 12°, which was the most chosen by other groups of evaluators. Although there was a difference between the groups, both profiles (8° and 12°) fit in the normality clinical standard. Still regarding the black male, the visual artists agreed with the surgeons and elected the most pronounced Class II profile as the least friendly. On the other hand, orthodontists and laypersons elected the most pronounced Class III (0°) as the least friendly profile, in agreement with the findings of Romani et al,[31] in which laypersons and orthodontists presented the same level of perception to sagittal changes of the mandible. For Arpino et al.[32], orthodontists are more tolerant to changes in facial profiles than surgeons.

Employability

In general, orthodontists and surgeons follow a similar line of thinking, agreeing, in most cases, on which profile they would hire for a job position. As for visual artists and laypersons, they have shown great heterogeneity in their opinions, when each group was observed separately.

The majority of orthodontists, laypersons and visual artists agree that the black male and the black and white females with a straight profile in 12° would be chosen for the job position. For the white male, the most chosen individual was that with the convexity angle in 8°, which represents a straight profile with slight protrusion, creating a more aggressive face with traces of seriousness. For surgeons, the profile in 12° was chosen as the most favorable for hiring, regardless of race or gender. All these profiles were described as harmonic to the point of view of facial attractiveness, since for the white male the slight mandibular protrusion may indicate a peculiar beauty characteristic.

It is noted, thus, the strict relation of facial attractiveness with the easiness to get a job position. Many authors[33-35] performed studies with some level of similarity and concluded that persons deemed as more attractive are also considered as more intelligent and competent, and thus, present higher chances of professional success. It is possible that these results may be associated to the assumption that intelligent people are more concerned with the impact of their image on society.

Socioeconomic condition

When evaluators were asked which of the profiles appear to have better socioeconomic condition, it was observed that, in general, the same profiles were chosen as the most attractive ones and deserving job positions.

This result presents some similarities with the findings of Kershaw, Newton and Williams,[36] in which individuals with dental changes, and thus with less harmonic faces, were indicated as belonging to lower social classes, when compared to individuals without alterations. Such association may be justified by the financial investment required for dental treatment.

As for the groups of evaluators, orthodontists and maxillofacial surgeons once more followed a similar line of thought, agreeing, in majority, on which profile presented a better socioeconomic condition.

Finally, it is important to note that there are limitations in this study, because the examiners made their judgment based only on photographs, without considering characteristics such as professional technical quality, personal skills, social class, among others. Therefore, the results presented in this study express only a first impression about the evaluated facial profiles.

CONCLUSIONS

Despite limitations of the methodology applied, it can be concluded that:

» The anteroposterior position of the mandible exerted strong influence on the level of facial attractiveness, but few significant differences were observed among the different groups of evaluators.

» The profiles pointed as the most attractive were also pointed as the most favorable to be hired for a job position, and also pointed as those that seemed to have a better socioeconomic condition.

» Orthodontists and maxillofacial surgeons showed greater concordance in their results.

REFERENCES

1. Kokich VO, Kokich VG, Kiyak HA. Perceptions of dental professionals and laypersons to altered dental esthetics: asymmetric and symmetric situations. Am J Orthod Dentofacial Orthop. 2006 Aug;130(2):141-51.
2. Griffin AM, Langlois JH. Stereotype directionality and attractiveness stereotyping: is beauty good or is ugly bad? Soc Cogn. 2006 Apr;24(2):187-206.
3. Choi WS, Lee S, McGrathe C, Samman N. Change inquality of life after combined orthodontic-surgical treatment of dentofacial deformities. Oral Surg Oral Med Oral Pathol Oral Radiol Endod. 2010;109(1):46-51.
4. Baldwin DC. Appearance and aesthetics in oral health. Community Dent Oral Epidemiol. 1980;8(5):244-56.
5. Jacobson A. Psychological aspects of dentofacial esthetics and orthognathic surgery. Angle Orthod. 1984;54(1):18-35.
6. Hamdan AM. The relationship between patient, parent and clinician perceived need and normative orthodontic treatment need. Eur J Orthod. 2004;26(3):265-71.
7. Maple JR, Vig KWL, Beck FM, Larsen PE, Shanker S. A comparison of providers' and consumers' perceptions of facial-profile attractiveness. Am J Orthod Dentofacial Orthop. 2005;128(6):690-6.
8. Kumar S, Gandhi S, Valiathan A. Perception of smile esthetics among Indian dental professionals and laypersons. Indian J Dent Res. 2012 Mar-Apr;23(2):295.
9. Cochrane SM, Cunningham SJ, Hunt NP. A comparison of the perception of facial profile by the general public and 3 group of clinicians. Int J Adult Orthodon Orthognath Surg. 1999;14(4):291-5.
10. Shelly AD, Southard TE, Southard KA, Casko JS, Jakobsen JR, Fridrich KL, et al. Evaluation of profi le esthetic change with mandibular advancement surgery. Am J Orthod Dentofacial Orthop. 2000 June;117(6):630-7.
11. Fabré M, Mossaz C, Christou P, Kiliaridis S. Orthodontists' and laypersons' aesthetic assessment of Class III subjects referred for orthognathic surgery. Eur J Orthod. 2009 Aug;31(4):443-8.
12. Kuroda S, Sugahara T, Takabatake S, Taketa H, Ando R, Takano-Yamamoto T. Influence of anteroposterior mandibular positions on facial attractiveness in Japanese adults. Am J Orthod Dentofacial Orthop. 2009 Jan;135(1):73-8.
13. Johnston C, Hunt O, Burden D, Stevenson M, Hepper P. The influence of mandibular prominence on facial attractiveness. Eur J Orthod. 2005 Apr;27(2):129-33.
14. Naini FB. Facial aesthetics: concepts and clinical diagnosis. Oxford: Wiley-Blackwell; 2011.
15. Proffit WR, Fields HW Jr, Sarver DM. Contemporary Orthodontics. St. Louis: Mosby Elsevier; 2012.
16. Legan HL, Burstone CJ. Soft tissue cephalometric analysis for orthognathic surgery. J Oral Surg. 1980;38(10):744-51.
17. Steiner CC. Cephalometrics as a clinical tool. In: Kraus BS, Riedel RA. Vistas in Orthodontics. Philadelphia: Lea & Febiger; 1962.
18. Farrow AL, Zarrinnia K, Azizi K. Bimaxillary protrusion in black Americans—an esthetic evaluation and the treatment considerations. Am J Orthod Dentofacial Orthop. 1993 Sept;104(3):240-50.
19. McLaren EA, Rifkin R. Macroesthetics: facial and dentofacial analysis. J Calif Dent Assoc. 2002 Nov;30(11):839-46.
20. Burstone CJ. Integumental contour and extension patterns. Angle Orthod. 1959;29 (2):93-104.
21. Subtelny JD. A longitudinal study of soft-tissue facial structures and their profile characteristics defined in relation to underlying skeletal structure. Am J Orthod. 1959 July;45 (7):481-507.
22. Soh J, Chew MT, Wong HB. Professional assessment of facial profile attractiveness. Am J Orthod Dentofacial Orthop. 2005 Aug;128(2):201-5.
23. Almeida MD, Farias ACR, Bittencourt MAV. Influence of mandibular sagittal position on facial esthetics. Dental Press J Orthod. 2010;15(2):87-96.
24. Naini FB, Donaldson AN, Cobourne MT, McDonald F. Assessing the influence of mandibular prominence on perceived attractiveness in the orthognathic patient, clinician, and layperson. Eur J Orthod. 2012 Dec;34(6):738-46.
25. Naini FB, Donaldson F, McDonald F, Cobourne MT. Assessing the influence of chin prominence on perceived attractiveness in the orthognathic patient, clinician and layperson. Int J Oral Maxillofac Surg. 2012;41(7):839-46.
26. Bullen RN, Kook Y, Kim K, Park JH. Self-perception of the facial profile: an aid in treatment planning for orthognathic surgery. J Oral Maxillofac Surg. 2014;72(4):773-8.
27. Mcketa N, Rinchuse, JD, Close, JM. Practitioner and patient perceptions of orthodontic treatment: is the patient always right? J Est Restor Dent. 2012;24(1):40-50.
28. Orsini MG, Huang GJ, Kiyak HA, Ramsay DS, Bollen AM, Anderson NK, et al. Methods to evaluate profile preferences for the anteroposterior position of mandible. Am J Orthod Dentofacial Orthop. 2006 Sept;130(3):283-91.
29. Sushner NI. A photographic study of the soft-tissue profile of the Negro population. Am J Orthod. 1977 Oct;72(4):373-85.
30. Czarnecki ST, Nanda RS, Currier GF. Perceptions of a balanced facial profile. Am J Orthod Dentofacial Orthop. 1993 Aug;104(2):180-7.
31. Romani KL, Agahi F, Nanda R, Zernik JH. Evaluation of horizontal and vertical differences in facial profiles by orthodontists and lay people. Angle Orthod. 1993 Fall;63(3):175-82.
32. Arpino VJ, Giddon DB, BeGole EA, Evans CA. Presurgical profile preferences of patients and clinicians. Am J Orthod Dentofacial Orthop. 1998 Dec;114(6):631-7.
33. Henson ST, Lindauer SJ, Gardner WG, Shroff B, Tufekci E, Best AM. Influence of dental esthetics on social perceptions of adolescents judged by peers. Am J Orthod Dentofacial Orthop. 2011 Sept;140(3):389-95.
34. Malkinson S, Waldrop TC, Gunsolley JC, Lanning SK, Sabatini R. The effect of esthetic crown lengthening on perceptions of a patient's attractiveness, friendliness, trustworthiness, intelligence, and self-confidence. J Periodontol. 2013 Aug;84(8):1126-33.
35. Pithon MM, Nascimento CC, Barbosa GC, Coqueiro RS. Do dental esthetics have any influence on finding a job? Am J Orthod Dentofacial Orthop. 2014 Oct;146(4):423-9.

9

Effects of cervical headgear appliance

Fernanda Pinelli Henriques[1], Guilherme Janson[2], Jose Fernando Castanha Henriques[2], Daniela Cubas Pupulim[1]

Objective: Although much has been investigated about the effects of cervical headgear, there remains some controversy. Therefore, the objective of this systematic review is to disclose the actual effects of the cervical headgear appliance, based on articles of relevant quality. **Methods:** A literature review was conducted using PubMed, Web of Science, Embase, Scopus and Cochrane databases. Inclusion criteria consisted of human studies written in English; published between 1970 and 2014; in which only the cervical headgear was used to correct Class II malocclusion; prospective or retrospective; with a clear description of cervical headgear effects; with a sample size of at least 15 individuals. No comparative studies, clinical cases or cases with dental extractions were included and the sample should be homogeneous. **Results:** Initially, 267 articles were found. A total of 42 articles were selected by title and had their abstracts read. Finally, 12 articles were classified as with high quality and were used in this systematic review. **Conclusions:** The cervical headgear appliance proved efficient to correct Class II, Division 1 malocclusion. Its effects consisted in correction of the maxillomandibular relationship by restriction of maxillary anterior displacement; distalization and extrusion of maxillary molars; and slight maxillary expansion.

Keywords: Angle Class II malocclusion. Extraoral traction appliances. Orthodontic appliances. Removable orthodontic appliances. Orthopedic appliances.

[1] PhD resident, Universidade de São Paulo, School of Dentistry, Bauru, São Paulo, Brazil.
[2] Full professor, Universidade de São Paulo, School of Dentistry, Bauru, São Paulo, Brazil.

Fernanda Pinelli Henriques
Al. Octavio Pinheiro Brisolla 9-75
E-mail: fernandapinelli@yahoo.com.br

» The authors report no commercial, proprietary or financial interest in the products or companies described in this article.

INTRODUCTION

Growing patients can benefit from the use of the cervical headgear appliance to correct Class II, Division 1 malocclusion, although treatment effect is intimately related to patient's compliance and motivation. This protocol has been used for decades and has shown good results, providing orthopedic and orthodontic effects depending on the magnitude of force, time of daily use and patient's age.[1,2]

Although the use of cervical headgear has been currently decreasing, especially because of the development of mini-implants[3] and the increase in the use of fixed functional appliances,[4-7] it is still useful for specific Class II malocclusions with predominance of maxillary and/or dentoalveolar maxillary protrusion.

Studies have reported a variety of dentoskeletal effects produced by the cervical headgear, which are somewhat diverging. Therefore, this systematic review aimed to elucidate which are the actual effects of this treatment on Class II malocclusions.

MATERIAL AND METHODS

By using the terms 'effects', 'cervical' and 'headgear', a computerized search was performed on the following electronic databases: PubMed, Scopus, Web of Science, Embase, and Cochrane (Table 1).

Only the articles meeting the following criteria were selected for inclusion and analysis: human studies published in English between 1970 and 2014; prospective or retrospective studies, with a clear description of the effects of cervical headgear with sample size of at least 15 individuals; a homogeneous sample; studies in which only the cervical headgear appliance was used to correct Class II malocclusion. Exclusion criteria comprised comparison studies between appliances; case reports; studies on patients who used fixed appliances concurrently with cervical headgear and on patients who were treated with extractions. Duplicate articles were eliminated.

Initially, the articles were selected by titles. Subsequently, the abstracts of these articles were read to refine selection. If the abstracts did not contain enough information for the selection criteria, the article was fully read (Tables 2 and 3).

The selection process was independently conducted by two researchers in the same order. Interexaminer conflicts were solved by discussion on each article so as to reach a consensus regarding which articles fulfilled the main selection criteria.

The selected articles were ultimately classified according to the following quality characteristics:[8] number of observations, sample homogeneity, method of cervical headgear use and initial occlusal malocclusion severity.

The selected studies should present at least 15 individuals comprising the sample.[3,8] Therefore, studies that had 15 to 20 individuals were scored as 5, those with more than 30 individuals were scored as 7, and those with more than 40 individuals were scored as 10.

Studies with a more homogeneous group were scored as 10, whereas studies lacking homogeneity were scored as 5.

Additionally, we assessed how the cervical headgear was used: studies with proper installation and adequate daily use were scored as 10, whereas failures were scored as 7 or 5.

Articles that described malocclusion severity received higher scores. However, this was not an exclusion criterion. Therefore, if the type of malocclusion was described, the article was considered acceptable (Table 4).

The quality level of articles was assigned as follows:[8] high = total score from 30 to 40; medium = total score from 20 to 30 points; low = total score from 0 to 20.

RESULTS

After the database searching, 72 articles were found on PubMed, 7 on Cochrane, 68 on Web of Science, 36 on Embase, and 84 on Scopus (Table 1). Two articles were found by hand searching and 10 articles met the initial inclusion criteria (Fig 1). A synthesis of the information comprising the 12 selected articles is presented in Tables 2 and 3. After all analyses, 12 articles were classified with high level quality and were used in this systematic review (Table 4).

Table 1 - Database research results.

Database	Results	Articles selected	Articles included
PubMed	72	19	07
Cochrane	07	00	00
Web of Science	68	02	00
Embase	36	01	00
Scopus	84	10	03
Hand searching		10	02
Subtotal		42	
Duplicate articles		30	
Total			12

Table 2 - Details of studies included in the analysis.

Author	Initial age	Daily use	n	Malocclusion
Wieslander L, Buck DL[10] (1974)	9 years	12 to 14 h	28	Class II, division 1
Wieslander L[1] (1975)	8 years	12 to 14 h	23	Class II, division 1
Kirjavainen M, Kirjavainen T, Haavikko K[13] (1997)	9.3 years	12 to 14 h	40	Class II, division 1
Kirjavainen M, Kirjavainen T, Humrmerinta K, Haavikko K[14] (2000)	9.3 years	12 to 14 h	40	Class II, division 1
Ashmore JL, et al[17] (2002)	Not described	14 h	36	Class II, division 1
Kirjavainen M, Kirjavainen T[12] (2003)	9.1 years	12 to 14 h	40	Class II, division 1
Lima Filho RM, Lima AL, Oliveira Ruellas AC[8] (2003)	10.5 years	12 to 14 h	40	Class II, division 1
Mantysaari R, Kantomaa T, Pirttiniemi P, Pykalainen A[9] (2004)	7.6 years	8 to 10 h	68	Class II, division 1
Godt A, Kalwitzki M, Goz G[16] (2007)	10.9 years	Not described	247	Class II, division 1
Kirjavainen M, Hurmerinta K, Kirjavainen T[11] (2007)	9.1 years	12 to 14 h	40	Class II, division 1
Godt A, Berneburg M, Kalwitzki M, Göz G[15] (2008)	11 years	14 h	119	Class II, division 1
Alió-Sanz J, et al[18] (2012)	8 years	12 to 14 h	79	Class II, division 1

Table 3 - Justification for inclusion of selected articles.

Author	Article	Effects
Wieslander L, Buck DL[10] (1974)	Physiologic recovery after cervical traction therapy	Class II malocclusion corrected by distal movement of maxillary molars. Mandibular rotation was also present and maxillary growth was redirected. Changes remained stable.
Wieslander L[1] (1975)	Early or late cervical traction therapy of Class II malocclusion in the mixed dentition	The use of cervical headgear was more efficient in terms of skeletal changes in early mixed dentition. ANB angle decreased during the same period.
Kirjavainen M, Kirjavainen T, Haavikko K[13] (1997)	Changes in dental arch dimensions by use of an orthopedic cervical headgear in Class II correction	Class II malocclusion corrected by improving overjet and keeping overbite unchanged. There was an increase in upper arch width and, as a result, lower arch as well. Upper arch length also increased.
Kirjavainen M, Kirjavainen T, Humrmerinta K, Haavikko K[14] (2000)	Orthopedic cervical headgear with an expanded inner bow in Class II correction	All patients had Class II malocclusion successfully corrected. There was restriction of forward maxillary displacement and normal mandibular growth expression.
Ashmore et al[17] (2002)	A 3-dimensional analysis of molar movement during headgear treatment	Class II malocclusion corrected by distalization with extrusion of maxillary molars and arch expansion.
Kirjavainen M, Kirjavainen T[12] (2003)	Maxillary expansion in Class II correction with orthopedic cervical headgear. Posteroranterior cephalometric study	Malocclusion was corrected and Class I relationship reestablished in all cases. There was maxillary expansion. As a result of maxillary expansion, there was spontaneous mandibular increase.
Lima Filho RM, Lima AL, Oliveira Ruellas AC[8] (2003)	Mandibular changes in skeletal Class II patients treated with Kloehn cervical headgear	Skeletal Class II malocclusion correction was effective and stable. The ANB angle improved, there was restriction of maxillary displacement and mandibular rotation, in addition to extrusion of maxillary molars.
Mantysaari R, Kantomaa T, Pirttiniemi P, Pykalainen A[9] (2004)	The effects of early headgear treatment on dental arches and craniofacial morphology: a report of 2 years randomized study.	There was an increase in maxillary and mandibular arch length and width. The use of cervical headgear proved effective to treat moderate crowding during early mixed dentition.
Godt A, Berneburg M, Kalwitzki M, Göz G[15] (2008)	Cephalometric analysis of molar and anterior tooth movement during cervical headgear treatment in relation to growth patterns	There was extrusion of maxillary molars and mandibular rotation in patients with good growth pattern.
Kirjavainen M, Hurmerinta K, Kirjavainen T[11] (2007)	Facial profile changes in early Class II correction with cervical headgear	Cervical headgear proved effective to correct Class II malocclusion, as it minimized overbite regardless of patient's growth pattern.
Godt A, Kalwitzki M, Goz G[16] (2007)	Effects of cervical headgear on overbite against the background of existing growth patterns	Class II malocclusion was corrected by the cervical headgear. There was extrusion of maxillary molars. Treatment was followed by a decrease in maxillary convexity. There was an increase in lip seal.
Alió-Sanz J et al[18] (2012)	Effects on the maxilla and cranial base caused by cervical headgear: A longitudinal study	There was restriction of maxillary displacement in relation to the cranial base, in addition to retrusion of the A point.

Table 4 - Assessment of the quality of articles selected.

Author	Sample size	Homogeneity	Protocol for cervical headgear use	Initial malocclusion	Total
Wieslander L, Buck DL[10] (1974)	Appropriate 10	Appropriate 10	Appropriate 7	Appropriate 10	37
Wieslander L[1] (1975)	Appropriate 10	Appropriate 10	Appropriate 7	Appropriate 10	37
Kirjavainen M, Kirjavainen T, Haavikko K[13] (1997)	Appropriate 10	Appropriate 10	Appropriate 10	Appropriate 10	40
Kirjavainen M, Kirjavainen T, Humrmerinta K, Haavikko K[14] (2000)	Appropriate 10	Appropriate 10	Appropriate 10	Appropriate 10	40
Ashmore et al[17] (2002)	Appropriate 10	Appropriate 10	Appropriate 10	Appropriate 10	40
Kirjavainen M, Kirjavainen T[12] (2003)	Appropriate 10	Appropriate 10	Appropriate 7	Appropriate 10	37
Lima Filho RM, Lima AL, Oliveira Ruellas AC[8] (2003)	Appropriate 10	Appropriate 10	Appropriate 7	Appropriate 10	37
Mantysaaari R, Kantomaa T, Pirttiniemi P, Pykalainen A[9] (2004)	Appropriate 10	Appropriate 10	Appropriate 10	Appropriate 10	40
Godt A, Berneburg M, Kalwitzki M, Göz G[15] (2008)	Appropriate 10	Appropriate 10	Appropriate 10	Appropriate 10	40
Godt A, Kalwitzki M, Goz G[16] (2007)	Appropriate 10	Appropriate 10	Appropriate 10	Appropriate 10	40
Kirjavainen M, Hurmerinta K, Kirjavainen T[11] (2007)	Appropriate 10	Appropriate 10	Appropriate 10	Appropriate 10	40
Alió-Sanz J et al[18] (2012)	Appropriate 10	Appropriate 10	Appropriate 10	Appropriate 10	40

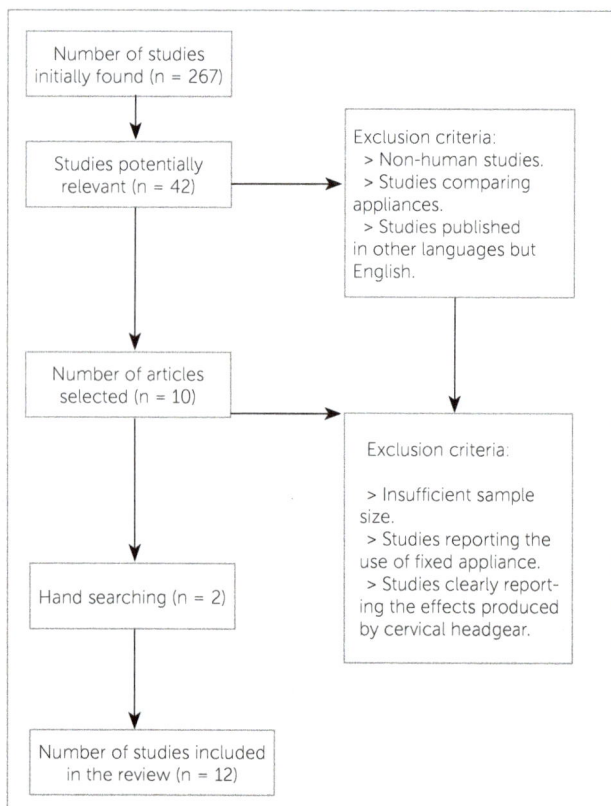

Number of studies initially found (n = 267)
→
Studies potentially relevant (n = 42)
→ Exclusion criteria:
> Non-human studies.
> Studies comparing appliances.
> Studies published in other languages but English.
→
Number of articles selected (n = 10)
→ Exclusion criteria:
> Insufficient sample size.
> Studies reporting the use of fixed appliance.
> Studies clearly reporting the effects produced by cervical headgear.
→
Hand searching (n = 2)
→
Number of studies included in the review (n = 12)

Figure 1 - Fluxogram of database research.

DISCUSSION

All patients selected in the articles presented Class II, Division 1 malocclusion with a protrusive maxilla that would benefit from correction with an orthopedic cervical headgear as the only appliance.[1,8-18]

However, most articles did not describe the initial occlusal malocclusion severity and, therefore, the information in this review will be limited regarding this issue.

Class II malocclusion treatment is very difficult not only because several types of appliances can be used, but also because numerous combinations of dental and/or skeletal relationships established between the maxilla and the mandible can cause Class II malocclusion.

To avoid combined effects of several appliances, only patients treated exclusively with cervical headgear should have been considered in the selected studies.

It has also been suggested that the age at treatment onset is another critical factor.[8] Most studies suggest starting treatment at the late mixed dentition or at the beginning of the permanent dentition to increase treatment efficiency.

The cervical headgear is supported on tubes fixed on maxillary molars bands with force ranging from 450 to 500 g on each side, and it is recommended to be used for 12 to 14 hours a day.

In the selected articles, there was extrusion of maxillary first molars, as it had been described in the 70's.[19,20] For this reason, the use of cervical headgear alone induces bite opening and increase in vertical parameters in patients with a vertical growth pattern at the beginning of treatment.[15] Due to molar extrusion, the cervical headgear would not be indicated for dolichofacial patients with extremely long faces, because it could worsen a profile that is already considered unpleasant.[8,11,13,15,16] Notwithstanding, this would not be a reason to avoid the use of cervical headgear in patients with vertical growth.[16]

Consequently to molar extrusion, there is also mandibular clockwise rotation.[11,15,16,17] Many researchers have found that the mandible rotates backwards and the mandibular plane angle increases with the use of cervical headgear.

Additionally, the cervical headgear promoted slight expansion of the upper arch, obtained by the expansion introduced in the inner bow of about 8 to 10 mm, which favors alignment of maxillary teeth.[13,14] This maxillary expansion may be eventually accompanied by mandibular arch expansion[12] and creates excellent conditions for the mandible to grow to a full extent, helping to correct Class II malocclusion.

Another headgear effect, described by the articles, was the improvement of the maxillomandibular relationship by means of maxillary repositioning.[1,9-17]

In other words, there was restriction of forward and downward maxillary displacement and normal mandibular growth expression, compensating the initial overjet that patients presented before treatment.[1,9,14] This was especially observed in the early mixed dentition.[1,9]

All articles also showed improvements of molar relationship, that is, all patients initially found with Class II molar relationship ended up with Class I molar relationship. Therefore, there was actual distalization of maxillary molars. However, because initial anterior-posterior malocclusion severity was not specified in most articles, the amount of distalization could not be determined.[1,8-18]

All articles selected showed that patient's compliance and motivation are essential to correct Class II malocclusion.[1,8,15,16] Nevertheless, no article reported patient exclusion due to lack of compliance, which is especially difficult with an extraoral appliance due to esthetic implications.

The orthodontist plays a great role in motivating the patients to use the appliance.[2] If there is a good level of compliance, the favorable results demonstrated by this review can be obtained.

CONCLUSIONS

The effects of the cervical headgear were as follows:

» Effective correction of Class II, Division 1, malocclusion.

» Correction of maxillomandibular relationship by restriction of maxillary anterior displacement.

» Distalization and extrusion of maxillary molars.

» Slight maxillary expansion.

REFERENCES

1. Wieslander L. Early or late cervical traction therapy of Class II malocclusion in the mixed dentition. Am J Orthod. 1975;67(4):432-9.

2. Allan T, Hodgson E. The use of personality measurements as a determinant of patient cooperation in an orthodontic practice. Am J Orthod. 1968;54(6):433-40.

3. Grec RH, Janson G, Branco NC, Moura-Grec PG, Patel MP, Castanha Henriques JF. Intraoral distalizer effects with conventional and skeletal anchorage: a meta-analysis. Am J Orthod Dentofacial Orthop. 2013;143(5):602-15.

4. Angelieri F, Almeida RR, Janson G, Castanha Henriques JF, Pinzan A. Comparison of the effects produced by headgear and pendulum appliances followed by fixed orthodontic treatment. Eur J Orthod. 2008;30(6):572-9.

5. Bolla E, Muratore F, Carano A, Bowman SJ. Evaluation of maxillary molar distalization with the distal jet: a comparison with other contemporary methods. Angle Orthod. 2002;72(5):481-94.

6. Fortini A, Lupoli M, Parri M. The First Class Appliance for rapid molar distalization. J Clin Orthod. 1999;33(6):322-8.

7. Jones RD, White JM. Rapid Class II molar correction with an open-coil jig. J Clin Orthod. 1992;26(10):661-4.

8. Lima Filho RM, Lima AL, Oliveira Ruellas AC. Mandibular changes in skeletal Class II patients treated with Kloehn cervical headgear. Am J Orthod Dentofacial Orthop. 2003;124(1):83-90.

9. Mantysaari R, Kantomaa T, Pirttiniemi P, Pykalainen A. The effects of early headgear treatment on dental arches and craniofacial morphology: a report of a 2 year randomized study. Eur J Orthod. 2004;26(1):59-64.

10. Wieslander L, Buck DL. Physiologic recovery after cervical traction therapy. Am J Orthod. 1974;66(3):294-301.

11. Kirjavainen M, Hurmerinta K, Kirjavainen T. Facial profile changes in early Class II correction with cervical headgear. Angle Orthod. 2007;77(6):960-7.

12. Kirjavainen M, Kirjavainen T. Maxillary expansion in Class II correction with orthopedic cervical headgear. A posteroanterior cephalometric study. Angle Orthod. 2003;73(3):281-5.

13. Kirjavainen M, Kirjavainen T, Haavikko K. Changes in dental arch dimensions by use of an orthopedic cervical headgear in Class II correction. Am J Orthod Dentofacial Orthop. 1997;111(1):59-66.

14. Kirjavainen M, Kirjavainen T, Hurmerinta K, Haavikko K. Orthopedic cervical headgear with an expanded inner bow in Class II correction. Angle Orthod. 2000;70(4):317-25.

15. Godt A, Berneburg M, Kalwitzki M, Göz G. Cephalometric analysis of molar an anterior tooth movement during cervical headgear treatment in relation growth patterns. J Orofac Orthop. 2008;69(3):189-200.

16. Godt A, Kalwitzki M, Goz G. Effects of cervical headgear on overbite against the background of existing growth patterns. A retrospective analysis of study casts. Angle Orthod. 2007;77(1):42-6.

17. Ashmore JL, Kurland BF, King GJ, Wheeler TT, Ghafari J, Ramsay DS. A 3-dimensional analysis of molar movement during headgear treatment. Am J Orthod Dentofacial Orthop. 2002;121(1):18-30.

18. Alió-Sanz J, Iglesias-Conde C, Lorenzo-Pernia J, Iglesias-Linares A, Mendoza-Mendoza A, Solano-Reina E. Effects on the maxilla and cranial base caused by cervical headgear: a longitudinal study. Med Oral Patol Oral Cir Bucal. 2012;17(5):e845-51.

19. King EW. Cervical anchorage in Class II, division 1 treatment, a cephalometric appraisal. Angle Orthod. 1957;27(2):98-104.

20. Klein PL. An evaluation of cervical traction on the maxilla and upper first permanent molar. Angle Orthod. 1957;27(1):61-8.

10

Efficiency of different protocols for enamel clean-up after bracket debonding: an *in vitro* study

Lara Carvalho Freitas Sigilião[1], Mariana Marquezan[2], Carlos Nelson Elias[3],
Antônio Carlos Ruellas[4], Eduardo Franzotti Sant'Anna[4]

Objective: This study aimed to assess the efficiency of six protocols for cleaning-up tooth enamel after bracket debonding. **Methods:** A total of 60 premolars were divided into six groups, according to the tools used for clean-up: 12-blade bur at low speed (G12L), 12-blade bur at high speed (G12H), 30-blade bur at low speed (G30L), DU10CO ORTHO polisher (GDU), Renew System (GR) and Diagloss polisher (GD). Mean roughness (Ra) and mean roughness depth (Rz) of enamel surface were analyzed with a profilometer. Paired t-test was used to assess Ra and Rz before and after enamel clean-up. ANOVA/Tukey tests were used for intergroup comparison. The duration of removal procedures was recorded. The association between time and variation in enamel roughness (ΔRa, ΔRz) were evaluated by Pearson's correlation test. Enamel topography was assessed by scanning electron microscopy (SEM). **Results:** In Groups G12L and G12H, original enamel roughness did not change significantly. In Groups G30L, GDU, GR and GD, a smoother surface ($p < 0.05$) was found after clean-up. In Groups G30L and GD, the protocols used were more time-consuming than those used in the other groups. Negative and moderate correlation was observed between time and (ΔRa, ΔRz); Ra and (ΔRa, ΔRz); Rz ($r = -0.445$, $r = -0.475$, $p < 0.01$). **Conclusion:** All enamel clean-up protocols were efficient because they did not result in increased surface roughness. The longer the time spent performing the protocol, the lower the surface roughness.

Keywords: Orthodontic brackets. Dental enamel. Dental debonding.

[1] Dentist, Brazilian Navy, Rio de Janeiro, Rio de Janeiro, Brazil.
[2] Postdoc resident in Orthodontics, Universidade Federal do Rio de Janeiro
(UFRJ), Rio de Janeiro, Rio de Janeiro, Brazil.
[3] Professor, Instituto Militar de Engenharia (IME),
Rio de Janeiro, Rio de Janeiro, Brazil.
[4] Professor, Universidade Federal do Rio de Janeiro (UFRJ), Rio de Janeiro, Rio
de Janeiro, Brazil.

» The authors report no commercial, proprietary or financial interest in the products
or companies described in this article.

Eduardo Franzotti Sant'Anna
Av. Professor Rodolpho Paulo Rocco, 325, Ilha do Fundão, Rio de Janeiro/RJ
E-mail: eduardo.franzotti@gmail.com

INTRODUCTION

Direct bracket bonding to tooth surface became possible with the advent of acid etching which revolutionized the orthodontic practice.[1] On completion of orthodontic treatment, the residual resin left behind after bracket debonding must be cleaned efficiently and rapidly while preserving enamel surface; in addition, enamel surface must be smoothed and polished to prevent plaque accumulation. Several factors are involved in these procedures, including the tools used for debonding, protocols for residual resin removal, the type of adhesive used[2] and the operator's skill.

Although there is no consensus in the literature regarding this matter, one of the most common methods of removing residual adhesive from the enamel surface is using a tungsten carbide bur at low speed.[3-6] Several new and more conservative multiple and one-step systems for enamel clean-up, such as fiber-reinforced composites,[7] polishers with diamond particles, aluminum oxide rubber and sandblasting,[6] have been developed and gained popularity among orthodontists. However, many of these tools have not been tested as a method of providing characteristics similar to those of the original enamel.

The aims of this study were to compare *in vitro* enamel surface roughness by using six protocols for removal of adhesive remnant and enamel polishing after bracket debonding; assess the time spent to remove residual resin in each one of them; and assess the correlation between roughness and removal time.

MATERIAL AND METHODS

This study was approved by the Research and Ethics Committee of the Institute of Public Health and Research at Universidade Federal do Rio de Janeiro, Brazil (#05/2012).

A total of 60 human caries-free premolars extracted for orthodontic purposes were stored in aqueous solution of thymol (0.1%) to prevent bacterial growth and dehydration. Teeth were selected based on visual observation of soundness of the buccal surfaces, absence of caries and cracks in the coronal portion, and no previous exposure to adhesive agents. The teeth roots were removed and the crowns were embedded in self-polymerizing acrylic resin with the buccal surfaces facing upwards.

The bond area was limited by marks made on the base of the specimens to ensure that roughness assessments were made in the same area.

Samples were randomly divided into six equal groups (n = 10) to compare different protocols for removal of adhesive remnant and enamel polishing (Table 1). Sample size was calculated at a level of significance set at 5% and test power of 80%, based on data from a previous study.[8]

Teeth were cleaned with fine pumice slurry using a rubber cup in a low-speed handpiece for approximately 10 seconds, followed by rinsing and drying with moisture-free air spray. Subsequently, teeth were etched for 20 seconds with 37% phosphoric acid gel (Magic Acid Vigodent®, Rio de Janeiro, RJ, Brazil), rinsed for 20 seconds and dried. Premolar metal brackets (Morelli®, Sorocaba, SP, Brazil) were bonded to teeth with Transbond XT (3M Unitek, Monrovia, Calif, USA), following the manufacturer's instructions. Brackets were placed on teeth surfaces and firmly pressed into position for the base to fit perfectly, providing uniform resin layer in all specimens. After removing excess resin from the edges of bracket bases with the aid of a dental probe, teeth were light-polymerized for 10 seconds on each side of the bracket by means of a conventional LED curing unit (Optilight Max - Gnatus®, Ribeirão Preto, SP, Brazil). Specimens were then stored in artificial saliva at 37 °C for 24 hours to facilitate maximum polymerization and hydration of the material.

Brackets were then removed by gently squeezing their mesial and distal wings with How Reto pliers.[9] Enamel surfaces were evaluated under Olympus SZ40 stereomicroscope (Olympus, Japan) under 15X magnification.[10] They were classified according to the Adhesive Remnant Index (ARI)[11]: score 0 = no adhesive on enamel, score 1 = less than 50% adhesive on enamel, score 2 = more than 50% adhesive on enamel, score 3 = all adhesive remaining on enamel. Teeth were included in the experiment only if the most of resin remained on enamel surface after debonding (score 2 or 3), in order to allow adequate evaluation of all finishing protocols. Fortunately, none of the samples were excluded. Groups G12L, G12H, G30L and GD had five specimens classified as ARI score 2 and five specimens classified as ARI score 3. Groups GDU and GR had four specimens classified as score 2 and six specimens classified as score 3.

The same operator performed debonding and adhesive removal without water cooling, and with a new bur or rubber used after treating every two teeth. The overall extent of resin removal was determined by visual inspection under the light of an operative lamp. The time required for completion of each resin removal protocol was recorded in seconds with a digital chronometer.

Quantitative and qualitative enamel evaluations were performed. For quantitative evaluation, roughness was measured at two time points: before bonding, to establish initial roughness; and after debonding and removal of adhesive remnants with finishing and polishing protocols, to establish final roughness. A profilometer (Mitutoyo Surftest SJ-400, Japan), with a cut-off value of 0.8 mm, was used to measure the roughness profile of each surface. Two measurements were performed on each specimen, parallel to one another, traversing the entire 4-mm bonding surface. The mean value of the two measurements of each specimen was recorded. This process involved recording two roughness parameters: 1) Mean roughness (Ra), in μm, determined as the arithmetic mean of all absolute distances of the roughness profile from the center line within the measuring length; and 2) Mean roughness depth (Rz) which describes the average maximum peak-to-valley height of five consecutive sampling lengths.[5,12] Variation in roughness was calculated by the equations: ΔRa = final Ra − initial Ra and ΔRz = final Rz − initial Rz.

For qualitative evaluation of enamel surface, scanning electron microscopy (Quanta Feg 250, FEI Company, Oregon, USA) was performed to compare enamel surface of experimental groups.

STATISTICAL ANALYSIS

Results were collected and statistically analyzed by means of SPSS version 20.0 software (Statistical Package for Social Sciences, SPSS Inc., Chicago, IL, USA). Distribution of variables was assessed for normality by Kolmogorov-Smirnov and Shapiro-Wilk tests. Paired t-test was used to assess the mean values of roughness parameters (Ra and Rz) before and after enamel surface clean-up, and verify whether this processes altered enamel surface roughness. Intergroup differences for ΔRa, ΔRz and time required for cleaning the residual resin after bracket debonding were assessed by ANOVA/Tukey

tests. Pearson's correlation test was performed to assess the association between ΔRa and ΔRz and time spent on each enamel clean-up protocol. A level of significance of 0.05 was used for all analyses.

RESULTS

Results showed that all protocols tested for removal of adhesive remnant from enamel did not lead to increase in the original surface roughness significantly.

Ra results for measurements taken before bracket bonding and after residual resin removal are summarized in Table 2. Groups G12H and G12L, in which a 12-blade tungsten carbide bur was used at low and high speed, respectively, showed no significant differences before bonding and after debonding. Groups G30L, GDU, GR and GD showed a smoother surface after 30-blade tungsten carbide bur (low speed), DU10CA ORTHO points, 12-blade tungsten carbide bur (high speed) + Renew™ Finishing System, and Diagloss polisher were used, respectively ($p < 0.05$).

Rz results for measurements taken before bracket bonding and after residual resin removal are summarized in Table 3. Groups G12H and G12L showed no significant differences before bonding and after debonding, and so did Group GDU. Groups G30L, GR and GD showed a reduction in maximum peak-to-valley height ($p < 0.05$).

When ΔRa was compared by means of ANOVA/Tukey tests, there was no statistically significant difference among the six groups (Table 4). All values were negative because the final Ra value was lower than the initial Ra value. When the six groups were compared in terms of ΔRz, some statistical differences were observed (Table 4). Groups G30L and GD presented a decrease in vertical irregularities, while the positive value of ΔRz for G12H implied an increase in vertical irregularities.

The time spent for resin remnant removal is shown in Table 5. The protocols used in Groups G30L and GD were more time-consuming than those used in the other groups ($p < 0.05$). Correlation between time-ΔRa and time-ΔRz was negative and moderate (Table 6). Scatter plots illustrate these results (Figs 1 and 2).

Inspection in scanning electron microscopy shows the enamel surface before bonding (Fig 3) as well as

Table 1 - Distribution of groups according to the protocol applied for removal of adhesive remnant.

Groups	N	Protocols
G12L	10	12-blade tungsten carbide bur (low speed)[a]
G12H	10	12-blade tungsten carbide bur (high speed)[b]
G30L	10	30-blade tungsten carbide bur (low speed)[c]
GDU	10	DU10CA ORTHO Points[d]
GR	10	12-blade tungsten carbide bur (high speed) + Renew™ Finishing System Point[e]
GD	10	Diagloss polisher[f]

[a] Ref. H23R.21.012 (Brasseler®, Savannah, GA, USA), 20,000 rpm;
[b] Ref. H23R.31.012 (Brasseler®, Savannah, GA, USA);
[c] Ref. FF9714 (Jet - Beavers Dental®, Ontario, Canada), 20,000 rpm;
[d] DU10CA ORTHO (DhPro®, Paranaguá, PR, Brazil), 9,000 rpm;
[e] Renew™ Finishing System (Reliance Orthodontics® – Illinois, USA);
[f] Diagloss polisher (Edenta, Switzerland), 10,000 a 12,000 rpm

Table 2 - Mean and standard deviation (SD) for initial and final Ra and results of paired t-test.

Groups	Initial Ra (μm) Mean (SD)	Final Ra (μm) Mean (SD)	p-value
G12L	1.60 (0.50)	1.39 (0,15)	0.289
G12H	1.99 (0.34)	1.79 (0.38)	0.187
G30L	1.96 (0.50)	1.45 (0.43)	0.003 *
GDU	1.65 (0.34)	1.45 (0.24)	0.045 *
GR	1.64 (0.32)	1.31 (0.32)	0.025 *
GD	2.04 (0.43)	1.45 (0.22)	0.001 *

* Indicates statistical significance ($p < 0.05$).

Table 3 - Mean and standard deviation (SD) for initial and final Rz and results of paired t-test.

Groups	Initial Rz (μm) Mean (SD)	Final Rz (μm) Mean (SD)	p-value
G12L	6.03 (3.04)	5.48 (0.59)	0.595
G12H	8.16 (2.16)	8.66 (1.75)	0.634
G30L	7.90 (2.33)	5.16 (1.77)	0.001*
GDU	6.26 (2.31)	5.82 (1.62)	0.404
GR	6.04 (1.50)	4.65 (1.00)	0.023*
GD	8.07 (2.47)	5.35 (1.06)	0.002*

* Indicates statistical significance ($p < 0.05$).

Table 4 - Mean and standard deviation (SD) for ΔRa and ΔRz and results of ANOVA/Tukey.

Groups	ΔRa Mean (SD)	ΔRz Mean (SD)
G12L	- 0.20 (0.58)[a]	- 0.55 (3.15)[AB]
G12H	- 0.19 (0.43)[a]	0.49 (3.17)[B]
G30L	- 0.51 (0.39)[a]	- 2.74 (1.82)[A]
GDU	- 0.20 (0.27)[a]	- 0.44 (1.59)[AB]
GR	- 0.32 (0.38)[a]	- 1.39 (1.60)[AB]
GD	- 0.59 (0.38)[a]	- 2.71 (2.00)[A]

Each column indicates an independent statistical analysis.
Different letters indicate statistically significant difference ($p < 0.05$) for ANOVA/Tukey.

Table 5 - Time required for cleaning residual resin after debracketing (seconds) $p < 0.05$.

	G12L	G12H	G30L	GDU	GR	GD
Mean	34.0	23.5	57.5	31.8	31.9	63.5
(SD)	(5.73)	(5.01)	(19.9)	(4.56)	(5.85)	(13.8)
	A	A	B	A	A	B

SD - Standard deviation.
Different letters indicate statistically significant difference.

Table 6 - Pearson's Linear Correlation Coefficient between the time required and the variations in roughness.

	ΔRa (95% confidence interval)	ΔRz (95% confidence interval)
Time	- 0.445 ** - (-0.685 _ -0.143)	-0.475 ** (- 0.627 _ -0.214)

** $p \leq 0.01$.

after debonding and enamel clean-up (Fig 4). Scratches produced by the 12-blade burs at low speed are presented in Figure 4A. Deeper scratches were produced by the burs at high speed (Fig 4B). The highest degree of surface smoothness was obtained in Group G30L (Fig 4C) This group presented surface more similar to the original tooth, as shown in Figure 3. In Groups GDU and GR, there was loss of perikymata with fine scratches caused by polishers of varying abrasiveness (Fig 4D and Fig 4E). Fine scratches, which appeared to be well-marked and deep, caused by the diamond particles embedded in rubber, were also seen in Group GD (Fig 4F).

DISCUSSION

In this study, six protocols for removal of adhesive remnant from enamel after bracket debonding were assessed. The choice of burs and abrasive points was based on the protocols most used by orthodontists, in other words, tungsten carbide burs in low and high-speed handpieces,[3-6] and products launched on the market in recent years.

Many studies use the parameter Ra as the only indicator of surface smoothness. However, this universally accepted parameter has limitations when

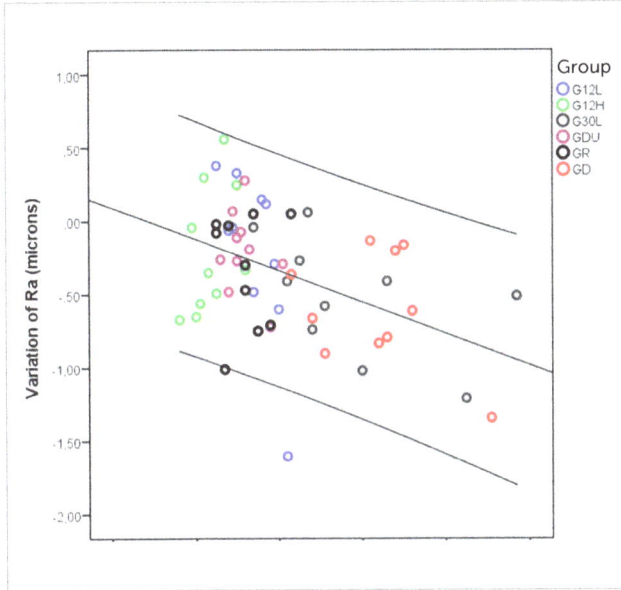

Figure 1 - Scatter plot of variation in roughness (ΔRa) in relation to time in all groups.

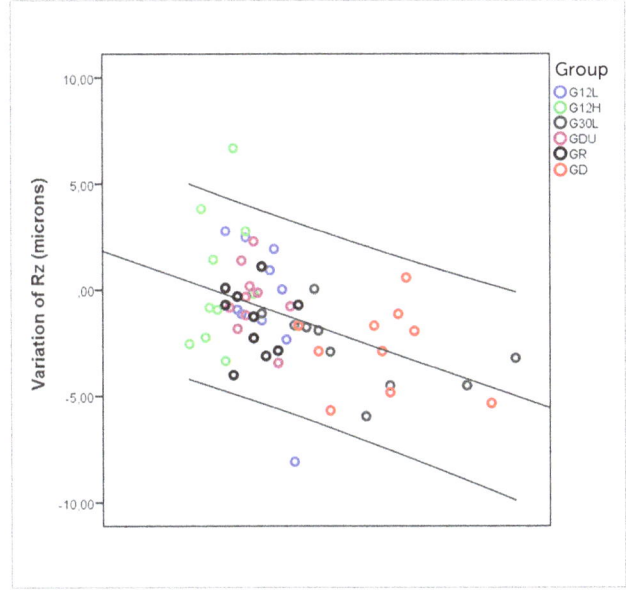

Figure 2 - Scatter plot of variation in roughness (ΔRz) in relation to time in all groups.

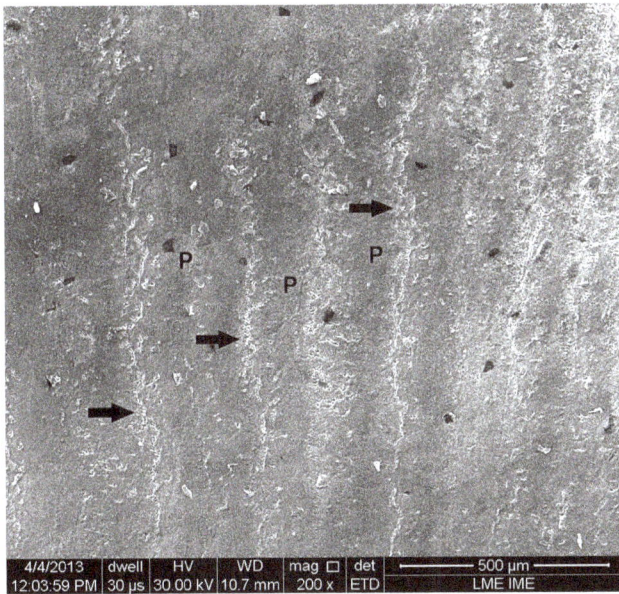

Figure 3 - Scanning electron microscopy (200 X magnification) of original enamel; perikymata (P); prism end openings (arrows).

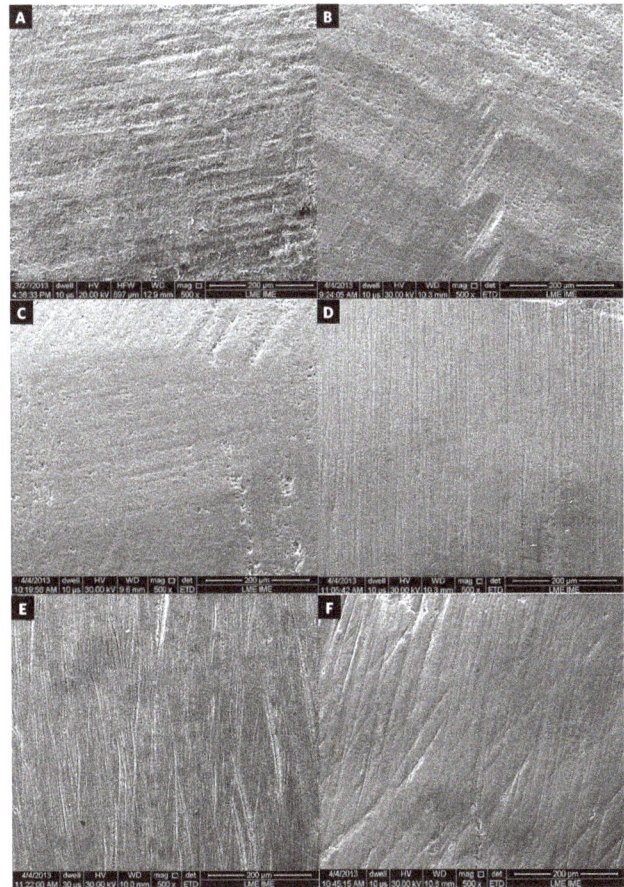

Figure 4 - Scanning electron microscopy (500 X magnification) showing the effect of enamel clean-up procedures on the surface. A) 12-blade tungsten carbide bur (low speed) (G12L); B) 12-blade tungsten carbide bur (high speed) (G12H); C) 30-blade tungsten carbide bur (low speed) (G30L); D) DU10CA ORTHO polisher; E) Renew Finishing System; F) Diagloss polisher.

used alone[5,7] because it does not determine the profile of irregularities and makes no distinction between peaks and valleys. The association of other parameters used in this study, such as Rz, enabled us to study the shape of the vertical profile.

In this study, the protocols involving 12-blade tungsten carbide burs at low and high speed produced similar results considering Ra. The Rz parameter, however, was markedly affected when the 12-blade tungsten carbide bur was used at high speed. A ΔRz value of 0.49 was the only positive value (indicating increase in roughness) and statistically different from Groups G30L and GD. This outcome demonstrated the increase in irregularities with sporadic deep scratches, which were not detected by ΔRa, because Ra is an indicator of mean roughness and does not account for the presence of an occasional peak or valley. In SEM evaluation, the 12-blade bur produced deeper scratches at high speed. However, no statistically significant difference was observed for both roughness parameters (ΔRa and ΔRz) between G12L and G12H.

The literature reports that the use of tungsten carbide burs at high speed to remove resin remnant after debonding leaves the surface similar to that of intact enamel;[2,8,13,14] however, at the cost of a substantial loss in enamel thickness (19.2 μm).[2,15] Other studies recommend the use of tungsten carbide burs at low speed[3,16-18], which create fine scratches[19] with a lower level of enamel loss (7.9 μm to 11.3 μm)[2,10].

In this study, enamel loss was not measured, although this factor should be an important consideration when choosing the method for resin removal. According to Smith et al,[21] the average enamel thickness of a maxillary central incisor is approximately 0.6 mm (600 μm). Considering a single bracket/resin removal, a loss of 10 or 20 μm might seem harmless, but it is necessary to consider the possibility of multiple rebondings due to bracket loss (caused by the patient) or bonding errors (caused by the orthodontist). Therefore, the orthodontist should minimize enamel damage and loss.

The use of high-speed burs without water cooling has been previously described by Bicakci et al.[22] They observed heating in the pulp chamber, leading to vascular hyperemia and occasional breakage of odontoblasts. However, this condition is transient, thereby indicating that the damage caused by this protocol is reversible, and pulp repair occurs within about 20 days. The authors recommend removing most of the resin under water cooling and turning the water cooling off when removing the last layer of resin, so that it is possible to successfully distinguish between enamel and resin, thereby preventing further damage to enamel. Considering the results of the present study, low-speed burs without water cooling could be used to remove the last layer of resin, so the risk of enamel scratches might be reduced. In this study, all resin remnant was removed without water cooling. It is suggested that future studies assess enamel roughness and loss when following the aforementioned recommendations.

Group GR, which involved the use of 12-blade tungsten carbide burs at high speed followed by Renew polisher, showed a significant ($p < 0.05$) decrease in the two roughness parameters between the two time points, indicating the importance of gently eliminating the last layer of resin with polishers after using burs at high speed.[1,6,8] The literature shows that the sequential use of multiple tools for polishing is more efficient than one-step procedures[2,3,17,20,23,24] in terms of reduction in surface roughness. In this study, GR resulted in a low level of surface roughness, with negative values for ΔRa and ΔRz. However, the final variation in ΔRz roughness of GR was not statistically different from the majority of the other groups, except for G12L (Table 4).

Roughness values obtained after clean-up in Groups G30L, GDU, GR and GD were lower than the initial roughness values. Similar results were found in other studies,[7,18,20] in which abrasive points and 30-blade tungsten carbide burs were used to eliminate adhesive remnant. In a previous study, microscopic evaluation showed that the use of abrasive points (Optimize Discs – TDV – and Onegloss Discs – Shofu) maintained the enamel surface of the study groups in a similar condition to the enamel surface of the control groups.[25]

The time required for removing resin differed among the six groups, mainly due to differences in the cutting power of tools used,[7] which was mainly determined by the speed of rotation,[17] type of bur, number of blades, composition, particle size, and pressure applied to the handpiece.[2] The latter variable was minimized because the same operator performed all resin removal procedures. The time required in the groups in which Diagloss polishers (63.5 seconds) and 30-blade tungsten carbide burs at low speed (57.5 seconds) were used, was significantly longer than that required in the other groups ($p < 0.05$). The protocol used in GD involved two steps: use of rubber with a high gradient of diamond particle concentration, which ensured resin reduction, followed by another point for polishing. Hence, the procedure consumed more chair time. In Group G30L, the higher number of blades of the bur used at low speed decreased its cutting power and removed the resin layer by layer, which results in a smoother and scratch-free surface; however, it increased the time required for resin removal.

The fastest protocol was the use of the 12-blade tungsten carbide bur at high speed (23.5 seconds), followed by DU10CA ORTHO polisher (31.8 seconds), and the Renew system (31.9 seconds), which also made use of 12-blade tungsten carbide burs at high speed, however, in a two-step procedure. Ryf et al[20] assessed the Renew system, and showed it required a considerably longer time to remove and polish the enamel (83.6 seconds); however, the burs were used were at low speed. The potential reasons for this difference were the use of lower-speed handpieces (under 20,000 rpm) and the use of the same bur every 10 specimens; thus, the bur became worn and had its cutting power diminished.

Our findings corroborate those of other studies,[3,14,19,20,25,26] indicating that all rotary instruments cause varying changes in enamel surface. The association between the time spent and change in roughness (ΔRa, ΔRz) showed a negative and moderate correlation: the longer the time spent on removing the remaining resin, the lower was the roughness left on the enamel surface, which is in agreement with a previous study.[1] Instruments with low cutting power perform slower resin removal,

leaving a smoother surface less prone to plaque adhesion and pigmentation.

–

After orthodontic treatment, it is impossible to re store the surface of teeth to their original condition. Prophylaxis with pumice, acid etching, debonding and aggressive resin removal procedures cause enamel loss.[15] Rotating instruments create some degree of enamel irregularities, and when rebonding is frequently necessary, the surface is modified and the perikymata pattern of young teeth is probably damaged.[3] Therefore, fine scratches, such as those made when using the protocols tested in this study, appear to cause minimum damage and must be placed in an expected clinical perspective. It is up to the orthodontist to apply methods to minimize damage to tooth enamel.[25] Thorough resin removal and polishing after debonding is entirely dependent on the operator[27] who is responsible for selecting the instruments, using points with particles with a lower degree of hardness than enamel to minimize iatrogenic abrasions and scratches;[2] for the pressure applied to the handpiece and for eliminating resin from the tooth surface.

CONCLUSIONS

1) All finishing and polishing protocols were considered satisfactory for residual resin removal without increasing enamel roughness.

2) The time spent on enamel clean-up varied from 23.5 (12-blade tungsten carbide bur at high speed) to 63.5 seconds (Diagloss polishers).

3) The longer the time spent on removing the remaining resin, the smaller the variation in roughness level.

Author contributions

EFS: Supervised the project, guiding the experiments and text reviewing. LCFS: Performed the experiments and wrote the master's thesis of which this article was originated. MM: Performed the statistical analysis and wrote the article. CNE: Guided shearing's testing and supplied the equipment and location for the experiments. ACOR: Guided microscopy analysis.

REFERENCES

1. Ulusoy C. Comparison of finishing and polishing systems for residual resin removal after debonding. J Appl Oral Sci. 2009;17(3):209-15.

2. Zarrinnia K, Eid NM, Kehoe MJ. The effect of different debonding techniques on the enamel surface: an in vitro qualitative study. Am J Orthod Dentofacial Orthop. 1995;108(3):284-93.

3. Zachrisson BU, Arthun J. Enamel surface appearance after various debonding techniques. Am J Orthod. 1979;75(2):121-7.

4. Hong YH, Lew KK. Quantitative and qualitative assessment of enamel surface following five composite removal methods after bracket debonding. Eur J Orthod. 1995;17(2):121-8.

5. Eliades T, Gioka C, Eliades G, Makou M. Enamel surface roughness following debonding using two resin grinding methods. Eur J Orthod. 2004;26(3):333-8.

6. Brauchli LM, Baumgartner EM, Ball J, Wichelhaus A. Roughness of enamel surfaces after different bonding and debonding procedures: an in vitro study. J Orofac Orthop. 2011;72(1):61-7.

7. Karan S, Kircelli BH, Tasdelen B. Enamel surface roughness after debonding. Angle Orthod. 2010;80(6):1081-8.

8. Albuquerque GS, Filho MV, Lucato AS, Boeck EM, Degan V, Kuramae M. Evaluation of enamel roughness after ceramic bracket debonding and clean-up with different methods. Braz J Oral Sci. 2010;9(2):81-4.

9. Bennett CG, Shen C, Waldron JM. The effects of debonding on the enamel surface. Am J Orthod Dentofacial Orthop. 1995;108(3):284-93.

10. Montasser MA, Drummond JL. Reliability of the adhesive remnant index score system with different magnifications. Angle Orthod. 2009;79(4):773-6.

11. Artun J, Bergland S. Clinical trials with crystal growth conditioning as an alternative to acid-etch enamel pretreatment. Am J Orthod. 1984;85(4):333-40.

12. 4287 ANI. Geometrical Product Specifications (GPS) - Surface texture: Profile method -Terms, definitions and surface texture parameters; 2002.

13. Rouleau BD Jr, Marshall GW Jr, Cooley RO. Enamel surface evaluations after clinical treatment and removal of orthodontic brackets. Am J Orthod. 1982;81(5):423-6.

14. Pignatta LMB, Duarte Júnior S, Santos ECA. Evaluation of enamel surface after bracket debonding and polishing. Dental Press J Orthod. 2012;17(4):77-84.

15. Hosein I, Sherriff M, Ireland AJ. Enamel loss during bonding, debonding, and cleanup with use of a self-etching primer. Am J Orthod Dentofacial Orthop. 2004;126(6):717-24.

16. Eliades T, Kakaboura A, Eliades G, Bradley TG. Comparison of enamel colour changes associated with orthodontic bonding using two different adhesives. Eur J Orthod. 2001;23(1):85-90.

17. Radlanski RJ. A new carbide finishing bur for bracket debonding. J Orofac Orthop. 2001;62(4):296-304.

18. Giampaolo ET, Machado AL, Pavarina AC, Vergani CE. Different methods of finishing and polishing enamel. J Prosthet Dent. 2003;89(2):135-40.

19. Macieski K, Rocha R, Locks A, Ribeiro GU. Effects evaluation of remaining resin removal (three modes) on enamel surface after bracket debonding. Dental Press J Orthod. 2011;16(5):146-54.

20. Ryf S, Flury S, Palaniappan S, Lussi A, van Meerbeek B, Zimmerli B. Enamel loss and adhesive remnants following bracket removal and various clean-up procedures in vitro. Eur J Orthod. 2012;34(1):25-32.

21. Smith TM, Olejniczak AJ, Zermeno JP, Tafforeau P, Skinner MM, Hoffmann A, et al. Variation in enamel thickness within the genus Homo. J Hum Evol. 2012;62(3):395-411.

22. Bicakci AA, Kocoglu-Altan B, Celik-Ozenci C, Tekcan M, Babacan H, Gungor E. Histopathologic evaluation of pulpal tissue response to various adhesive cleanup techniques. Am J Orthod Dentofacial Orthop. 2010;138(1):12.e1-e7; discussion 12-3.

23. Campbell PM. Enamel surfaces after orthodontic bracket debonding. Angle Orthod. 1995;65(2):103-10.

24. Joo HJ, Lee YK, Lee DY, Kim YJ, Lim YK. Influence of orthodontic adhesives and clean-up procedures on the stain susceptibility of enamel after debonding. Angle Orthod. 2011;81(2):334-40.

25. De Marchi R, De Marchi LM, Terada RSS, Terada HH. Comparison between two methods for resin removing after bracket debonding. Dental Press J Orthod. 2012;17(6):130-6.

26. Retief DH, Denys FR. Finishing of enamel surfaces after debonding of orthodontic attachments. Angle Orthod. 1979;49(1):1-10.

27. Pont HB, Ozcan M, Bagis B, Ren Y. Loss of surface enamel after bracket debonding: an in-vivo and ex-vivo evaluation. Am J Orthod Dentofacial Orthop. 2010;138(4):387.e1-e9; discussion 387-9.

11

In vitro evaluation of force degradation of elastomeric chains used in Orthodontics

André Weissheimer[1], Arno Locks[2], Luciane Macedo de Menezes[3],
Adriano Ferreti Borgatto[4], Carla D'Agostini Derech[5]

Objective: To analyze the *in vitro* force degradation of four different brands of elastomeric chains: American Orthodontics, Morelli, Ormco and TP Orthodontics. **Methods:** The sample consisted of 80 gray elastomeric chains that were divided into four groups according to their respective manufacturers. Chain stretching was standardized at 21 mm with initial force release ranging from 300 g to 370 g. The samples were kept in artificial saliva at a constant temperature of 37°C and the degradation force was recorded at the following time intervals: initial, 1, 3, 5, 7 and 9 hours, and 1, 7, 14, 21, 28, and 35 days. **Results:** There was a statistically significant difference between the groups regarding the force degradation, mainly within the first day, as a force loss of 50-55% was observed during that time in relation to the initial force. The force delivered at 35 days ranged from 122 g to 148 g. **Conclusion:** All groups showed force degradation over time, regardless of their trademarks, a force loss of 59-69% was observed in the first hour compared to baseline. However, because the variation in force degradation depends on the trademark, studies such as the present one are important for guiding the clinical use of these materials.

Keywords: Elastomers. Shear bond strength. Biomedical and dental materials.

[1] PhD Student in Orthodontics, PUC-RS.
[2] Professor of Orthodontics, UFSC.
[3] Professor of Orthodontics, PUC-RS.
[4] Professor of Statistics, UFSC.
[5] Professor of the Specialization Course in Orthodontics, UFSC.

» The authors report no commercial, proprietary or financial interest in the products or companies described in this article.

Carla D'Agostini Derech
Av. Rio Branco, 333/306 – Centro – CEP: 88.015-201 – Florianópolis/SC – Brazil
E-mail: carladerech@hotmail.com

INTRODUCTION

Elastomers are materials that have the ability to quickly return to their original size after substantial deformation, acting similarly to the coil spring. They are structurally classified as polymers, i.e., materials which are characterized by the formation of a repeating chain with simpler chemical structure. Since they are thermoplastic, it is possible to create devices with different shapes.[5]

They are widely used in promoting dental movement, correction of rotations, midline discrepancies, space closure, canine distalization and dental arch constriction.[1,4,6] The main advantages are: They are easy to handle, patient cooperation is not required, and they are comfortable, hygienic and economic.[4,7]

However, the forces released by these materials are unstable and alter due to time, the addition of dyes, chain configuration (open or closed), pre-stretch, speed and amount of stretch, the oral environment, saliva, enzymes, changes in Ph, exposure to light, air, water, ozone, oxidants, food, chemical hygiene and the physical action of chewing and tooth brushing.[8,11,13,15,16,18-22,25]

In Orthodontics, synthetic elastomers are polymers based on polyurethane, with superior physicochemical properties than those derived from natural rubber. The derivatives of polyurethane elastomers, after chemical reaction which causes polymerization, present as a shapeless mass, with polymeric chains presenting relatively weak forces of attraction between them. The vulcanization process is then used to improve the mechanical properties of the material through the lateral union between chains by covalent cross-linking. Thus, three-dimensional structures are formed, converting the flexible product into a resistant material, elastic, with lower solubility to organic solvents and greater resistance to deterioration by heat, light and natural aging. Another phenomenon responsible for improving the final properties of these materials is assigned to tie points distributed along the polymer formed by linear chains, called cross virtual chains.[17] These chains are non-covalent chemical bonds formed within the same molecule or between different molecules. Chemically are referred to as hydrogen bonding and van der Waals forces.[10] What makes this information important is the fact that the power assigned to the material, which is from virtual cross-links, is not obtained by the addition of loads as in conventional rubber, but chemically determined by the internal composition of materials. This internal composition is determined by the technology, the refinement of the technique and the quality of raw materials used in the manufacture of this material.[17] Therefore, the final quality of the elastomer critically depends on the manufacturing process, which makes the conduction of periodic surveys essential to verify the quality and the physical properties behavior of the elastomeric chains available on the market.

Therefore, the objective of this study was to evaluate *in vitro* the magnitude of the force degradation of different elastomeric chains of four trademarks.

MATERIAL AND METHODS

Eighty gray elastomeric chain segments were evaluated in the closed configuration, divided into four groups of different brands, each with 20 segments:

» Am Group (Memory chain; ref.: 854-252, American Orthodontics, Sheboygan, WI, USA);

» Mo Group (Short gray Rubber chain, ref.: 60.05.501 - Morelli, Sorocaba, SP, Brazil);

» Or Group (Power chain generation II, ref.: 639-0001, Ormco Corporation, Glendora, CA, USA) and

» TP Group (E-chain, ref.: 383-050, TP Orthodontics Inc, La Porte, IN, USA).

It was standardized that the elastomeric chain segments were drawn to a distance of 21 mm, producing average initial force of 318.85 g/f. Thus, the required number of links in each elastomeric chains to produce such strength, varied according to the manufacturer (Table 1). However, the stretching of elastomeric segments in the chain did not exceed 50% of its original length because they can generate excessive forces.[15]

The elastomers tested were kept in their original packaging until the moment of testing. To avoid possible damage to the structure of the elastomeric chain during the cutting procedure, the same was done in the half of the next link that was not part of the elastomeric chain to be analyzed. Eighty maintainer devices were made to keep the elastomeric chain segments stretched at a distance of 21 mm throughout the experiment. The devices were attached to acrylic plates and placed in plastic containers with artificial saliva at a constant temperature of 37° C (98.6° F) (Fig 1).

To assess the behavior of the elastomeric chains, a universal mechanical testing machine (Instron Corporate - Norwood, MA, USA) was configured to stretch the elastomeric chains with a constant speed of 50 mm / min to the distance of 21 mm. Each segment of the elastomer was pulled to the ends of the machine and stretched to 21 mm. After 15 seconds, the time needed for stabilization of the material, the initial force value was recorded.

Next, the samples were carefully transferred to the maintainer device, which returned to the acrylic plate and immersed in artificial saliva at 37 °C (98.6 °F).

For subsequent measurements, the universal testing machine was programmed to maintain fixed at 21 mm the distance between their edges (Fig 2). Next, the elastomers were placed on the device, and the force values were recorded after 5 seconds.[7] Again the elastomeric chains were transferred to the maintainer, and stored under the conditions described above, until the next measurement. Besides the initial measurement, the samples were evaluated at intervals of 1, 3, 5, 7, 9 and 24 hours, and 7, 14, 21, 28 and 35 days.

The 15 seconds waiting to record the initial force was adopted as a result of fluctuations in the value of the force after the initial stretching of the elastomeric chains. After that time, the force value remained stable allowing its registration. During the revaluation of elastomeric chains, the time required to stop the force stabilization was 5 seconds.

To assess the different behaviors of the elastomeric chain according to the time, we used the Analysis of Variance (ANOVA), according to a completely randomized design with factorial arrangement and further tested the normal distribution of data. The F test was

Table 1 - Characterization of sample groups, with the number of links before stretching, original length without stretching (in millimeters), amount of stretching (in millimeters and in percentage), till the extent of 21 mm.

Group	Number of links	Initial (mm)	Stretching (mm/%)
Am	5	14.5	6.5/44.8
Mo	7	17.5	3.5/20.0
Or	5	14.5	6.5/44.8
TP	6	15.5	5.5/35.4

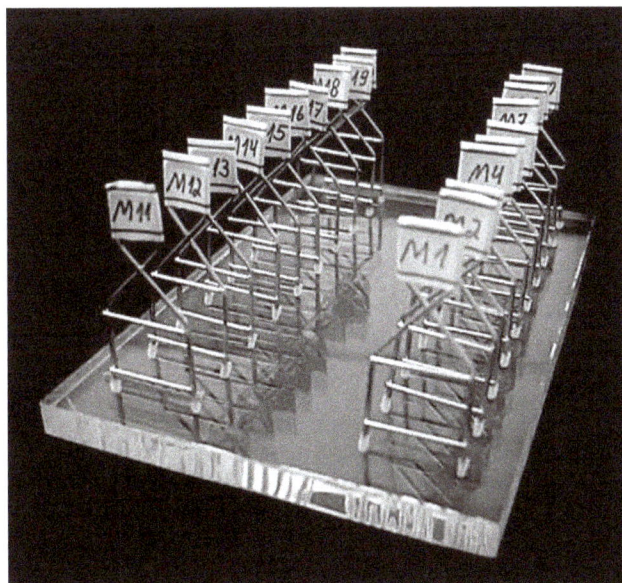

Figure 1 - Maintainer devices, attached to an acrylic plate, with tips fixed at a distance of 21 mm.

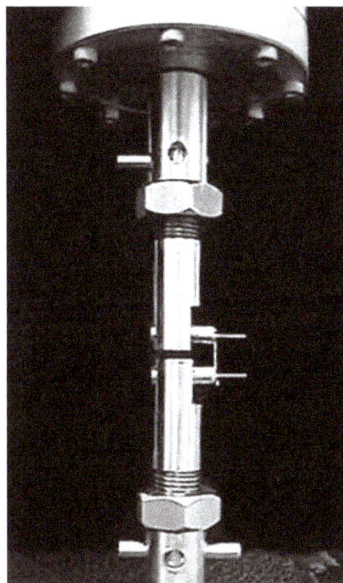

Figure 2 - Detail of the device attached to the universal testing machine with a fixed distance of 21 mm between the metallic rods.

used to determine differences between groups in the time interval. To compare the averages two by two in the analyzed time, the Tukey test was used, complemented by the Scott-Knott test, to avoid ambiguity due to the large amount of time in the analysis. For both tests, $p \leq 0.05$ was considered statistically significant.

RESULTS

The average values of the forces released by elastomeric chain group Am, Mo, Or and TP during the 35 days of the experiment are shown in Table 2. In general, the greater degradation of force occurred during the first day. From that on, the level of force continued to decrease, but slowly and gradually until the end of the third week. From the 21st to 35th days, there were no statistically significant changes ($p \leq 0.05$) in the force release.

At the end of the experiment, elastomers from the TP Group had the highest average force (148.5 g) it was statistically significant ($p \leq 0.05$) when compared to groups Am, Mo and Or. However, it's noted that the average initial force of the TP Group was also higher than the other groups.

It was noticed that on the first day of evaluation, there was no difference between groups, but this feature did not stand, for example, within one assessment week the average force is equal between the groups Am, Mo, Or and differ from the TP group, which is maintained up to 28 days of evaluation.

Given the initial force discrepancy of TP Group and to facilitate the understanding, the force degradation was also examined as a percentage of the initial strength in each time interval, irrespective of the initial value of the force in grams (Table 3). Considering that in the beginning, the absolute force values amounted to 100%. The data showed that after 1 h, the percentage of strength remaining ranged between 59% to 69%, ending up at the end of the first day with values in the order 45% to 50%. The remaining force found in day 21st was 40-45% depending on the group. At the end of the experiment, groups TP and Or had the highest percentage of force remaining, with no differences between them, while the lowest percentage of initial force were found in groups Mo and Am. There was no statistically significant difference between the groups Mo and Am.

DISCUSSION

The specification of the polyurethane used as raw material in the processing of elastomeric chains is not provided by the manufacturer, therefore the physical properties of these materials is only available through published studies.[2,4,6,7,11,14,16,20,21,22]

The frequency and diversity in the methodology of these studies provides the clinician an important parameter of quality, perhaps the only one, supplying data to make the best choice in purchasing the product, among the many trademarks, and once that is in clinical use, to know the physical behavior of the material you are using.

Table 2 - Mean (g) and standard deviation of the forces in each time period of four groups tested.

	Am	Mo	Or	TP
	mean ± SD	mean ± SD	mean ± SD	mean ± SD
Initial	307.2 ± 5.6 a,E	298.7 ± 4,5 a,G	296.2 ± 4.2 a,F	373.3 ± 42.0 b,G
1 hour	185.5 ± 9.6 a,D	204.7 ± 9.0 b,F	182.7 ± 7.3 a,E	220.4 ± 31.7 c,F
3 hours	165.7 ± 8.5 a,C	188.6 ± 5.4 b,E	170.0 ± 6.2 a,D	202.0 ± 30.7 c,E
5 hours	161.0 ± 6.7 a,C	176.0 ± 7.5 b,D	169.5 ± 6.9 ab,D	188.9 ± 29.5 c,D
7 hours	158.0 ± 6.2 a,C	169.3 ± 6.7 ab,D	157.3 ± 6.1 a,C	175.0 ± 28.6 b,C
9 hours	148.1 ± 6.4 ab,B	154.5 ± 6.9 b,C	140.2 ± 5.5 a,B	157.8 ± 28.3 b,A
1 day	142.1 ± 5.1 a,B	143.5 ± 5.8 a,B	143.1 ± 4.4 a,B	152.0 ± 27.8 a,A
7 days	146.4 ± 4.9 ab,B	144.8 ± 6.1 a,B	158.0 ± 5.1 bc,C	170.4 ± 25.6 c,C
14 days	139.6 ± 3.5 ab,B	136.7 ± 5.0 a,B	149.9 ± 6.0 b,B	162.8 ± 26.1 c,B
21 days	127.2 ± 4.7 ab,A	118.3 ± 3.9 a,A	135.0 ± 4.3 b,A	150.9 ± 25.1 c,A
28 days	123.6 ± 4.2 ab,A	118.4 ± 5.1 a,A	135.2 ± 5.7 b,A	148.3 ± 24.5 c,A
35 days	127.0 ± 9.2 a,A	122.0 ± 6.2 a,A	132.3 ± 4.9 a,A	148.5 ± 22.7 b,A

In the rows, means followed by same lowercase letters do not differ significantly ($p > 0.05$) by Tukey test. In columns, means followed by same capital letters do not differ significantly ($p > 0.05$) by Scott-Knott test.

The optimal force required for space closure in orthodontics is controversial. Ren et al[19] published a meta-analysis study of optimal force for tooth movement and concluded that there is no scientific evidence as to recommend the optimal force level in orthodontic practice. The few studies in humans suggest that the magnitude of force required for the body movement of the canines ranging from 100 to 350 g for mechanics with friction and approximately 60 g mechanical friction-free.[19] In the present work an initial force of approximately 300 g was selected because according to the literature,[1,4,14,21,23] during the first 24 hours the highest rate of force decay would occur (ranging from 45% to 75%), and thus the remaining force level would be consistent with the movement of the canines.

Commonly, orthodontic consultations occur every 3 or 4 weeks, when the replacement of the elastomeric chain happens. Thus, most studies[2,12,21] evaluated the behavior of these materials for a period of 28 days. However, the return of the patient, in certain cases may be in a larger interval. Therefore, this study evaluated the behavior of elastic chains for five weeks, to complement the data already existing in the literature.

The null hypothesis that the elastomeric ligatures remain dimensionally stable and do not lose strength during the stretch was rejected based on the results of this experiment.

The behavior of the elastomers in groups Am, Mo, Or, and TP during the first 9 hours and 5 weeks of this experiment can be seen in Figures 3 and 4. All the samples showed a similar degradation curve, varying only in intensity according to the tested group.

The results demonstrated that the highest level of force degradation occurred during the first day of the experiment, especially in the first hour in all groups (Table 3, Figs 3 and 4), which is in agreement with other studies.[1,3,9,12,14,23,24]

In general, the initial loss of strength during the first hour ranged from 31 to 41%. In the first 24 hours the loss of strength was between 50 and 55% (Table 3, Fig 4). The literature reports similar results with a decrease of strength ranging from 50% to 75% during the first day.[1,4,14,21,23] From the first 24 hours on, the level of force continued to decrease, but slowly and gradually until the third week, where it remained almost constant. Because of this, it seems prudent to pre-stretch the elastomeric chains prior to clinical application.

The fact that the TP group has shown the highest average ultimate force (148 g) probably happened because the group had the greatest force at the beginning when compared to other groups. In addition, TP group showed the highest average of the initial forces, differing from the other groups ($p \leq 0.05$), and a great variability in the values of these forces at the beginning, which was evidenced by the large standard deviation (42 g) groups when compared to the groups Am (5.6 g), Mo (4.5 g) and Or (4.2 g).

Table 3 - Mean and standard deviation of the percentage of the initial period of time in each of the four groups tested.

	Am mean ± SD	Mo mean ± SD	Or mean ± SD	TP mean ± SD
Initial	100 %	100%	100%	100%
1 hour	59 ± 3 [a]	69 ± 3 [c]	63 ± 3 [b]	66 ± 9 [b]
3 hours	53 ± 3 [a]	63 ± 2 [c]	59 ± 2 [b]	60 ± 9 [b]
5 hours	51 ± 2 [a]	59 ± 3 [b]	59 ± 2 [b]	56 ± 9 [b]
7 hours	50 ± 2 [a]	57 ± 2 [b]	55 ± 2 [b]	52 ± 9 [a]
9 hours	47 ± 2 [a]	52 ± 2 [b]	49 ± 2 [a]	47 ± 8 [a]
1 day	45 ± 2 [a]	48 ± 2 [b]	50 ± 2 [b]	45 ± 8 [a]
7 days	47 ± 2 [a]	49 ± 2 [a]	55 ± 2 [c]	51 ± 8 [b]
14 days	44 ± 1 [a]	46 ± 2 [a]	52 ± 2 [c]	48 ± 8 [b]
21 days	40 ± 2 [a]	40 ± 1 [a]	47 ± 1 [b]	45 ± 7 [b]
28 days	39 ± 1 [a]	40 ± 2 [a]	47 ± 2 [b]	44 ± 7 [b]
35 days	40 ± 3 [a]	41 ± 2 [a]	46 ± 2 [b]	44 ± 7 [b]

In the rows, mean followed by the same letters do not differ significantly (p > 0.05) by Scott-Knott test.

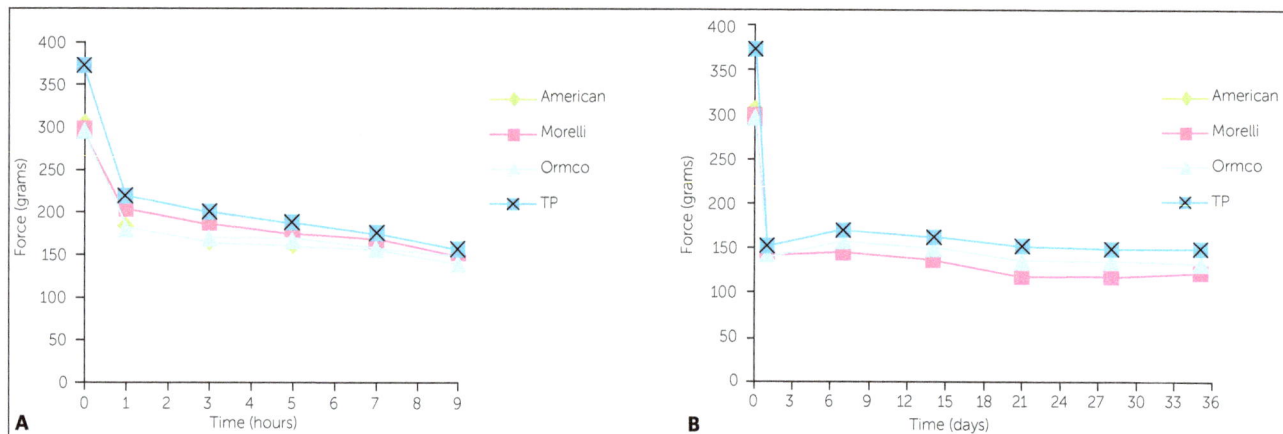

Figure 3 - **A)** Force degradation in the first 9 hours. **B)** Force degradation during 35 days of the experiment.

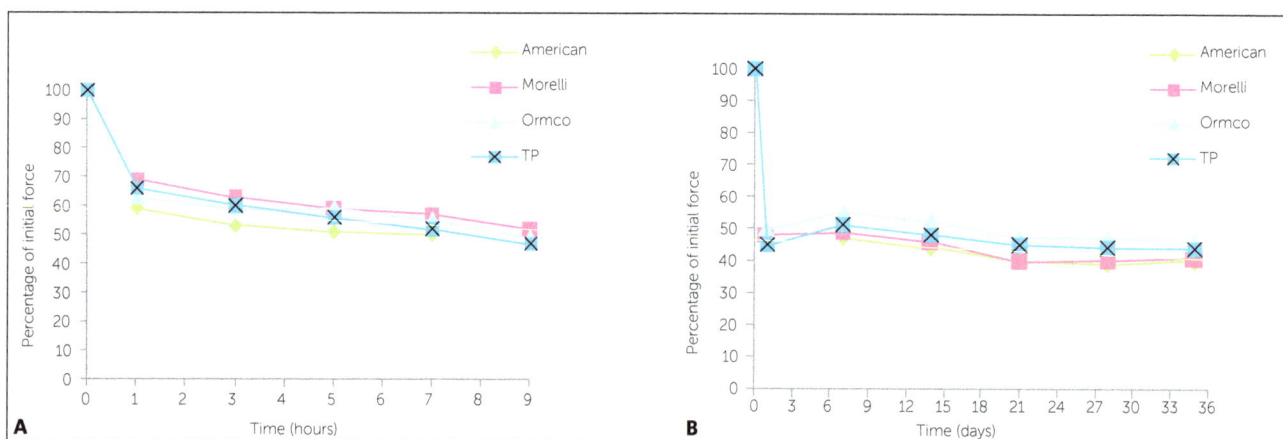

Figure 4 - **A)** Percentage of initial force during the first 9 hours. **B)** Percentage of the initial force during 35 days of the experiment.

It is important to mention that even using elastomeric chains with similar characteristics, i.e. number of links, cut by the same operator, stretched the same distance for the same period of time, elastomers from TP Group showed great variability in initial force values (300 g to 434 g). Similar findings were found in another study, where we observed standard deviation of 39.5 g of the initial forces in elastomers from TP Orthodontics.[12]

Groups Or and TP showed the same amount of force decay in percentage terms, from the beginning to the end of the experiment. Thus, although the Group TP had larger initial and final strength, when compared to Oregon, there was no statistical difference in the amount of force decay in proportion to their initial strength (Table 3).

De Genova et al[6] found on the 21st day of the study, percentages of remaining force of Ormco elastomers (39%) and TP Orthodontics (49%) who keep similar to those found in the present work, where the values for the group Or were 47% and Group TP of 45%. However, Jossel et al[12] found a higher percentage of force remaining on the 28th day (TP 78%, 68% Ormco; American 58%) than those found in this study, possibly because of the methodology used by the authors, the elastomers were maintained in room temperature and not at 37° C, which may have contributed to the decreased strength deterioration.

The results showed that by the end of the experiment, groups TP and Or had the highest percentage of initial force while Mo and Am groups had the lowest. No statistical difference in the percentage of initial force was demonstrated, between the groups Mo and Am at the end of the evaluation. However, it should be considered that the samples of the Mo Group stretched only 20% of its original length while the Am Group was drawn at 44.8% (Table 1). According to the literature,[25] the greater the stretching, the greater the deterioration of the strength. The smallest stretch, and consequently lower plastic deformation of Mo Group sample compared to the Am Group sample, may have contributed to the similar performance between these groups. Therefore, Morelli's elastomeric chains that stretch above 20% may have further deterioration of strength.

In the study by Araujo and Ursi,[2] initial forces were used ranging from 178 to 249 g whereas in the present work initial forces from 296 to 374 g were used. The use of lower initial forces may have contributed to the authors finding less degradation of strength. However, elastomers creating lower initial forces, although under less degradation, tend to produce lower final strengths. After four weeks the absolute values of force obtained by Araújo and Ursi[2] (Morelli 72 g, Ormco 68 g, TP 114g) were lower than those found in this study (Morelli 118g, Ormco 135g, TP 148g). Considering that both studies were performed *in vitro*, where there is less degradation of force in the oral cavity,[3] it is questioned whether lower forces would be clinically compatible with canine tooth movement.

Measuring the clinically used force of an elastomer with a precision instrument is strongly advisable when using any commercial brand. In the case of TP Orthodontics elastomers, the high standard deviation does not disqualify it for clinical use, because the degradation of force standard is similar when compared to the other ones tested, but the difference of the initial strength with the same number of links is mandatory for measurement in all its clinical application.

Therefore, since the raw material used and the manufacturing process of the elastomer is not available, it is important to know the theoretical material published in the literature and to measure routinely the applied force.

CONCLUSION

Based on the results of this study, it can be concluded that: There was a force degradation over time in all groups, being greatest on the first day of the experiment, especially in the first hour; From the third to the fifth week there was no noticeable force degradation in either group; By the end of the experiment, the brands Ormco and TP Orthodontics showed the highest percentage of remaining force.

REFERENCES

1. Andreasen GF, Bishara S. Comparison of alastik chains to elastics involved with intra-arch molar-to-molar forces. Am J Orthod. 1971;60(2):200-1.
2. Araujo FB, Ursi WJ. Estudo da degradação de força gerada por elásticos ortodônticos sintéticos. Rev Dental Press Ortod Ortop Facial. 2006;11(6):52-61.
3. Ash JL, Nikolai RJ. Relaxation of orthodontic elastomeric chains and modules in vitro and in vivo. J Dent Res. 1978;57(5-6):685-90.
4. Baty DL, Storie DJ, von Fraunhofer JA. Synthetic elastomeric chains: a literature review. Am J Orthod Dentofacial Orthop. 1994;105(6):536-42.
5. Billmeyer FW. Textbook of polymer science. 3rd ed. New York: John Wiley & Sons; 1984.
6. De Genova DC, McInnes-Ledoux P, Weinberg R, Shaye R. Force degradation of orthodontic elastomeric chains: a product comparison study. Am J Orthod. 1985;87(5):377-84.
7. Eliades T, Eliades G, Silikas N, Watts DC. In vitro degradation of polyurethane orthodontic elastomeric modules. J Oral Rehabil. 2005;32(1):72-7.
8. Ferriter JP, Meyers CE Jr, Lorton L. The effect of hydrogen ion concentration on the force-degradation rate of orthodontic polyurethane chain elastics. Am J Orthod Dentofacial Orthop. 1990;98(5):404-10.
9. Hershey HG, Reynolds WG. The plastic module as an orthodontic tooth-moving mechanism. Am J Orthod. 1975;67(5):554-62.
10. Huget EF, Patrick KS, Nunez LJ. Observations on the elastic behavior of a synthetic orthodontic elastomer. J Dent Res. 1990;69(2):496-501.
11. Jeffries CL, von Fraunhofer JA. The effects of 2% alkaline glutaraldehyde solution on the elastic properties of elastomeric chain. Angle Orthod. 1991;61(1):25-30.
12. Josell SD, Leiss JB, Rekow ED. Force degradation in elastomeric chains. Semin Orthod. 1997;3(3):189-97.
13. Kovatch JS, Lautenschlager EP, Apfel DA, Keller JC. Load extension time behavior of orthodontic alastiks. J Dent Res. 1976;55(5):783-6.
14. Lu TC, Wang WN, Tarng TH, Chen JW. Force decay of elastomeric chain - a serial study. Part II. Am J Orthod Dentofacial Orthop. 1993;104(4):373-7.
15. Matta ENR, Chevitarese O. Avaliação laboratorial da força liberada por elásticos plásticos. Rev SBO. 1997;3(4):131-6.
16. Matta ENR, Chevitarese O. Deformação plástica de elásticos ortodônticos em cadeia: estudo in vitro. Rev SOB. 1998;3(5):188-92.
17. Morton M. Rubber technology. 3rd ed. Londres: Chapman & Hall; 1995.
18. Nattrass C, Ireland AJ, Sherriff M. The effect of environmental factors on elastomeric chain and nickel titanium coil springs. Eur J Orthod. 1998;20(2):169-76.
19. Ren Y, Maltha JC, Kuijpers-Jagtman AM. Optimum force magnitude for orthodontic tooth movement: a systematic literature review. Angle Orthod. 2003;73(1):86-92.
20. Stevenson JS, Kusy RP. Force application and decay characteristics of untreated and treated polyurethane elastomeric chains. Angle Orthod. 1994;64(6):455-64.
21. Taloumis LJ, Smith TM, Hondrum SO, Lorton L. Force decay and deformation of orthodontic elastomeric ligatures. Am J Orthod Dentofacial Orthop. 1997;111(1):1-11.

22. Teixeira L, Pereira B do R, Bortoly TG, Brancher JA, Tanaka OM, Guariza-Filho O. The environmental influence of Light Coke, phosphoric acid, and citric acid on elastomeric chains. J Contemp Dent Pract. 2008;9(7):17-24.

23. von Fraunhofer JA, Coffelt MT, Orbell GM. The effects of artificial saliva and topical fluoride treatments on the degradation of the elastic properties of orthodontic chains. Angle Orthod. 1992;62(4):265-74.

24. Wong AK. Orthodontic elastic materials. Angle Orthod. 1976;46(2):196-205.

25. Young J, Sandrik JL. The influence of preloading on stress relaxation of orthodontic elastic polymers. Angle Orthod. 1974;49(2):104-9.

12

Comparison of space analysis performed on plaster vs. digital dental casts applying Tanaka and Johnston's equation

Júlia Olien Sanches[1], Lourdes Aparecida Martins dos Santos-Pinto[2],
Ary dos Santos-Pinto[3], Betina Grehs[1], Fabiano Jeremias[4]

Objective: The purpose of this study was to compare dental size measurements, their reproducibility and the application of Tanaka and Johnston regression equation in predicting the size of canines and premolars on plaster and digital dental casts. **Methods:** Thirty plaster casts were scanned and digitized. Mesiodistal measurements of the teeth were then performed with a digital caliper on the plaster and digital casts using O3d software system (Widialabs©). The sum of the sizes of the lower incisors was used to obtain predictive values of the sizes of the premolars and canines using the regression equation, and these values were compared with the actual sizes of the teeth. The data were statistically analyzed by applying to the results Pearson's correlation test, Dahlberg's formula, paired t-test and analysis of variance (p<0.05). **Results:** Excellent intraexaminer agreement was observed in the measurements performed on both dental casts. No random error was present in the measurements obtained with the caliper and systematic error (bias) was more frequent in the digital casts. Space prediction obtained by applying the regression equation was greater than the sum of the canines and premolars on the plaster and digital casts. **Conclusions:** Despite an adequate reproducibility of the measurements performed on both casts, most measurements on the digital casts were higher than those on the plaster casts. The predicted space was overestimated in both models and significantly higher in the digital casts.

Keywords: Three-dimensional image. Dental casts. Test reproducibility.

[1] Undergraduate student, Araraquara Dental School, São Paulo State University (UNESP).
[2] Full Professor, Children's Clinic Department, Araraquara Dental School (UNESP).
[3] Associate Professor, Children's Clinic Department, Araraquara Dental School (UNESP).
[4] Graduate student, Araraquara Dental School (UNESP).

» The authors report no commercial, proprietary or financial interest in the products or companies described in this article.

Lourdes Aparecida Martins dos Santos-Pinto
Rua Humaitá, 1680 – Araraquara/SP
CEP: 14801-930 – Email: lspinto@foar.unesp.br

INTRODUCTION

Determining the mesiodistal size of unerupted permanent teeth is an important procedure in the diagnosis and treatment planning of patients in the mixed dentition as it is instrumental in predicting the required space in the dental arch where the teeth — usually canines and premolars — will be positioned.

Some methods use the adequate correlation found between the width of the permanent lower incisors and unerupted canines and premolars to predict space in mixed dentition. One such example is Moyer's analysis.[1] Space prediction in mixed dentition can also be carried out using regression equations for each side of the upper $[Y = 11 + 0.5 \ (X)]$ and lower $[Y = 10.5 + 0.5 \ (X)]$ dental arches, where Y is the sum of the unerupted canines and premolars and X the sum of the four unerupted permanent incisors.[2] This analysis is considered one of the most practical for clinical use as it requires no x-rays or tables to predict the size of the teeth.[1]

Traditionally, these diagnostic tests have been performed on plaster casts, where one can (a) assess the occlusal relationships of patients without interfering with soft tissues, (b) determine the issues to be addressed and (c) define which orthodontic mechanics will be applied. However, some of the disadvantages inherent in the use of plaster casts[3,4] are their weight and volume, time spent on their fabrication, the need for a physical storage space, the risk of breakage and difficulty in exchanging information with other professionals. Currently, digital casts offer orthodontists a convenient alternative to routine plaster casts. Their greater attractiveness is related to the speed to store patient diagnoses in a computer, instant accessibility and convenient sharing of information with colleagues.[5] A variety of methods have been developed to digitize plaster casts. Digitization is performed on casts or alginate impressions with the aid of a scanner or digital camera. The software used can electronically store the images and perform three-dimensional measurements.[4,6,7] Digital casts can be overviewed in a 360º view, in all planes of space, and can also be viewed singly, i.e., only the upper or only the lower dental arch.[5] Most digital image analysis software available on the market are not developed in Brazil, which results in high costs since patient impressions or plaster casts must be shipped overseas for scanning. O3d is a software system developed by Widialabs© (Goiânia, Brazil), a pioneering Brazilian company in the development of technologies geared to the digitization and analysis of dental casts for use in orthodontics. Orthodontists can access their digitized casts on the company's website, download these data to their computer and perform measurements and analyses.

Recent studies show that measurements of dental arch sizes, arch width, overjet and overbite on digital models are valid and can be reproduced.[8,9] Measuring tooth size on the arch itself is influenced by several factors such as tooth inclination, rotation, proximal contact, anatomical variations and interexaminer variability. Thus, the accuracy and reliability of these software need to be evaluated prior to clinical implementation.[10] Within the context outlined above, the aim of this study was to compare the measurements of dental sizes, their reproducibility and prediction of the sizes of the upper and lower canines and premolars by applying Tanaka and Johnston's[2] regression equation on plaster dental casts and digital models.

MATERIAL AND METHODS

After approval by the Ethics Committee of Araraquara Dental School (UNESP) (Protocol #33/07) thirty plaster casts were selected from the diagnostic records of patients that were receiving treatment with fixed appliances. All casts were scanned in the Orthodontic Records Service (SDO) in Araraquara, São Paulo State, and standardized by the same professional.

The criteria for inclusion of plaster casts in the study were: Presence of incisors, canines, premolars and permanent first molars in both the maxillary and mandibular arches; all cast teeth showing normal morphology; absence of irregularities in the plaster caused by carious lesions and restorations, which might affect the mesiodistal or buccolingual diameter of dental crowns; no prior orthodontic treatment.

The models were replicated to prevent damage to the patient records. The impressions were taken by the same professional using plastic trays (Morelli Orthodontics, Sorocaba, SP, Brazil) and alginate (Jeltrate, Dentsply, Petrópolis, RJ, Brazil). The casts were fabricated with special dental stone (Durone V, Dentsply, Petrópolis, RJ, Brazil) vacuum mixed at a ratio of 19 ml water to 100 g of powder and poured onto a vibrator to decrease the likelihood of bubbles.

Two casts were used as standard and had 12 points marked on their upper arch and 20 points on their lower arch as reference for the largest mesiodistal diameter of the crowns of the maxillary and mandibular canines and premolars, and mandibular incisors. Ten casts were randomly selected to be measured with a digital caliper (Mitutoyo Digimatic®, Mitutoyo Ltd., Suzano, SP, Brazil). The measurements were repeated within a one-week interval for examiner calibration. Reliability of the variable measuring process was evaluated by Pearson's correlation coefficient, which was 0.96.

After calibration, the measurements reflecting the greatest distance between the mesial and distal surfaces of crowns of all mandibular teeth and of all maxillary canines and premolars were obtained using a digital caliper. In the posterior teeth, these distances were obtained with an occlusal view of the model, and in anterior teeth, with a labial view.

Once the measurements with the digital caliper were completed, the models were forwarded for non-destructive laser scanning, with the reading done by surface scanning using a R-700 Orthodontic 3D Scanner (Copenhagen, Denmark) without touching the cast, and with an accuracy of 0.005-in and 400 dots per inch (DPI). Using O3d software (Widialabs, Goiânia, Brazil) with three-dimensional images, measurements were carried out by drawing a transverse line across the largest mesiodistal width of the posterior teeth examined in occlusal view and labial view of the anterior teeth as described in the literature.[6,9,11,12]

Teeth prediction values calculated by applying Tanaka and Johnston's[2] regression equation were compared to the actual sizes of maxillary and mandibular premolars and canines measured directly on the plaster models and three-dimensional images. All measurements were repeated within a one-week interval to test intraexaminer reliability, confirmed by Pearson's correlation test. Dahlberg's formula was applied to estimate the magnitude of casual errors and the paired t-test was applied to identify systematic errors, according to Houston.[13] The difference between the measurements obtained in the plaster vs. digital casts was evaluated by means of analysis of variance at a 5% significance level (p<0.05).

RESULTS

Assessment of intraexaminer reliability was performed for all dental measurements and in all models, yielding an excellent correlation between the first and second measurements performed both using a caliper on the plaster casts and the O3d software system on digital models. Application of Dahlberg's formula showed no random error in measurements performed with a caliper on the plaster casts. Systematic error was found only in the measurements of teeth 24 and 43, which showed a difference of one hundredth of a millimeter (-0.06 and -0.05 mm, respectively), considered clinically insignificant. The measurements carried out on digital casts using the O3d System showed random error in teeth 13, 23 and 33. In assessing systematic error statistical differences occurred in measuring teeth 13, 14, 15, 23, 33, 35, 43 and 44 (Table 1).

In comparing the measuring instruments it was noted that the mesiodistal measurements of teeth 13, 14, 23, 33 and 35 were statistically significantly higher for measurements carried out by the O3d software system compared with a digital caliper (Table 1). The values for required space obtained by applying the regression equation were larger than the sum of the measurements of the premolars and canines on the plaster casts (mean of 3.35 mm for the maxillary arch and 2.84 mm for the mandibular arch, and digital casts (mean of 1.11 mm for the maxillary arch and 0.72 mm for the mandibular arch). Statistically significant differences were found in the measurements performed in all segments of the dental arch (Table 2).

DISCUSSION

The measurements of dental sizes obtained both by caliper and by the O3d system presented excellent intraexaminer reliability, established by the correlation (r), which ranged from 0.87 to 0.99 for the caliper and 0.96 to 0.99 for the O3d System (Table 1). A similar intraexaminer reliability — found for both the plaster and digital casts — was reported by Quimby et al[8]. However, Dalstra and Melsen[14], after measuring the maxillary right central incisor and first molar on the right side, reported that the intraexaminer variation was lower for the measurements performed on digital casts. Moreover, El-Zanaty et al[15] found little correlation between the two methods and attributed the error to (a) difficulties in accurately identifying the contact points and (b) lack of experience of the examiner to conduct measurements on three-dimensional computer images. Random error was not noted in the measurements performed with a caliper.

Table 1 - Means, standard deviations (SD) and differences (dif) between the first and second mesiodistal measurements of the teeth, in millimeters. Random error (Dahlberg's Formula), systematic error (p<0.05), correlation (r) obtained from plaster and digital casts and comparison between methods (ANOVA: p<0.05).

Teeth	Caliper						O3d						Caliper	
	mean	SD	dif.	Dahlberg	p	r	mean	SD	dif.	Dahlberg	p	r	dif.	ANOVA
15	5.69	0.46	-0.02	0.06	0.28	0.98	6.47	0.50	0.01	0.09	0.57	0.99	-0.78	0.31
14	5.83	0.48	0.01	0.04	0.18	0.99	6.59	0.34	-0.08	0.14	0.02*	0.99	-0.77	0.01*
13	7.17	0.48	-0.04	0.08	0.10	0.97	7.49	0.69	-0.17	0.27	0.01*	0.97	-0.32	0.05*
23	7.09	0.46	-0.01	0.06	0.57	0.98	7.63	0.69	-0.16	0.29	0.04*	0.96	-0.54	0.05*
24	5.85	0.52	-0.06	0.07	0.00*	0.98	6.76	0.50	-0.05	0.15	0.22	0.99	-0.92	0.91
25	5.62	0.52	-0.03	0.06	0.11	0.98	6.44	0.41	0.00	0.11	0.98	0.99	-0.81	0.49
35	6.25	0.57	0.01	0.05	0.34	0.99	7.10	0.44	-0.09	0.14	0.02*	0.99	-0.85	0.01*
34	6.20	0.52	-0.05	0.15	0.18	0.92	6.87	0.53	-0.06	0.16	0.21	0.98	-0.67	0.91
33	6.35	0.56	0.00	0.05	0.98	0.99	6.77	0.61	-0.20	0.29	0.01*	0.96	-0.43	0.03*
32	5.72	0.41	-0.02	0.06	0.17	0.98	5.75	0.42	-0.04	0.15	0.35	0.98	-0.03	0.60
31	5.31	0.35	-0.03	0.14	0.48	0.87	5.09	0.42	-0.06	0.14	0.14	0.98	0.21	0.53
41	5.27	0.32	0.00	0.05	0.85	0.98	5.16	0.35	-0.05	0.19	0.47	0.96	0.11	0.41
42	5.67	0.44	0.01	0.04	0.61	0.91	5.60	0.40	-0.04	0.13	0.38	0.98	0.06	0.28
43	6.25	0.49	-0.05	0.09	0.03	0.97	6.45	0.60	-0.08	0.16	0.07*	0.98	-0.20	0.39
44	6.05	0.59	-0.01	0.09	0.76	0.97	6.91	0.51	-0.06	0.12	0.05*	0.99	-0.85	0.12
45	6.18	0.46	-0.01	0.06	0.62	0.98	7.06	0.49	-0.03	0.13	0.53	0.99	-0.88	0.62

* Statistical significance.

Table 2 - Measurement values (mm) of the required space (RS) obtained by Tanaka and Johnston's regression equation, existing space (ES), difference between the two (RS-ES) and comparison between the methods (Anova: p<0.05).

Arch	Measurements	Side	Caliper		O3d		Caliper	
			mean	SD	mean	SD	dif.	ANOVA
Superior	RS	Right	21.98	0.68	21.81	0.67	0.18	0.02*
	ES		18.68	1.25	20.55	1.24	-1.87	0.00*
	RS-ES		3.30	0.82	1.25	0.95	2.05	0.00*
	ES	Left	18.55	1.33	20.82	1.24	-2.27	0.00*
	RS-ES		3.43	0.98	0.98	0.96	2.45	0.00*
Inferior	RS	Right	21.48	0.68	21.31	0.67	0.18	0.02*
	ES		18.49	1.35	20.42	1.39	-1.93	0.00*
	RS-ES		2.99	0.90	0.89	0.96	2.11	0.00*
	ES	Left	18.79	1.47	20.74	1.37	-1.95	0.00*
	RS-ES		2.69	1.03	0.56	1.01	2.12	0.00*

* Statistical significance.

However, in the measurements carried out with the O3d System, random error was found in teeth 13, 23 and 33, which can be explained by a difficulty in determining the angle between the proximal surfaces and the cusps as reference for the largest mesiodistal diameter in three-dimensional images.

The mean value of the differences observed between the first and second measurement of the size of the teeth ranged from 0.00 to 0.06 mm on the plaster casts and from 0.01 to 0.20 mm on the digital casts (Table 1). These values have no clinical relevance as they are below the acceptable values, i.e., 0.20 mm[16] or 30 mm.[17]

Despite the excellent intraexaminer reliability of the measurements carried out with the O3d system, systematic error was present in teeth 13, 14, 15, 23, 33, 35 and 43. The error found in the canines was probably due to the position of these teeth, i.e., on the curvature of the dental arch, thereby hindering the movement of the digitized model in the program and the identification of reference points used to perform the measurements.

While performing the measurements, it was noted that the tool used to locate the first reference point was similar to an arrowhead while the second point was defined by a tool shaped like a filled circle, which is less accurate. The points are important in setting the distance that must be measured by the program, which may have affected the measurements of the premolars.

In comparing the measurements obtained with the two instruments, digital caliper and O3d System, it was observed that the values yielded by the latter were higher for all teeth except teeth 31, 41 and 42, where the difference between measurements was very low, ranging from 0.06 to 0.21 mm. The results of this study do not corroborate the findings of Santoro et al[6] and Dalstra and Melsen,[14] who found higher values for the teeth measured with the caliper, and Aguiar and Freitas[18] and Redlich et al,[12] in whose research the tooth sizes were underestimated for both dental arches in the measurements performed on digital casts. Keating et al[3] and Jedlinska[19] reported that the measurements obtained with a digital caliper on plaster and digital casts were similar.

In applying Tanaka and Johnston's regression equations to each side of the maxillary arch [Y=11+0.5 (X)] and mandibular arch [Y=10.5+0.5 (X)] using the sum of the four erupted permanent mandibular incisors (X) to predict the sum of the non-erupted canines and premolars(Y), it was noted that the predicted spaces were larger than the spaces actually present in the arches. A statistically significant difference was observed in all segments of both arches. Due to the fact that the measurements performed on the digital casts yielded larger values than the measurements obtained from the plaster casts, the difference found by the O3d System between the required space and the existing space were lower than those obtained by the caliper. Thus, in both the plaster and digital casts, the space predicted by Tanaka and Johnston's equation overestimated the size of the premolars and canines in both arches, corroborating the findings of Bishara and Jakobsen,[20] nikTahere et al,[21] Arslan et al,[22] and unlike Melgaço et al,[23] who found underestimated values, although with no clinical significance.

The measurements obtained from the digital casts in this study were reproducible, although some difficulties were encountered during measuring. The viewing of contact points, the excessive brightness in the models, the determination of reference points with the locating tool in the shape of a filled circle and the frequent failure in saving the data are some of the issues that need to be addressed by those who use the digital measurement analysis. This measuring instrument proved to be a promising tool in the analysis of dental casts. The system, however, calls for improvement while professionals must be trained to ensure proper use.

CONCLUSIONS

Based on the method employed in this study, one can conclude that dental size measurements showed good reproducibility in both plaster and digital casts. However, the measurements taken by the O3d software system proved superior to those obtained by caliper, and Tanaka and Johnston's equation[2] overestimated the sizes of premolar and canine teeth in the maxillary and mandibular arches with both measurement instruments.

REFERENCES

1. Alhaija ESJ, Qudeimat, MA. Mixed dentition space analysis in a Jordanian population: comparison of two methods. Int J Paediatr Dent. 2006;16(2):104-10.

2. Tanaka MM, Johnston LE. The prediction of the size of unerupted canines and premolars in a contemporary orthodontic population. J Am Dent Assoc. 1974;88(4):798-801.

3. Keating AP, Knox J, Bibb R, Zhurov AI. A comparison of plaster, digital and reconstructed study model accuracy. J Orthod. 2008;35(3):191-201.

4. Redmond WR. Digital models: a new diagnostic tool. J Clin Orthod. 2001;35(6):386-7.

5. Paredes V, Gandia JL, Cibrián R. Digital diagnosis records in orthodontics. An overview. Med Oral Patol Oral Cir Bucal. 2006;11(1):e88-93.

6. Santoro M, Galkin S, Teredesai M, Nicolay OF, Cangialosi TJ. Comparison of measurements made on digital and plaster models. Am J Orthod Dentofacial Orthop. 2003;124(1):101-5.

7. Whetten JL, Williamson PC, Heo G, Varnhagen C, Major PW. Variations in orthodontic treatment planning decisions of Class II patients between virtual 3-dimensional models and traditional plaster study models. Am J Orthod Dentofacial Orthop. 2006;130(4):485-91.

8. Quimby ML, Vig KW, Rashid GR, Firestone AR. The accuracy and reliability of measurements made on computer-based digital models. Angle Orthod. 2004;74(3):298-303.

9. Zilberman O, Huggare JA, Parikakis KA. Evaluation of the validity of tooth size and arch width measurements using conventional and three-dimensional virtual orthodontic models. Angle Orthod. 2003;73(3):301-6.

10. Leifert MF, Leifert MM, Efstratiadis SS, Cangialosi TJ. Comparison of space analysis evaluations with digital models and plaster dental casts. Am J Orthod Dentofacial Orthop. 2009;136(1):16.e1-4.

11. Mayers M, Firestone AR, Rashid R, Vig KW. Comparison of peer assessment rating (PAR) index scores of plaster and computer-based digital models. Am J Orthod Dentofacial Orthop. 2005;128(4):431-4.

12. Redlich M, Weinstock T, Abed Y, Schneor R, Holdstein Y, Fischer A. A new system for scanning, measuring and analyzing dental casts based on a 3D holographic sensor. Orthod Craniofac Res. 2008;11(2):90-5.

13. Houston WJB. The analysis of error in orthodontics measurements. Am J Orthod. 1983;83(5):382-90.

14. Dalstra M, Melsen B. From alginate impression to digital virtual models: accuracy and reproducibility. J Orthod. 2009;36(1):36-41.

15. El-Zanaty HM, El-Beialy AR, Abou El-Ezz AM, Attia KH, El-Bialy AR, Mostafa YA. Three-dimensional dental measurements: an alternative to plaster models. Am J Orthod Dentofacial Orthop. 2010;137(2):259-65.

16. Schirmer UR, Wiltshire WA. Manual and computer-aided apace analysis: a comparative study. Am J Orthod Dentofacial Orthop. 1997;112(6):676-80.

17. Hirogaki Y, Sohmura T, Satoh H, Takahashi J, Takada K. Complete 3-D reconstruction of dental cast shape using perceptual grouping. IEEE Trans Med Imaging. 2001;20(10):1093-101.

18. Aguiar RM, Freitas BV. Confiabilidade da análise de Moyers em indivíduos de São Luís-MA. Ortho Sci Orthod Sci Pract. 2008;1(2):147-52.

19. Jedlinska A. The comparison analysis of the line measurements between plaster and virtual orthodontic 3D models. Ann Acad Med Stetin. 2008;54(2):106-13.

20. Bishara SE, Jakobson JR. Comparison of two non radiographic methods of predicting permanent tooth size in the mixed dentition. Am J Orthod Dentofacial Orthop. 1998;114(5):573-6.

21. nikTahere H, Majid S, Fateme M, Kharazi F, Javad M. Predicting the size of unerupted canines and premolars of the maxillary and mandibular quadrants in an Iranian population. J Clin Pediatr Dent. 2007;32(1):43-7.

22. Arslan SG, Dildes, N, Kama JD, Genc C. Mixed-dentition analysis in a Turkish population. World J Orthod. 2009;10(2):135-40.

23. Melgaço CA, Araújo MT, Ruellas AC. Applicability of three tooth size prediction methods for white Brasilians. Angle Orthod. 2006;76(4):644-9.

13

Effects of mandibular protraction appliance associated to fixed appliance in adults

Bruno D'Aurea Furquim[1], José Fernando Castanha Henriques[2], Guilherme Janson[2], Danilo Furquim Siqueira[3], Laurindo Zanco Furquim[4]

Objective: This retrospective study aimed to conduct a cephalometric evaluation of the skeletal, dental and soft tissue effects resulting from treatment of adult patients presenting Class II malocclusion, performed with a Mandibular Protraction Appliance (MPA) combined with a fixed orthodontic appliance. **Methods:** The sample consisted of teleradiographs obtained before and after treatment of 9 adult patients (initial mean age of 22.48 years) with bilateral Class II, division 1, malocclusion. Paired t test (p < 0.05) was applied to compare initial and final values. **Results:** t test revealed an increase in anteroinferior facial height and posterior facial height. The dental changes include: extrusion of upper incisors, buccal inclination, protrusion of lower incisors, mesialization and extrusion of mandibular molars. Regarding the soft tissue component, there was an increase in nasolabial angle in addition to upper lip retrusion. **Conclusions:** The effects of treating Class II malocclusion adult patients, by means of using Mandibular Protraction Appliance (MPA) combined with a fixed appliance were mostly observed in the mandibular arch, and consisted of buccal inclination, protrusion and intrusion of incisors, and mesialization and extrusion of the molars.

Keywords: Angle Class II Malocclusion. Functional orthodontic appliances. Mandibular advancement. Adult.

[1] PhD Student in Oral Rehabilitation, School of Dentistry of Bauru, University of São Paulo (FOB-USP).

[2] Full and Head Professor, University of São Paulo (USP).

[3] PhD in Orthodontics, FOB-USP. Professor, UNICID.

[4] PhD in Oral Pathology, FOB-USP. Associate Professor, State University of Maringá (UEM).

» The authors report no commercial, proprietary or financial interest in the products or companies described in this article.

Bruno D'Aurea Furquim
Rua Arthur Thomas, 999 - Maringá/PR – CEP: 87013-250 – Brazil
Email: brunofurquim@hotmail.com

INTRODUCTION

Treatment of adult patients has become a reality in orthodontic practice for many years.[1,2,3] For cases of adult patients with mandibular deficiency, two treatment approaches are usually available. The first is compensatory, involving premolar extractions, allowing retraction of upper incisors and, as a result, overjet correction, while the second is surgical, repositioning the mandible more anteriorly.[4]

In addition to these two more traditional treatment options, functional fixed appliances constitute yet a third alternative to treat Class II malocclusion without extraction or surgery.[4-12]

The Herbst appliance was the first fixed functional appliance designed for the correction of Class II malocclusion, and also the first one described for this purpose in adult patients.[8] Besides the Herbst appliance, there are other fixed functional appliances effective in the correction of Class II malocclusion such as the Jasper Jumper, the MARA, the AMF and MPA.[5,6,7,13] The Mandibular Protraction Appliance (MPA) stands out for its easy fabrication, low cost and swift installation.[14]

Some studies have compared the treatment of Class II malocclusion with MPA associated to other appliances in adolescent patients.[13,15] Clinical cases of adult patients treated with MPA can be found in the literature.[16,17,18] But no research has yet been conducted to investigate treatment with MPA in a group of adult patients. Thus, this retrospective study aimed to conduct a cephalometric evaluation of the skeletal, dental and soft tissue effects resulting from treatment with MPA in combination with fixed appliance in adult patients presenting with Class II malocclusion.

MATERIAL AND METHODS

In selecting the sample, the following inclusion criteria were applied:

1. Presence of early bilateral Class II, division 1, malocclusion.
2. Absence of agenesis and no permanent teeth missing.
3. Absence of supernumerary teeth.
4. Treatment conducted exclusively with MPA combined with a fixed orthodontic appliance.
5. Class I molar relationship with a reduced overjet at the end of treatment.

Patients were defined as adults based on the cervical vertebral maturation method for evaluation of mandibular growth proposed by Baccetti et al.[21] Patients in the fifth cervical vertebral maturation stage (CVMS V) and above were considered adults. Evaluation was performed using the initial teleradiograph. Patients who raised any doubt as to their classification were excluded from the sample.

The sample consisted of nine Brazilian Caucasian adults (6 females and 3 males) presenting bilateral Class II division 1 malocclusion. The patients had an initial mean age of 22.48 years (S.D. = 5.64, ranging from 15.14 to 29.69 years.) The mean follow-up period was 4.01 years, and the final mean age of the patients was 26.50 years. The patients were treated by experienced professors.

As this was a retrospective study, the teleradiographs were taken at different centers. The anatomical tracing and landmarks were scanned on a flatbed Numonics AccuGrid XNT, model A30TL.F (Austin, Texas/ USA). Dentofacial Planner 7.02 software (Toronto, Ontario - Canada) was used for measuring the cephalometric variables since this computer program automatically corrects the radiographic image magnification. Midplane tracing was performed on bilateral structures, except for the molars, given that the more distally positioned molar was used as reference.

Intraexaminer error was determined by taking new measurements of 15 teleradiographs, either initial or final, after an interval of 30 days since the first measurement. Systematic errors were analyzed by dependent test as described by Houston.[19]

For evaluation of casual errors the Dahlberg test was utilized, which shows the average change between the first and second measurements. The test is performed by the formula $S^2 = \Sigma d^2/2n$, where S^2 is the error variance, d represents the difference between the first and second measurement, and n is the number of measurement pairs.[20] Random error was calculated using a Microsoft Excel XP spreadsheet.

Kolmogorov-Smirnov test was used to assess if the values had a normal distribution, thus allowing the dependent t test to be performed. The latter was performed to compare the mean cephalometric values at the beginning and end of treatment.

Statistical tests were carried out using Statistica software. Results where $p < 0.05$ were considered to be statistically significant.

RESULTS

Only two variables (1-PTV and 1-PP) exhibited systematic error approximately one month after the first measurement, and random errors ranged from 0.28 for SML to 2.80 for 1.PP (Table 1).

MPA revealed no significant changes in the maxilla or mandible. As regards growth pattern, only the linear variables (anteroinferior facial height and posterior facial height) changed.

Incisor extrusion was the only significant change noted in the maxillary dentoalveolar component. On the other hand, the mandibular dentoalveolar component showed buccal inclination, incisor protrusion, and molar mesialization and extrusion. The treatment achieved significant correction of overjet and overbite as well as molar relationship. Regarding the soft tissue component, the nasolabial angle increased and the upper lip retracted relative to line E.

DISCUSSION

This study evaluated the dental, skeletal and soft tissue effects of correcting Class II malocclusion in a group of adult patients using Mandibular Protraction Appliances (MPAs). The Cervical Vertebral Maturation Method for assessment of mandibular growth,[21] and the patient's chronological age were the criteria used to classify patients as adults. Given that no other researcher has ever evaluated the effects of MPA on adult patients, the results will be compared with those of other studies that evaluated fixed functional appliances other than MPAs for correction of Class II malocclusion in adults or young adults .

It is noteworthy that the effects observed in this study result from treatment carried out with MPAs and fixed appliances. Further studies are warranted to evaluate not only the overall effects of treatment, but also specific effects observed in the period when the MPA was in place.

Skeletal effects

Other studies are in agreement with the results in terms of MPA effects on the maxilla. Treatment with MPA in a group with initial mean age of 15 years and five months was also unable to produce effects in the maxilla.[6] Nalbantgil et al[7] assessed the effects of Jasper Jumper in a group with an initial mean age of 16.5 years, and reported it had limited effects on the

maxilla. Moreover, no significant differences were found between the beginning and end of treatment. However, in comparison with the control group, the authors suggested that Jasper Jumper inhibited the growth potential of the maxilla.

As in the present study, Nalbantgil et al[7] observed no significant effects on mandibular growth in patients with an initial mean age of 16.5 years treated with Jasper Jumper. However, significant changes were observed in the maxillomandibular relationship. Gönner et al[5] observed greater reduction (3 degrees) in the ANB angle, and in older patients (33.7 years / SD 7.9) treated with MARA.

With regard to growth pattern, only the linear variables (anteroinferior facial height and posterior facial height) increased, which can also be construed as a result of late changes in craniofacial growth. Nalbantgil et al[7] also observed no changes in the growth pattern. Ruf and Pancherz[12] observed that the SN.GoGn angle did not change during the Herbst phase, which is consistent with studies of Herbst in children. Decreases in the SN.GoGn angle during the fixed appliance phase and throughout the observation period as well as mandibular advancement caused a reduction in the convexity of the skeletal and soft tissue profile. The opposite seems to have occurred with controls, of which convexity increased over time.

Dental effects

In agreement with the present study, Nalbantgil et al[7] noted extrusion in upper incisors as a result of treatment with Jasper Jumper. They also observed retraction of the upper incisors and distal tipping of the molar crown, which was not observed in this study. This may have been due to the fact that patients in this study were older (22.41 years) than patients evaluated by Nalbantgil et al[7] (16.5 years.) Given that the lower lip droops with aging,[22] extrusion of upper incisors can be regarded as an advantage afforded by this treatment.

The lower dentoalveolar component exhibited significant changes in nearly all variables (buccal inclination, incisor protrusion and intrusion, mesialization and extrusion of molars), except for the vertical position of the incisors as these remained unchanged.

Ruf and Pancherz[11] showed the dental and facial adjustments they achieved in adolescents and young adults. In both groups, Class II and overjet correction

Table 1 - Results of paired t test and Dahlberg's formula applied to variables studied to estimate random and systematic errors, respectively.

VARIABLES	1st measurement Mean ± SD	2nd measurement Mean ± SD	Difference between means	Dahlberg	p
Maxillary Component					
SNA (degrees)	80.19 ± 4.28	80.77 ± 4.85	0.57	1.93	0.435
A-Nperp (mm)	2.40 ± 4.12	1.53 ± 4.37	-0.87	1.84	0.207
Co-A (mm)	85.93 ± 3.61	86.45 ± 4.00	0.52	0.90	0.118
Mandibular Component					
SNB (degrees)	76.23 ± 4.12	76.85 ± 4.52	0.61	1.26	0.193
Pog-Nperp (mm)	0 ± 5.91	-1.28 ± 6.29	-1.28	1.96	0.072
Co-Gn (mm)	108.21 ± 5.73	108.15 ± 5.75	-0.06	0.79	0.844
Go-Gn (mm)	72.86 ± 4.96	73.58 ± 5.02	0.72	1.87	0.308
Co-Go (mm)	53.21 ± 6.51	52.09 ± 6.16	-1.12	2.22	0.175
Maxillomandibular relationship					
ANB (degrees)	3.97 ± 2.48	3.92 ± 2.30	-0.05	0.90	0.893
NAP (degrees)	4.44 ± 6.74	4.14 ± 6.18	-0.30	1.17	0.501
Co-A/Co-Gn (mm)	79.47 ± 2.11	79.99 ± 1.77	0.51	0.93	0.137
Growth pattern					
FMA (degrees)	20.09 ± 7.74	21.21 ± 7.19	1.12	2.17	0.165
SN.GoGn (degrees)	29.28 ± 9.13	28.58 ± 8.84	-0.70	1.91	0.334
SN.PP (degrees)	7.75 ± 5.62	8.14 ± 4.59	0.39	1.73	0.559
AIFH (mm)	63.39 ± 3.73	62.63 ± 3.55	-0.76	1.54	0.184
S-GO (mm)	74.97 ± 7.81	74.55 ± 7.81	-0.43	1.10	0.306
Maxillary dentoalveolar component					
1.PP (degrees)	101.93 ± 9.72	106.75 ± 5.74	4.82	2.80	0.150
1-PP (mm)	28.26 ± 1.90	27.49 ± 2.01	-0.77	0.98	0.024*
1.NA (graus)	15.81 ± 9.34	17.86 ± 8.94	2.05	2.21	0.085
1-NA (mm)	2.77 ± 3.26	3.17 ± 3.21	0.40	1.03	0.304
1-PTV	56.10 ± 5.01	55.28 ± 5.90	-0.82	1.17	0.050
6-PP (mm)	22.54 ± 1.27	22.47 ± 1.23	-0.07	0.47	0.682
6-PTV	27.34 ± 4.21	26.33 ± 4.32	-1.01	1.75	0.116
Mandibular dentoalveolar component					
IMPA (degrees)	102.81 ± 6.60	102.71 ± 5.85	-0.10	1.54	0.892
1.NB (degrees)	31.39 ± 7.06	31.59 ± 6.18	0.21	1.50	0.720
1-NB (mm)	4.95 ± 2.21	4.74 ± 2.41	-0.21	0.79	0.479
1-PM (mm)	38.09 ± 2.19	38.11 ± 2.38	0.02	1.54	0.973
1-PTV	52.62 ± 4.80	51.59 ± 5.74	-1.03	1.28	0.021*
6-PM (mm)	29.86 ± 2.49	29.84 ± 2.72	-0.02	1.17	0.964
6-PTV	28.25 ± 4.45	27.31 ± 4.75	-0.94	1.67	0.126
Dental relationships					
T.H. (mm)	3.48 ± 0.74	3.69 ± 0.65	0.21	0.45	0.221
T.V. (mm)	3.33 ± 0.97	3.02 ± 1.21	-0.31	0.42	0.221
Molar relationship	-0.91 ± 1.65	-0.99 ± 1.62	-0.07	0.30	0.520
Soft tissue component					
ANL	111.29 ± 6.65	111.41 ± 5.52	0.12	2.88	0.914
SML	6.03 ± 0.97	6.02 ± 0.84	-0.01	0.28	0.950
UL-E	-4.21 ± 1.96	-4.14 ± 1.91	0.07	1.38	0.900
LL-E	-2.09 ± 2.91	-1.81 ± 2.70	0.28	1.68	0.663
UL-Pog'Sn	2.70 ± 1.14	2.92 ± 1.23	0.22	0.83	0.486
LL-Pog'Sn	1.41 ± 2.42	1.67 ± 2.22	0.26	1.26	0.588

*p < 0.05.

Table 2 - Comparison between initial and final mean values by paired t test.

VARIABLES	Initial (n = 9) Mean ± SD	Final (n = 9) Mean ± SD	Difference between means	p
Chronological age				
Age	22.48 ± 5.64	26.50 ± 6.32	4.01	0.000*
Maxillary component				
SNA (degrees)	79.83 ± 6.52	80.24 ± 6.87	0.41	0.255
A-Nperp (mm)	-0.54 ± 3.29	0.07 ± 4.16	0.61	0.215
Co-A (mm)	85.01 ± 8.06	85.20 ± 7.77	0.19	0.537
Mandibular component				
SNB (degrees)	76.70 ± 6.44	77.13 ± 5.93	0.43	0.279
Pog-Nperp (mm)	-3.28 ± 5.38	-1.92 ± 5.47	1.36	0.169
Co-Gn (mm)	109.82 ± 8.34	110.38 ± 7.74	0.56	0.219
Go-Gn (mm)	73.43 ± 4.75	73.90 ± 4.92	0.47	0.110
Co-Go (mm)	53.07 ± 7.85	53.49 ± 7.00	0.42	0.407
Maxillomandibular relationship				
ANB (degrees)	3.14 ± 2.57	3.12 ± 3.20	-0.02	0.959
NAP (degrees)	2.38 ± 6.94	2.33 ± 8.04	-0.04	0.957
Co-A/Co-Gn (mm)	77.41 ± 4.22	77.19 ± 4.30	-0.22	0.422
Growth pattern				
FMA (degrees)	23.18 ± 7.73	22.76 ± 7.75	-0.42	0.378
SN.GoGn (degrees)	30.41 ± 11.13	30.06 ± 10.53	-0.36	0.439
SN.PP (degrees)	7.64 ± 5.44	7.02 ± 5.36	-0.62	0.271
AIFH (mm)	63.18 ± 6.17	64.86 ± 5.36	1.68	0.010*
S-GO (mm)	74.14 ± 10.19	75.58 ± 9.50	1.43	0.011*
Maxillary dentoalveolar component				
1.PP (degrees)	114.51 ± 9.65	111.23 ± 5.94	-3.28	0.192
1-PP (mm)	26.71 ± 3.13	28.22 ± 3.00	1.51	0.027*
1.NA (degrees)	27.06 ± 12.10	23.94 ± 8.98	-3.11	0.220
1-NA (mm)	6.41 ± 4.24	4.79 ± 3.71	-1.62	0.064
1-PTV	57.21 ± 4.25	56.54 ± 5.30	-0.67	0.441
6-PP (mm)	22.69 ± 2.48	23.03 ± 2.37	0.34	0.339
6-PTV	27.07 ± 3.34	27.36 ± 4.19	0.29	0.809
Mandibular dentoalveolar component				
IMPA (degrees)	99.62 ± 4.77	105.37 ± 4.53	5.74	0.000*
1.NB (degrees)	29.14 ± 4.94	35.13 ± 4.48	5.99	0.000*
1-NB (mm)	4.93 ± 2.41	5.78 ± 2.02	0.84	0.023*
1-PM (mm)	39.10 ± 3.31	38.16 ± 2.92	-0.94	0.124
1-PTV	51.59 ± 5.36	53.32 ± 4.96	1.73	0.053*
6-PM (mm)	28.59 ± 3.56	30.87 ± 2.84	2.28	0.001*
6-PTV	26.63 ± 4.35	29.72 ± 4.13	-3.09	0.027*
Dental relationships				
T.H. (mm)	5.62 ± 2.76	3.22 ± 0.57	-2.40	0.035*
T.V. (mm)	3.08 ± 1.75	1.48 ± 1.24	-1.60	0.008*
Molar relationship	0.43 ± 2.06	-2.06 ± 0.30	-2.49	0.007*
Soft tissue component				
ANL	108.19 ± 11.05	109.32 ± 12.46	1.13	0.007*
SML	6.34 ± 1.22	6.12 ± 1.34	-0.22	0.548
UL-E	-3.36 ± 2.38	-4.36 ± 1.94	-1.00	0.006*
LL-E	-2.08 ± 2.84	-2.13 ± 2.42	-0.06	0.888
UL-Pog'Sn	3.27 ± 1.91	2.94 ± 1.77	-0.32	0.365
LL-Pog'Sn	1.37 ± 2.53	1.68 ± 2.04	0.31	0.539

*p < 0.05.

was promoted mostly by dental changes and to a lesser extent by skeletal changes.[10] Adolescent patients showed greater mandibular growth, whereas young adult patients exhibited greater molar mesialization and consequently greater protrusion of the lower incisors. Gönner et al[5] observed an increase of more than 5° in the IMPA of adult patients (33.7 years) treated with MARA combined with fixed appliances. Conversely, Nalbantgil et al[7] observed — in addition to lower incisor protrusion — intrusion of these same teeth, as was the case in the present study.

Buccal inclination of lower incisors and its impact on periodontal status is controversial. Some studies have seen protrusion as a risk factor for gingival recession since an association between recession and buccal movement has been observed.[22-25] Others did not note such association.[26,27,28] To Melsen and Allais,[29] other predisposing factors for gingival recession should be taken into account such as gingival biotype, visible plaque and inflammation.

A positive relationship between the patient's age and the severity of bone loss has been identified.[30,31] According to Ko-Kimura et al,[32] the prevalence of black spaces in post-orthodontic treatment is greater in patients over twenty years old, and these spaces are linked to resorption of the alveolar crest. The average prevalence of black spaces found in the adult orthodontic population post-treatment, regardless of the initial crowding, was 38%,[33] and 43% in adolescents after correction of incisor crowding, according to Burke.[34] Tanaka et al[35] demonstrated that due to crowding the interdental papilla can be crushed and it is only after the dental malocclusions have been corrected that black space may become evident. Tuverson[36] reported that since triangular teeth have no contact areas, but rather contact points, these teeth are more unstable

and more susceptible to crowding. According to Olsson and Lindhe,[37] patients with triangular maxillary central incisors (slender and tall) tend to develop more gingival recession than those patients with wider and shorter maxillary central incisors, since there seems to be a relationship between "gingival biotype" and shape of the upper central incisor.

How maxillary incisors are positioned determines to a great extent the motivation that drives adult patients to seek orthodontic treatment. Few of these patients even notice skeletal abnormalities.[38] Therefore, preventive care should be provided for as long as there is orthodontic movement, mainly protrusive movement, in patients with thin gum / triangular incisor "biotype." Special attention should be paid when these features are associated with some degree of crowding and/or visible plaque and inflammation.

Soft tissue effects

Retrusion of the upper lip in terms of variable LL-E and an increased nasolabial angle were observed. These changes may have been influenced by nose growth, since the upper lip remained unchanged in terms of variable UL-Pog'Sn, consistent with the unchanged position of upper incisors in the sagittal direction. Despite the fact that protrusion and labial inclination of the lower incisors did occur, the lower lip did not protrude.

CONCLUSIONS

The effects of treating Class II malocclusion in adults using a Mandibular Protraction Appliance combined with fixed orthodontic appliance were mostly observed in the mandibular arch, and consisted of buccal inclination, incisor protrusion, and mesialization and extrusion of the molars. Incisor extrusion was the only significant change observed in the maxillary arch.

REFERENCES

1. Harris EF, Vaden JL, Dunn KL, Behrents RG. Effects of patient age on postorthodontic stability in Class II, division 1 malocclusions. Am J Orthod Dentofacial Orthop. 1994;105(1):25-34.

2. Kokich V, Mathews D. Managing treatment for the orthodontic patient with periodontal problems. Semin Orthod. 1997;3(1):21-38.

3. LaSota E. Orthodontic considerations in prosthetic and restorative dentistry. Dent Clin North Am. 1988;32(3):447-56.

4. Ruf S, Pancherz H. Orthognathic surgery and dentofacial orthopedics in adult Class II division 1 treatment: mandibular sagittal split osteotomy versus Herbst appliance. Am J Orthod Dentofacial Orthop. 2004;126(2):140-52; quiz 254-5.

5. Gonner U, Ozkan V, Jahn E, Toll DE. Effect of the MARA appliance on the position of the lower anteriors in children, adolescents and adults with Class II malocclusion. J Orofac Orthop. 2007;68(5):397-412.

6. Kinzinger G, Diedrich P. Skeletal effects in Class II treatment with the functional mandibular advancer (FMA)? J Orofac Orthop. 2005;66(6):469-90.

7. Nalbantgil D, Arun T, Sayinsu K, Fulya I. Skeletal, dental and soft-tissue changes induced by the Jasper Jumper appliance in late adolescence. Angle Orthod. 2005;75(3):426-36.

8. Paulsen HU. Morphological changes of the TMJ condyles of 100 patients treated with the Herbst appliance in the period of puberty to adulthood: a long-term radiographic study. Eur J Orthod. 1997;19(6):657-68.

9. Paulsen HU, Karle A. Computer tomographic and radiographic changes in the temporomandibular joints of two young adults with occlusal asymmetry, treated with the Herbst appliance. Eur J Orthod. 2000;22(6):649-56.

10. Ruf S, Pancherz H. Dentoskeletal effects and facial profile changes in young adults treated with the Herbst appliance. Angle Orthod. 1999;69(3):239-46.

11. Ruf S, Pancherz H. Temporomandibular joint remodeling in adolescents and young adults during Herbst treatment: a prospective longitudinal magnetic resonance imaging and cephalometric radiographic investigation. Am J Orthod Dentofacial Orthop. 1999;115(6):607-18.

12. Ruf S, Pancherz H. Herbst/multibracket appliance treatment of Class II division 1 malocclusions in early and late adulthood. A prospective cephalometric study of consecutively treated subjects. Eur J Orthod. 2006;28(4):352-60. Epub 2006 Apr 27.

13. Siqueira D, de Almeira RR, Janson G, Brandão AG, Coelho Filho CM. Dentoskeletal and soft-tissue changes with cervical headgear and mandibular protraction appliance therapy in the treatment of Class II malocclusions. Am J Orthod. 2007;131(4):447.e 21-30.

14. Coelho Filho CM. Mandibular protraction appliances for Class II treatment. J Clin Orthod. 1995;29(5):319-36.

15. Alves P, Oliveira A, Silveira C, Oliveira J, Oliveira Júnior J, Coelho Filho C. Estudo comparativo dos efeitos esqueléticos, dentários e tegumentares, promovidos pelo tratamento da má oclusão Classe II mandibular com o aparelho de Herbst e com o Aparelho de Protração Mandibular. Rev Clin Ortod Dental Press. 2006;5(1):85-105.

16. Bicalho J, Bicalho R. Utilização do APM no tratamento da má oclusão de Classe II, 2ª divisão, em paciente adulto. Rev Clin Ortod Dental Press. 2007;6(1):99-106.

17. Coelho Filho C. Clinical application of the Mandibular Protraction Appliance in upper lateral agenesis and in asymmetric cases. Texas Dent J. 2002;119(7):618-26.

18. Coelho Filho C, White L. Treating adults with the Mandibular Protraction Appliance. Orthodontic Cyber J. 2003 jan [Access 2009 Jul 20]. Available from: http://orthocj.com/2003/01/treating-adults-with-the-mandibular-protraction-appliance/.

19. Houston WJ. The analysis of errors in orthodontic measurements. Am J Orthod. 1983;83(5):382-90.

20. Dahlberg G. Statistical methods for medical and biological students. Br Med J. 1940;2(4158):358-9.

21. Baccetti T, Franchi L, McNamara JA Jr. An improved version of the cervical vertebral maturation (CVM) method for the assessment of mandibular growth. Angle Orthod. 2002;72(4):316-23.

22. Dorfman HS. Mucogingival changes resulting from mandibular incisor tooth movement. Am J Orthod. 1978;74(3):286-97.

23. Fuhrmann R. Three-dimensional interpretation of labiolingual bone width of the lower incisors. Part II. J Orofac Orthop. 1996;57(3):168-85.

24. Hollender L, Ronnerman A, Thilander B. Root resorption, marginal bone support and clinical crown length in orthodontically treated patients. Eur J Orthod. 1980;2(4):197-205.

25. Wennstrom JL, Lindhe J, Sinclair F, Thilander B. Some periodontal tissue reactions to orthodontic tooth movement in monkeys. J Clin Periodontol. 1987;14(3):121-9.

26. Artun J, Krogstad O. Periodontal status of mandibular incisors following excessive proclination. A study in adults with surgically treated mandibular prognathism. Am J Orthod Dentofacial Orthop. 1987;91(3):225-32.

27. Djeu G, Hayes C, Zawaideh S. Correlation between mandibular central incisor proclination and gingival recession during fixed appliance therapy. Angle Orthod. 2002;72(3):238-45.

28. Hansen K, Pancherz H, Petersson A. Long-term effects of the Herbst appliance on the craniomandibular system with special reference to the TMJ. Eur J Orthod. 1990;12(3):244-53.

29. Melsen B, Allais D. Factors of importance for the development of dehiscences during labial movement of mandibular incisors: a retrospective study of adult orthodontic patients. Am J Orthod Dentofacial Orthop. 2005;127(5):552-61; quiz 625.

30. Van der Geld P, Oosterveld P, Kuijpers-Jagtman AM. Age-related changes of the dental aesthetic zone at rest and during spontaneous smiling and speech. Eur J Orthod. 2008;30(4):366-73.

31. Nelson PA, Artun J. Alveolar bone loss of maxillary anterior teeth in adult orthodontic patients. Am J Orthod Dentofacial Orthop. 1997;111(3):328-34.

32. Ko-Kimura N, Kimura-Hayashi M, Yamaguchi M, Ikeda T, Meguro D, Kanekawa M, et al. Some factors associated with open gingival embrasures following orthodontic treatment. Aust Orthod J. 2003;19(1):19-24.

33. Kurth JR, Kokich VG. Open gingival embrasures after orthodontic treatment in adults: prevalence and etiology. Am J Orthod Dentofacial Orthop. 2001;120(2):116-23.

34. Burke S, Burch JG, Tetz JA. Incidence and size of pretreatment overlap and posttreatment gingival embrasure space between maxillary central incisors. Am J Orthod Dentofacial Orthop. 1994;105(5):506-11.

35. Tanaka OM, Furquim BD, Pascotto RC, Ribeiro GL, Bosio JA, Maruo H. The dilemma of the open gingival embrasure between maxillary central incisors. J Contemp Dent Pract. 2008;9(6):92-8.

36. Tuverson DL. Anterior interocclusal relations. Part I. Am J Orthod. 1980;78(4):361-70.

37. Olsson M, Lindhe J. Periodontal characteristics in individuals with varying form of the upper central incisors. J Clin Periodontol. 1991;18(1):78-82.

38. Maltagliati L, Montes L. Análise dos fatores que motivam os pacientes adultos a buscarem o tratamento ortodôntico. Rev Dental Press Ortod Ortop Facial. 2007;12(6):54-60.

14

Severe root resorption resulting from orthodontic treatment: Prevalence and risk factors

Caroline Pelagio Raick Maués[1], Rizomar Ramos do Nascimento[2], Oswaldo de Vasconcellos Vilella[3]

Objective: To assess the prevalence of severe external root resorption and its potential risk factors resulting from orthodontic treatment. **Methods:** A randomly selected sample was used. It comprised conventional periapical radiographs taken in the same radiology center for maxillary and mandibular incisors before and after active orthodontic treatment of 129 patients, males and females, treated by means of the Standard Edgewise technique. Two examiners measured and defined root resorption according to the index proposed by Levander et al. The degree of external apical root resorption was registered defining resorption in four degrees of severity. To assess intra and inter-rater reproducibility, kappa coefficient was used. Chi-square test was used to assess the relationship between the amount of root resorption and patient's sex, dental arch (maxillary or mandibular), treatment with or without extractions, treatment duration, root apex stage (open or closed), root shape, as well as overjet and overbite at treatment onset. **Results:** Maxillary central incisors had the highest percentage of severe root resorption, followed by maxillary lateral incisors and mandibular lateral incisors. Out of 959 teeth, 28 (2.9%) presented severe root resorption. The following risk factors were observed: anterior maxillary teeth, overjet greater than or equal to 5 mm at treatment onset, treatment with extractions, prolonged therapy, and degree of apex formation at treatment onset. **Conclusion:** This study showed that care must be taken in orthodontic treatment involving extractions, great retraction of maxillary incisors, prolonged therapy, and/or completely formed apex at orthodontic treatment onset.

Keywords: Epidemiology. Root resorption. Orthodontics.

» The authors report no commercial, proprietary or financial interest in the products or companies described in this article.

[1] DDS in Dentistry, Fluminense Federal University (UFF).
[2] Specialist in Orthodontics, UFF.
[3] Professor, Postgraduate program in Orthodontics, UFF.

Rizomar Ramos do Nascimento
Departamento de Ortodontia Faculdade de Odontologia
Universidade Federal Fluminense, Niterói, Rio de Janeiro — Brazil
E-mail: rizonascimento@gmail.com

INTRODUCTION

External apical root resorption (EARR) is an undesirable side effect commonly associated with orthodontically induced tooth movement.[1-6] As it is considered a borderline phenomenon between cost-benefit and iatrogenesis, such resorptions gain importance not only due to being highly frequent, with potential biological damage to the patient, but also due to potential legal implications in daily orthodontic practice.

Root shortening results from a combination of complex biological activities in the region of the periodontal ligament, which will interact with force exerted during orthodontic treatment.[7] Factors such as dental trauma prior to orthodontic treatment, bone density and morphology, shape of teeth roots,[5,6,8] patient's age at orthodontic treatment onset,[9] treatment duration,[5,6,8,10] as well as orthodontic mechanics and magnitude of force[2,10-15] have been reported as significant for the occurrence of EARR.

Lateral cephalograms associated with panoramic radiograph or complete periapical radiographs are routinely requested for pretreatment planning. Studies highlight better precision of periapical radiograph when compared to panoramic radiograph when determining the magnitude of root resorption, due to lower distortion and accuracy of fine details. Therefore, an increasing number of professionals request complete periapical examination for treatment of adult orthodontic patients.[16]

The aim of this retrospective study was to determine, by means of periapical radiographs, the prevalence of severe EARR (exceeding 1/3 of the original root length) and its relationship with orthodontic treatment variables in patients treated with Edgewise Standard technique. It also assessed potential risk factors.

MATERIAL AND METHODS

The present study was submitted to Fluminense Federal University (UFF) Institutional Review Board (protocol #188780) and performed in accordance to its norms.

A randomly selected sample was used. It comprised conventional periapical radiographs taken in the same radiology center for all incisors of 129 patients (males and females) before and after active orthodontic treatment. Patients were treated by means of the Standard Edgewise technique in the last fifteen years at the Orthodontics Department of Fluminense Federal University (UFF). As inclusion criteria, only patients presenting periapical radiographs pre and post-treatment, and those who had completed orthodontic treatment were selected. Exclusion criteria excluded teeth with periapical lesions, history of dental trauma or endodontic treatment, patients with severe crowding in which overlap hindered visualization of roots and subsequent measurements. Low-quality radiographs were also eliminated.

All subjects were treated with conventional metallic non pre-adjusted appliances (Edgewise Standard) with 0.022 x 0.028-in bracket slots, and followed a predetermined archwire sequence during levelling and alignment: For initial leveling, 0.014-in and 0.016-in nickel-titanium (NiTi) archwires were selected, followed by 0.017 × 0.025-in, 0.019 × 0.025-in nickel-titanium (NiTi), and 0.019 × 0.025-in stainless-steel archwires. In cases involving extractions, straight 0.019 × 0.025-in stainless-steel archwires with "T" loops were used to close extraction spaces. No temporary skeletal anchorage devices were used in the selected sample.

Due to applicability and broad acceptance, the index proposed by Malmgren et al[17] was used to assess the degree of root changes yielded in this study. Zero degree was added to this index, as proposed by Levander et al,[9] in order to point out unaltered teeth in the root apex (Fig 1).

Tooth length was measured as the distance from the root apex tip to the midpoint of the incisal edge. A digital caliper (Lee Tools, Brazil) with an accuracy of ±0.02 mm and reproducibility of ±0.01 mm was used following the long axis of the tooth. Root contour of maxillary and mandibular incisors assessed before and after treatment were compared, positioning the long axis of the tooth/root parallel to the index image. The degree of EARR was assessed according to the index proposed, using a 0-4 scale of severity, as follows:

» Score 0: Absence of changes in the root apex;
» Score 1: Irregular root contour;
» Score 2: EARR of less than 2 mm;
» Score 3: EARR from 2 mm to one-third of the original root length;
» Score 4: EARR exceeding one-third of the original root length.

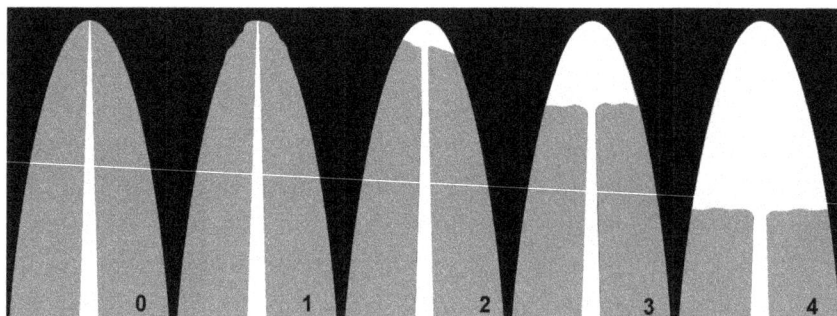

Figure 1 - Degrees of external root resorption based on Levander et al[9] adding (zero) degree in order to point out unaltered root apex.

Evaluations were carried out by two observers using an x-ray viewer with standard light intensity, equipped with a 5-x magnification loop (Cristófoli Equipamentos de Biossegurança Ltda., Campo Mourão, Paraná, Brazil). After a 15–day interval, measurements were reassessed by the observers using periapical radiographs of 20 patients (160 teeth)randomly selected before and after orthodontic treatment.

A total of 1,032 teeth were evaluated; out of which 73 were excluded, thereby totaling 959 teeth. The prevalence of EARR was calculated for each tooth. In order to identify potential risk factors, the following variables were assessed: sex, dental arch (maxillary or mandibular), treatment with or without extractions, treatment duration, root apex stage (open or closed), root shape, as well as overjet and overbite at treatment onset. Severity of resorption was scored as follows: 0-3 (none to mild EARR); 4 (severe EARR).

STATISTICAL ANALYSIS

Results were formatted in a Microsoft Office Excel (version 2007, Microsoft Office Corporation) spreadsheet. Sample size calculation was performed, and the final sample was within the recommendations established for this study.

To assess intra and inter-rater reproducibility, kappa coefficient and chi-square test were used for comparison among groups. Level of probability was set at 5% (P < 0.05).

Both statistical tests and sample size calculation were performed with the aid of QuickCalcs GraphPad software (version 2013), available at www.graphpad.com/quickcalcs.

RESULTS

Sample distribution is shown in Table 1. The means of treatment duration, overbite, overjet and changes between pre and post-treatment are demonstrated in Table 2. Overbite and overjet were measured by pre and post-treatment lateral cephalograms obtained in the same radiology center.

According to the results shown in Table 3, maxillary central incisors had the highest percentage of severe EARR, followed by maxillary lateral incisors and mandibular lateral incisors. Out of 959 teeth, 28 (2.9%) had severe EARR.

Table 4 shows the factors that could contribute to severe EARR. Anterior maxillary teeth, dental extraction for orthodontic purposes, treatment extended to more than three years, closed root apex at treatment onset and cases presenting overjet greater than or equal to 5 mm were statistically significant and, for this reason, were considered risk factors of EARR.

Kappa coefficient revealed that agreement between the two measurement times was excellent (k = 0.84). Inter observer agreement was also excellent (k = 0.81).

DISCUSSION

Periapical radiograph has been the examination most frequently used to evaluate EARR resulting from orthodontic treatment due to its higher accuracy compared to panoramic radiograph and better cost-benefit relationship compared to CT scans.[16]

In this study, apical dental alterations were classified according to the widely applicable and accepted index proposed by Malmgren et al,[17] and modified by Levander et al.[9] This method is predominantly used in

Table 1 - Sample distribution.

Variable		n
Sex	Male	397
	Female	562
Extraction	Yes	413
	No	546
Treatment duration	≤ 3 years	174
	> 3 years	785
Angle's classification	Class I	452
	Class II	428
	Class III	79

Table 2 - Continuous variables.

Variable	Mean + SD	Minimum	Maximum
Initial overbite (mm)	2.37 ± 3.4	-4	9
Initial overjet (mm)	5.37 ± 4.14	-4	14
Change in overbite (mm)	1.86 ± 1.51	0	7
Change in overjet (mm)	2.57 ± 2.32	0	11
Treatment duration (years)	7.15 ± 3.97	1	14

Table 3 - Prevalence of external apical root resorption (EARR) according to each tooth.

| Tooth | Total | | Degree of final resorption | | | | | | | | | | | | |
| | n | (%) | Degree 0 | | Degree 1 | | Degree 2 | | Degree 3 | | Degree 0-3 | | Degree 4 | |
			n	(%)	n	(%)	n	(%)	n	(%)	n	(%)	n	(%)
11	121	100	24	(19.8)	19	(15.7)	55	(45.4)	15	(12.3)	113	(93.4)	8	(6.6)
12	118	100	22	(18.6)	16	(13.5)	56	(47.4)	19	(16.1)	113	(95.8)	5	(4.2)
21	120	100	26	(22.1)	20	(16.6)	51	(42.5)	15	(12.5)	112	(93.3)	8	(6.6)
22	118	100	26	(22.0)	18	(15.2)	49	(41.5)	20	(16.9)	113	(95.7)	5	(4.2)
31	120	100	43	(35.8)	41	(34.2)	30	(25.0)	6	(5.0)	120	100	0	(0.0)
32	120	100	53	(44.1)	33	(27.5)	30	(25.0)	3	(2.5)	119	(99.2)	1	(0.8)
41	121	100	49	(40.5)	40	(33.0)	27	(22.3)	5	(4.1)	121	100	0	(0.0)
42	121	100	60	(49.6)	29	(23.9)	27	(22.3)	4	(3.3)	120	(99.2)	1	(0.8)
Total	959	100	303	(31.6)	216	(22.5)	325	(33.9)	87	(9.0)	931	(97.1)	28	(2.9)

Table 4 - Analysis of variables related to severe external root resorption (EARR).

| Variable | | Severe root resorption | | Total (%) | χ² | P-value |
		Absent n (%)	Present n (%)			
Sex	Male	389 (98.0)	8 (2.0)	397 (100)	1.95	0.162
	Female	542 (96.4)	20 (3.5)	562(100)		
Dental arch	Upper	451 (94.5)	26(5.4)	477 (100)	22.3	0.000
	Lower	480 (99.6)	2 (0.4)	482 (100)		
Extraction	Yes	389 (94.1)	24 (5.8)	413 (100)	21.3	0.000
	No	542 (99.2)	4 (0.7)	546 (100)		
Treatment duration	< 3 years	174 (100)	0 (0)	174 (100)	6.4	0.011
	> 3 years	757 (96.4)	28 (3.6)	785 (100)		
Apex	Open	264 (100)	0 (0)	264 (100)	10.9	0.000
	Closed	667 (96.6)	28 (4.0)	695 (100)		
Root shape*	Romboidal	325 (96.7)	11 (3.3)	336 (100)	0.97	0.324
	Triangular	342 (95.2)	17 (4.7)	359 (100)		
Overjet	< 5 mm	516 (98.7)	7 (1.3)	523 (100)	10.4	0.001
	≥ 5 mm	415 (95.2)	21 (4.8)	436 (100)		
Overbite	< 5 mm	693 (96.9)	22 (3.1)	715 (100)	0.24	0.624
	≥ 5 mm	238 (97.5)	6 (2.5)	244 (100)		

*The sum of root shapes T and R (695) corresponding to the number of teeth with closed apex.

root resorption studies performed after orthodontically induced tooth movement, and has the major advantage of not depending on standardization of initial radiographs.[13,18,19] An important factor that must be considered in studies involving variables is the adequate review of the error of the method . The method used herein seems reliable, showing an excellent correlation between the two measurements. Intra and inter observer error of method was considered of little importance. These results validate the methods used to collect data in this research.

In the present investigation, the risk factors associated with severe EARR were teeth located in the anterior region of the maxillary arch, treatment involving extractions, treatment duration (over 3 years), overjet greater than or equal to 5 mm at treatment onset, and complete root formation (closed apex) also at treatment onset. It was not possible to relate the degree of resorption to root shape, the amount of overbite at treatment onset, or to patient's sex.

In agreement with the results of other researches,[1,5,6,12,18,20,21] the present study found a low number of teeth with severe EARR (2.9%), while 97.1% showed no resorption or resorption classified as moderate, i.e., clinically accepted as part of the biological costs of orthodontic treatment. Marques et al[22] analyzed 1,049 patients treated by means of the Edgewise technique alone. The authors found high percentages of severe resorption (14.5%). However, they reported difficulties in comparing the prevalence found in their research with the findings of other studies because their sample was larger than those found in the literature, which allowed the inclusion of more variables. Furthermore, they cited differences in methods and techniques as a factor that could help explain this discrepancy. Lim et al[23] found differences in procedures used in routine clinical practice, such as the use of light forces and/or rest periods (discontinuous forces) every two to three months. Thus, groups of patients treated by different professionals, allied to the relatively recent advent of superelastic material enabling the use of light and progressive forces especially in the early stages of treatment,[4,11,20] tend to show different final results.[5,6,23]

Anterior maxillary teeth proved more likely to present severe EARR than teeth located in the mandibular arch, which is in agreement with

other studies.[5,10,22,24,25,26] Previous research on intrusion and retraction movements of anterior teeth with lingual root torque,[2,12] required to reduce overjet[7] and to close extraction spaces, might support this finding. According to Martins et al,[19] patients treated with intrusion mechanics combined with anterior retraction had statistically greater maxillary incisor root resorption than those treated with anterior retraction without intrusion. This finding is probably related to greater tooth movement necessary to close extraction spaces,[8,27] specially when associated with intrusive mechanics[25] and torque movement,[2,10,12] which overburdens the dental apex. In addition, proximity between the roots of maxillary central incisors and the cortical bone of the socket, the incisive canal and the alveolar bone on the buccal surface, combined with the type of movement may explain the higher incidence of severe EARR in these teeth.[24] On the other hand, if the extraction space is used to relieve crowding,[28] which is usual in the mandibular arch, incisors might not be submitted to major retractions. This could explain the discrepancy between maxillary and mandibular teeth in this study.

The present investigation found that treatment duration was significantly correlated with severe EARR. Extended treatment duration is cited as a risk factor in the development of severe EARR,[5,6,10,26] although some authors do not agree with this finding.[1,8,13,19,21] Confounding factors, such as more difficult treatment plans, appointment intervals and lack of patient's cooperation, can increase treatment time and also be related to EARR.[26] Moreover, longer treatment time might reflect more severe malocclusion and the need for different treatment mechanics, thereby resulting in extended period of time for treatment finishing. For example, by assessing the influence of metal and ceramic brackets on root resorption, some authors reported a higher incidence of EARR in patients treated with ceramic brackets. According to these authors, treatment with ceramic brackets lasts longer, which may explain these findings.[29] Harris and Baker[30] stated that there is a threshold time at which the dynamic process is overwhelmed and significant resorption takes place. Therefore, it can be hypothesized that continuous stimulation of the root leads to increased root resorption, and accumulation of surface root resorption over a long period of time can lead to the onset of severe EARR.[24]

We did not assess the association between inter-maxillary elastics and EARR in this study. However, several authors have related the use of elastics and EARR,[8,24,25] while others have not found this association in their studies.[6] In our sample, all patients used elastics for treatment finishing. Those who showed less cooperation usually had treatment time and the use of elastics increased. It seems reasonable to assume that long-term jiggling forces caused by intermittent use of elastics can be a contributing factor in the prevalence of EARR.[24]

Most studies have found an association between orthodontic treatment with extraction and the presence of severe EARR.[5,6,24,27] In the present study, cases with extraction presented significantly more severe EARR than those treated without extractions. Increased movement and retraction of the apex of incisors are necessary to close extraction spaces. Additionally, extraction cases usually require longer treatment time for orthodontic treatment finishing. Thus, it could be assumed that tooth extraction can increase the amount of movement and the duration of treatment, thereby playing an important role as a risk factor.

With respect to overjet, significant association between its magnitude and the presence of severe EARR was observed, which is in agreement with other researches.[3,5,6,8,28] Brin et al[3] reported similar association in incisor retraction used to reduce overjet during fixed-appliance treatment. Nevertheless, this type of tooth movement was reduced in patients who underwent early therapy to reduce Class II malocclusion (e.g., headgear and/or functional appliances as a first phase of treatment). The authors stated that early growth modification, which reduces the severity of overjet in Class II malocclusions, might play an important role in reducing the likelihood of severe EARR.

It was found that teeth with complete root formation at treatment onset are more likely to develop severe EARR, which is in agreement with other researches.[28,29] Teeth with incomplete root formation at orthodontic treatment onset continue to develop their roots during therapy.[29] In adults, the periodontal ligament becomes less vascularized, aplastic and narrow; the bone becomes denser, avascular and aplastic; and the cementum wider.[28] These physiological changes could explain the higher susceptibility to severe EARR found in this study.

In contrast to other studies, our study revealed no correlation between patient's sex, root shape, the amount of overbite at treatment onset and the amount of severe EARR. Table 2 shows that our sample presented lower mean values of overbite than those found for overjet, for values measured before treatment and the reduction values of these variables. This may explain the poor relationship between overbite and EARR found in our study.

The results of this study suggest that care must be taken in orthodontic treatment with extraction, in which great retraction of maxillary incisors is planned; treatment that exceeds three years; and specially treatment involving anterior maxillary teeth with completely formed apex at orthodontic treatment onset. Considering that severity of malocclusion, rather than its type (e.g. Angle's classification),[8] is a determining factor in the amount and type of tooth movement as well as in the orthodontic mechanics used and the duration of orthodontic treatment, it can be assumed that EARR has a multifactorial cause, regardless of the sagittal characteristics of malocclusion.

CONCLUSION

The prevalence of severe EARR resulting from orthodontic treatment was considered low in this study (2.9%). Risk factors involved were as follows: treatment with extraction, anterior maxillary teeth, overjet greater than or equal to 5 mm at treatment onset, prolonged therapy and teeth with complete root formation at treatment onset; all of which suggest that EARR is a multifactorial phenomenon.

REFERENCES

1. Artun J, Van't Hullenaar R, Doppel D, Kuijpers-Jagtman AM. Identification of orthodontic patients at risk of severe apical root resorption. Am J Orthod Dentofacial Orthop. 2009;135(4):448-55.

2. Bartley N, Türk T, Colak C, Elekdag-Türk S, Jones A, Petocz P, et al. Physical properties of root cementum: Part 17. Root resorption after the application of 2.50 and 150 of buccal root torque for 4 weeks: a micro computed tomography study. Am J Orthod Dentofacial Orthop. 2011;139(4):e353-60.

3. Brin I, Tulloch JC, Koroluk L, Philips C. External apical root resorption in Class II malocclusion: a retrospective review of 1- versus 2-phase treatment. Am J Orthod Dentofacial Orthop. 2003;124(2):151-6.

4. Montenegro VJ, Jones A, Petocz P, Gonzales C, Darendeliler MA. Physical properties of root cementum: Part 22. Root resorption after the application of light and heavy extrusive orthodontic forces: a microcomputed tomography study Am J Orthod Dentofacial Orthop. 2012;141(1):e1-9.

5. Sameshima GT, Sinclair PM. Predicting and preventing root resorption: Part I. Diagnostic factors. Am J Orthod Dentofacial Orthop. 2001;119(5):505-10.

6. Sameshima GT, Sinclair PM. Predicting and preventing root resorption: Part II. Treatment factors. Am J Orthod Dentofacial Orthop. 2001;119(5):511-5.

7. Krishnan V, Davidovitch Z. Cellular, molecular, and tissue-level reactions to orthodontic force. Am J Orthod Dentofacial Orthop. 2006;129(4):469.e1-32.

8. Mirabella AD, Artun J. Risk factors for apical root resorption of maxillary anterior teeth in adult orthodontic patients. Am J Orthod Dentofacial Orthop. 1995;108(1):48-55.

9. Levander E, Malmgren O, Stenback K. Apical root resorption during orthodontic treatment of patients with multiple aplasia: a study of maxillary incisors. Eur J Orthod. 1998;20(4):427-34.

10. Liou EJW, Chang PMH. Apical root resorption in orthodontics patients with en-masse maxillary anterior retraction and intrusion with miniscrews. Am J Orthod Dentofacial Orthop. 2010;137(2):207-12.

11. Chan E, Darendeliler MA. Physical properties of root cementum: Part 5. Volumetric analysis of root resorption craters after application of light and heavy orthodontic forces. Am J Orthod Dentofacial Orthop. 2005;127(2):186-95.

12. Parker RJ, Harris EF. Directions of orthodontic tooth movements associated with external apical root resorption of the maxillary central incisor. Am J Orthod Dentofacial Orthop. 1998;114(6):677-83.

13. Levander E, Malmgren O. Evaluation of the risk of root resorption during orthodontic treatment: a study of upper incisors. Eur J Orthod. 1988;10(1):30-8.

14. Weltman B, Vig KL, Fields HW, Shanker S, Kaizar EE. Root resorption associated with orthodontic tooth movement: a systematic review. Am J Orthod Dentofacial Orthop. 2010;137(4):462-76.

15. Wu AJ, Tamer T, Colak C, Elekdag-Turk S, Jones AS, Petocz P, Darendeliler MA. Physical Properties of root cementum: Part 18. The extent of root resorption after the application of light and heavy controlled rotational orthodontic forces for 4 weeks: a microcomputed tomography study. Am J Orthod Dentofacial Orthop. 2011;139(5):E495-503.

16. Sameshima GT, Asgarifar KO. Assessment of root resorption and root shape: periapical vs panoramic films. Angle Orthod. 2001;71(3):185-9.

17. Malmgren O, Goldson L, Hill C, Orwin A, Petrini L, Lundberg M. Root resorption after orthodontic treatment of traumatized teeth. Am J Orthod. 1982;82(6):487-91.

18. Janson GP, Canto GL, Martins DR, Henriques JC, Freitas MR. A radiographic comparison of apical root resorption after orthodontic treatment with 3 different fixed appliance techniques. Am J Orthod Dentofacial Orthop. 1999;118(3):262-73.

19. Martins DR, Tibola D, Janson G, Maria FR. Effects of intrusion combined with anterior retaction on apical root resorption. Eur J Orthod. 2012;34(2):170-5.

20. Smale I, Artun J, Faraj B, Doppel D, van't Hof M, Kuijpers-Jagtman AM. Apical root resorption 6 months after initiation of fixed orthodontic appliance therapy. Am J Orthod Dentofacial Orthop. 2005;128(1):57-67.

21. Makedonas D, Lund H, Hansen K. Root resorption diagnosed with cone beam computed tomography after 6 months and at the end of orthodontic treatment with fixed appliances. Angle Orthod. 2013;83(3):389-93.

22. Marques LS, Ramos-Jorge ML, Rey AC, Armond MC, Ruellas AC. Severe root resorption in orthodontic patients treated with the edgewise method: Prevalence and predictive factors. Am J Orthod Dentofacial Orthop. 2010;137(3):384-8.

23. Lim E, Sameshima G, Petocz P, Darendeliler A.Comparison of Australian and American orthodontic clinical approaches towards root resorption. Aust Orthod J. 2012;28(2):181-9.

24. Motokawa M, Sasamoto T, Kaku M, Kawata T, Matsuda Y, Terao A, Tanne K. Association between root resorption incident to orthodontic treatment and treatment factors. Eur J Orthod. 2012;34(3):350-6.

25. Chiqueto K, Martins DR, Janson G. Effects of accentuated and reversed curve of Spee on apical root resorption. Am J Orthod Dentofacial Orthop. 2008;133(2):261-8.

26. Jung YH, Cho BH. External root resorption after orthodontic treatment: a study of contributing factors. Imaging Sci Dent. 2011;41:17-21.

27. Freitas MR, Beltrão RTS, Janson G, Henriques JF, Chiqueto K. Evaluation of root resorption after open bite treatment with and without extractions. Am J Orthod Dentofacial Orthop. 2007;132(2):143.e15-22.

28. Nanekrungsan K, Patanaporn V, Janhom A, Korwanich N. External apical root resorption in maxillary incisors in orthodontic patients: associated factors and radiographic evaluation. Imaging Sci Dent. 2012;42:147-54.

29. Lopatiene K, Dumbravait A. Risk factors of root resorption after orthodontic treatment. Stomatol Baltic Dent Maxillofac J. 2008;10:89-95.

30. Harris EF, Baker WC. Loss of root length and crestal bone height before and during treatment in adolescent and adult orthodontic patients. Am J Orthod Dentofacial Orthop. 1990;98(5):463-9.

15

Influence of treatment including second molars on final and postretention molar angulation

Luiz Filiphe Gonçalves Canuto[1], Karina Maria Salvatores de Freitas[2], Marcos Roberto de Freitas[3], Rodrigo Hermont Cançado[4]

Objective: Evaluate axial mesiodistal inclinations of the mandibular molars in orthodontically treated cases, analyzing whether inclusion of second mandibular molars in treatment mechanics has any influence on final and postretention molars angulations. **Methods:** The sample comprised 150 panoramic radiographs of 50 patients. Patients were treated with extraction of four first premolars and divided into 2 groups: Group 1 comprised 25 subjects without inclusion of mandibular second molars during orthodontic treatment, whereas Group 2 comprised 25 subjects with inclusion of mandibular second molars. Panoramic radiographs at three observation times were evaluated: pretreatment, post-treatment and postretention. The statistical analysis included one-way analysis of variance (ANOVA) for intragroup evaluation and independent t-tests for intergroup comparisons. **Results:** Intragroup analysis demonstrated significant uprighting of mandibular first and second molars during treatment in Group 2, which remained stable during the postretention stage. Intergroup comparison demonstrated that Group 2 presented first and second molars significantly more uprighted in relation to Group 1 in both post-treatment and postretention stages. **Conclusions:** It was concluded that inclusion of mandibular second molars in the orthodontic mechanics is relevant not only to correct the angulation of these teeth, but also to aid mandibular first molars uprighting.

Keywords: Panoramic X-ray. Tooth angulation. Tooth movement.

[1] Professor of graduate program in Orthodontics at the Brazilian Dental Association / Pernambuco (ABO-PE).
[2] Professor of the graduate program in Orthodontics at UNINGÁ.
[3] Full professor of Pediatric Dentistry, Orthodontics and Public Health at USP, Bauru Dental School.
[4] Associate professor at UNINGÁ.

» The authors report no commercial, proprietary or financial interest in the products or companies described in this article.

Luiz Filiphe Gonçalves Canuto
Rua José Bonifácio, 205 – Sl 109 – Madalena – Recife/PE, Brazil
CEP: 50.710-000 – E-mail: luizfiliphecanuto@yahoo.com.br

INTRODUCTION

The importance of appropriate mesiodistal teeth angulation in orthodontic patients has been emphasized by many clinicians. In 1972, Andrews reported that tooth angulation is one of the 6 keys to be evaluated in ideal static occlusions.[1]

It has been reported that the final spatial orientation of each tooth should be such that it can best withstand the forces during function. Corrected angulation is universally accepted, and other several related parameters have been studied. These include periodontal health,[1,2,3] even distribution of occlusal forces through contact points, tight posterior occlusion, no spaces as well as retention and stability of orthodontically closed extraction sites.[1,4-7] The American Board of Orthodontics has included assessment of mesiodistal angulation in panoramic radiographs as a parameter for evaluating finished cases for orthodontists aspiring to be board diplomate.

Adequate mesiodistal teeth angulations with roots parallel to each other are frequently mentioned in the literature[1,3,8,9-13] as a fact that not only improves teeth alignment stability in their apical bases, but also allows normal maxilomandibular occlusion.[6] Moreover, an adequate mesiodistal positioning allows a uniform distribution of occlusal forces through contact points and contributes to overall treatment stability.[3,6,10]

Given the importance of appropriate mesiodistal teeth angulation in orthodontic patients regarding quality and stability of treatment, the authors aimed to investigate the influence of mandibular second molars inclusion in orthodontic mechanics on final and postretention molar angulations.

MATERIAL AND METHODS

Material

The sample comprised 150 panoramic radiographs of 50 young patients of both genders. The radiographs were taken from the files of Pediatric Dentistry, Orthodontics and Public Health Department at University of São Paulo (USP), Bauru Dental School. Each case was evaluated at three stages: pretreatment (T_1), posttreatment (T_2) and after a minimum of 3 years of follow-up (T_3).

When selecting the sample, the following inclusion criteria were applied: cases initially presenting Class I or Class II malocclusion, treated with fixed Edgewise appliances and extraction of four first premolars. All subjects had all permanent teeth erupted except the third molars at the pretreatment stage. Other inclusion criteria were patients with no history of previous interceptive orthodontic treatment, absence of root dilaceration or mandibular skeletal asymmetries.

After active treatment, all patients wore a modified Hawley retainer in the maxillary arch, full time for the first 12 months and during sleep for the next 6 months. A lingual canine-to-canine mandibular bonded retainer was placed and left for a mean period of 3 years.

Methods

The sample was divided into two groups:

» Group 1: 25 patients (14 female; 11 male) in whom the mandibular second molars were not included in treatment mechanics.

» Group 2: 25 patients (15 female; 10 male) with mandibular second molars included in treatment mechanics.

The mean pretreatment age was 13.29 ± 1.44 years for Group 1 and 12.95 ± 1.26 years for Group 2. The mean treatment, retention and postretention evaluation times of each group are shown in Table 1.

First and second molar angulations were evaluated with panoramic radiographs (orthopantomography) traced manually by a single investigator, in acetate paper (Ultraphan Paper®, Berlin, Germany).

Table 1 - Descriptive statistics of treatment, retention and postretention evaluation mean times for Groups 1 and 2, with and without inclusion of second molars, respectively.

Time (years)	Group 1 2nd molar not included (n=25)	Group 2 2nd molar included (n=25)
	Mean ± SD	Mean ± SD
Treatment	2.41 ± 0.64	2.45 ± 0.53
Retention	1.33 ± 0.51	1.49 ± 0.76
Posttreatment	4.84 ± 2.38	4.18 ± 2.47

Tracing method

The tracing procedure of the initial, posttreatment and postretention radiographs was conducted in four phases: a) Delineation of dentoskeletal structures; b) Definition of reference points; c) Definition of horizontal and vertical reference lines; d) Measurement of tooth angulation (Fig 1).

a) Delineation of dentoskeletal structures:

The external outline of the mandible, mental foramen, and outlines of mandibular first and second molars roots and crowns were traced.

b) Definition of landmarks:

The definition of the landmarks was performed as proposed by Tavano et al:[14]

1) Right mental foramen (RMF) – The central point of the right mental foramen.
2) Left mental foramen (LMF) – The central point of the left mental foramen.

c) Tracing of horizontal and vertical reference lines:

1) Intermental line (IL): Line passing through the centers of the right and left mental foramens.
2) First and second molars long axes: The long axes of the mentioned teeth were determined as the mean of the images of mesial and distal root canals[13].

d) Angles measurement:

The angles formed by the Intermental line (IL) and the long axes of the first and second mandibular molars were then measured (Fig 1).

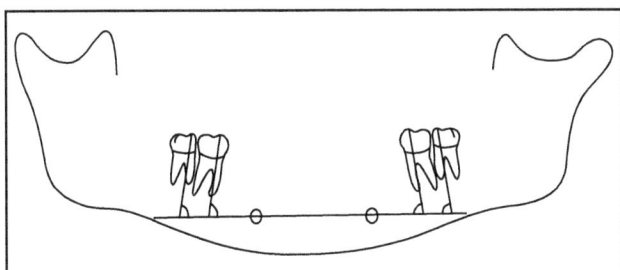

Figure 1 - Manual tracing performed at initial, final and posttreatment panoramic radiographs involving the delineation of dentoskeletal structures, demarcation of landmarks (RMF and LMF), vertical and horizontal reference lines and measurement of dental angulations.

Statistical analyses

Statistical analysis was performed with Statistica software (Statistica for Windows, version 7.0, StatSoft Inc).

To avoid type I error (probability of accepting the alternative hypothesis H1 and be wrong) sample was calculated considering $\alpha = 5\%$ (type I error), $\beta = 20\%$ (type II error), an estimated variability (s) of 5 degrees and a minimum detectable difference (d) of 5 degrees.

In each group, means and standard deviations for the mesiodistal inclination of the four evaluated teeth (left mandibular first molar-36; left mandibular second molar-37; right mandibular first molar-46; and right mandibular second molar-47) were determined. The intragroup comparison of these variables at the three observation stages was performed by one-way dependent ANOVA and Tukey tests as a second step. For intergroup comparison, t-tests were used. Prior to the use of ANOVA and t-tests, analyses of data normality and homoscedasticity of the groups was performed with Kolmogorov-Smirnov and Levene tests, respectively.

Method error

Within a week interval from the first measurement, 30 randomly selected radiographs were retraced and remeasured by the same examiner. The random error was calculated according to Dahlberg's formula $(Se^2 = \Sigma d^2/2n)$ and the systematic error was calculated with dependent t-tests, for $p < 0.05$.

RESULTS

Results for power analysis showed that a sample with 23 patients in each group would give a 80% ability to detect differences, whereas a sample comprising 26 patients in each group would give 85%.

Results for the data distribution evaluation performed by the Kolmogorov-Smirnov test showed $p > 0.05$ for both groups, for all variables evaluated, indicating that the data had normal distribution. Levene test was used to verify homoscedasticity. All results exhibited $p > 0.05$ for both groups, during the three stages evaluated. Thus, it was concluded that there was homogeneity of variables and that the ANOVA test could be applied for intragroup analysis.

The results for intragroup comparison in Group 1 (#37 and #47 teeth not included) demonstrated no statistically significant differences between the mean values for the mesiodistal inclinations of the teeth (36, 37, 46 and 47) at the three evaluated stages. On the other hand, results for the intragroup comparison in Group 2 (#37 and #47 teeth included) demonstrated significant uprighting of mandibular first and second molars throughout treatment, which remained stable during the postretention stage (Table 2).

Intergroup comparison demonstrated that Group 2 presented the first and second molars significantly uprighted in relation to Group 1 at both posttreatment and postretention stages (Table 3).

No significant systematic errors were detected and the major random error was of 1.27 degrees for the left mandibular first molar mesiodistal inclination.

DISCUSSION

Throughout this research, significant efforts were expended in order to minimize, or at least control the errors deriving from the procedures involved in panoramic radiograph tracings, demarcation of landmarks and measurement of the variables investigated. Knowledge of the methodology precision provided more reliable results. It was observed that the results obtained for random and systematic errors were within acceptable parameters, thus, not influencing the results and conclusions of the present study.

The methodology of this study was based on previous researches[9,13,14] that also used panoramic radiographs to obtain tooth angulation measurements. Panoramic radiographs are ordinarily used in orthodontic practice to provide significant information about teeth, axial inclinations, maturation periods, and surrounding tissues.[8,12,13,19] Some authors suggest that dental axial inclinations be radiographically checked at the beginning and end of orthodontic treatment.[3,5,7-10,13,16,17,19] Panoramic radiographs may be the technique of choice since it provides significant amount of diagnostic information obtained by viewing all teeth as well as the basal bone at once. In addition, it is the best option to evaluate teeth axial inclinations and root parallelism after orthodontic treatment.[2,5-7,11,12,13,15,17,24]

As occurring in other radiographic methods, the dimensions of structures in panoramic radiographs can be magnified[5,7,8,11,12,13,15-19] and due to distortions, hori-

Table 2 - Means and standard deviations of mesiodistal inclinations of the teeth (36, 37, 46 and 47) at the three evaluation stages (T_1, T_2 and T_3) for Groups 1 (second molars not included in treatment, n = 25) and 2 (second molars included, n = 25) and results of dependent ANOVA and Tukey tests.

Molar angulation	Initial (T_1) Mean ± SD	Posttreatment (T_2) Mean ± SD	Postretention (T_3) Mean ± SD	p
36 G1	59.60[A] ± 5.27	62.22[A] ± 6.57	62.56[A] ± 5.01	0.13
36 G2	56.80[A] ± 5.60	66.04[B] ± 4.87	66.26[B] ± 5.37	0.00*
37 G1	57.92[A] ± 8.07	56.66[A] ± 6.03	57.94[A] ± 8.35	0.79
37 G2	55.24[A] ± 6.70	65.56[B] ± 6.96	66.50[B] ± 6.94	0.00*
46 G1	62.92[A] ± 6.35	67.60[A] ± 6.94	65.08[A] ± 6.59	0.05
46 G2	64.68[A] ± 4.08	71.42[B] ± 3.97	70.88[B] ± 5.83	0.00*
47 G1	60.54[A] ± 8.01	62.98[A] ± 6.38	63.52[A] ± 9.90	0.39
47 G2	57.26[A] ± 10.24	70.08[B] ± 8.77	68.10[B] ± 6.03	0.00*

*Statistically significant for p < 0.05. Different letters mean a statistically significant difference between the phases.

Table 3 - Means and standard deviations of mesiodistal inclinations of the teeth (36, 37, 46 and 47) at the three evaluation stages (T_1, T_2 and T_3) for Group 2 (second molars included) and results of dependent ANOVA and Tukey tests.

Molar angulation	Initial (T_1) Mean ± SD	Posttreatment (T_2) Mean ± SD	Postretention (T_3) Mean ± SD	p
36	56.80[A] ± 5.60	66.04[B] ± 4.87	66.26[B] ± 5.37	0.00*
37	55.24[A] ± 6.70	65.56[B] ± 6.96	66.50[B] ± 6.94	0.00*
46	64.68[A] ± 4.08	71.42[B] ± 3.97	70.88[B] ± 5.83	0.00*
47	57.26[A] ± 10.24	70.08[B] ± 8.77	68.10[B] ± 6.03	0.00*

*Statistically significant for p < 0.05. Different letters mean a statistically significant difference between the phases.

zontal measurements are unreliable.[17,19] In this study, panoramic radiograph magnification did not influence the results, as the same radiographic equipment and similar techniques were used for both groups. Thus, when Groups 1 and 2 were compared, the possible influence of this variable was eliminated.

Accuracy of tooth length and angulation measurements on panoramic radiographs is thought to be highly dependent on head positioning technique.[18,20] Stramotas et al[18] noted a significant error (p < 0.05) in such measurements when the occlusal plane was tilted up anteriorly by 8 degrees. A lateral cant of the occlusal plane less than 10 degrees without an upward anterior rotation showed no significant effect on the measurements. Regarding angular measurements, the literature reports that the analysis of dental angulations through panoramic radiographs can be performed with good reliability[8,11,12,13,15,17,18,19] and that there is some tolerance of variation in head position.[18] During the radiographic examination, all patients who comprised the sample were positioned with both the occlusal plane parallel and the sagittal plane perpendicular to the ground.

Recent studies have compared the accuracy of assessing mesiodistal root angulations with posttreatment panoramic radiographs and with cone-beam computed tomography (CT). The results show that CT is the most accurate method for assessing dental angulation.[21,22] Thus, assessment of mesiodistal tooth angulations with panoramic radiograph should be approached with caution and reinforced by a thorough clinical examination of the dentition.[23] However, due to economic as well as biological reasons, CT should not be considered for clinical routine, but rather only for mesiodistal root angulations evaluation, before, during or after orthodontic treatment. The use of panoramic radiograph as data source may be considered a limitation of this study. The use of CT could result not only in a more accurate assessment of the mesiodistal root angulations, but it could also enable tridimensional evaluation of the teeth. Another limitation of this research is the fact that it evaluated the mandibular molars changes, only.

Results of Group 1 (#37 and #47 teeth not included) intragroup comparison demonstrated no statistically significant differences between the mean values for the mesiodistal inclinations of the teeth (36, 37, 46 and 47) at the three evaluation stages (T_1, T_2 and T_3) (Table 2). However, results of Group 2 (37 and 47 included) intragroup comparison demonstrated significant uprighting of mandibular first and second molars during treatment, which remained stable at the postretention stage (Table 2). Regarding the assessment of changes in mesiodistal dental inclination as a result of orthodontic treatment, there are few studies that could be used for comparisons, and most of them are related to patterns of normal occlusion.

In an attempt to establish a basis for quantitative evaluation of mesiodistal axial inclinations of permanent teeth after orthodontic treatment, Ursi et al[13] conducted a study that determined the normal mean values for dental angulations through panoramic radiographs. For the authors, the mesiodistal root angulations of high quality orthodontic treatment exhibited in the final panoramic radiographs should be similar to normal occlusion values. In the present study, it was noted that the mean values obtained for the mesiodistal inclinations of the teeth (36, 37, 46 and 47) at posttreatment and postretention phases in Group 2 (with inclusion of the second molars) were closer to the normal values proposed by Ursi et al.[13]

In 2002, Brandão[9] evaluated if alterations in the mesiodistal axial inclination of the mandibular anterior teeth would present any influence in the relapse of their crowding. The panoramic radiographic and dental casts of each patient were evaluated at the beginning (T_1), at the end (T_2) and five-year posttreatment (T_3) phases. Results showed that the mesiodistal axial inclinations of the teeth at the beginning of treatment were different from those observed in normal occlusion cases in 85% of the evaluated teeth. However, 45% of the teeth at the end, and 55% at the five-year posttreatment phase showed mean values similar to those of normal occlusion. Evaluation of mesiodistal axial inclination stability at the five-year posttreatment phase demonstrates that 75% of the teeth proved to maintain the angulation obtained at the end of the treatment, regardless of being similar or not to the normal values. The changes in the mesiodistal axial inclination between T_2 and T_3 did not influence the relapse of mandibular anterior crowding.

In 2006, Almeida-Pedrin et al[8] evaluated, through panoramic radiographs, the mesiodistal axial inclinations of the maxillary anterior teeth at the beginning and end of nonextraction orthodontic treatment. The experimental sample comprised 40 Caucasian patients who were treated orthodontically with a standard Edgewise technique, without extractions. The mesiodistal axial inclinations of the maxillary anterior teeth of

Table 4 - Intergroup comparison of mesiodistal inclinations of the teeth (36, 37, 46 and 47) at the three evaluation stages (T_1, T_2 and T_3) with t-test.

Molar angulation	Group 1 Second molar not included (n = 25) Mean ± SD	Group 2 Second molar included (n = 25) Mean ± SD	p
36 T_1	59.60 ± 5.27	56.80 ± 5.60	0.07
36 T_2	62.22 ± 6.57	66.04 ± 4.87	0.02*
36 T_3	62.56 ± 5.01	66.26 ± 5.37	0.01*
37 T_1	57.92 ± 8.07	55.24 ± 6.70	0.20
37 T_2	56.66 ± 6.03	65.56 ± 6.96	0.00*
37 T_3	57.94 ± 8.35	66.50 ± 6.94	0.00*
46 T_1	62.92 ± 6.35	64.68 ± 4.08	0.25
46 T_2	67.60 ± 6.94	71.42 ± 3.97	0.02*
46 T_3	65.08 ± 6.59	70.88 ± 5.83	0.00*
47 T_1	60.54 ± 8.01	57.26 ± 10.24	0.21
47 T_2	62.98 ± 6.38	70.08 ± 8.77	0.00*
47 T_3	63.52 ± 9.90	68.10 ± 6.03	0.05

*Statistically significant for p < 0.05.

the experimental group at T_1 were different from those of the control group for 50% of the evaluated teeth. In contrast, the inclinations at T_2 were consistent with the normal anatomical configuration of the controls. The authors concluded that panoramic radiograph is an effective tool for evaluating the mesiodistal axial inclinations of maxillary anterior teeth.

In 2009, Sella et al.[25] compared the normal mean values of mesiodistal axial angulations, proposed by Ursi et al,[13] with mesiodistal axial angulations of canine teeth, premolars and inferior molars in individuals aged between 18 and 25 years old, with and without the presence of the mandibular third molars. The authors concluded that the groups presented similar angular values for the canine teeth, premolars and inferior molars in such a way that the presence of the third molars did not influence dental angulations.

The intergroup comparison (Table 4) demonstrated statistically significant differences with regards to mesiodistal inclinations of mandibular first and second molars at T_2. Patients with mandibular second molars included in treatment mechanics presented mandibular first and second molars more uprighted. At T_3, mesiodistal inclinations of the molars remained significantly different be-

tween groups, except for the mean values for angulation of mandibular right second molars (#47 – T_3) that, despite not statistically significant (p = 0.05), were, on average, approximately 5 degrees more upright in comparison to Group 1. There are some limitations hindering comparison between these intergroup results with other studies, namely: the nonexistence of previous studies with similar objectives in the literature and their methodological differences. However, based on the results of this research, it may be inferred that the inclusion of second mandibular molars in orthodontic mechanics benefits not only the mandibular second molars, but also first molars uprighting, as the mandibular first molars in Group 2 were more uprighted at posttreatment and postretention stages (Tables 2 and 3). Additionally, the results suggest that the inclusion of second molars in orthodontic mechanics probably consists in a distal support that improves first molar uprighting.

There are some doubts and controversies about the necessity of second molars inclusion during orthodontic treatment. Two of the major goals of treatment consist in leveling the curve of Spee and correcting overbite. Thus, nothing is more rational than using the second molars to provide an anchorage that allows anterior teeth intrusion and correction of the curve of Spee. When using Class II elastics, the second molar inclusion increases arch length. Therefore, there is not only an increase in the horizontal component of force, but also a decrease of the vertical component. This fact is generally favorable because it facilitates sagittal interarch adjustment and prevents first molars extrusion. In extraction cases, mandibular second molars inclusion provides posterior anchorage improvement and avoids inclination and rotation of the first molars. It is also indicated for crossbites, proclined or rotated second molars cases as well as surgical cases. However, there are clinical situations in which inclusion of second molars may be contraindicated, such as in patients with initial anterior open bite and vertical facial growth tendency.

CONCLUSION

Inclusion of mandibular second molars in orthodontic mechanics is relevant not only for the correction of mandibular second molars mesiodistal inclination, but also for first molars uprighting.

REFERENCES

1. Andrews LF. The six keys to normal occlusion. Am J Orthod. 1972;62(3):296-309.
2. Dempster WT, Adams WJ, Duddles RA. Arrangement in the jaws of the roots of the teeth. J Am Dent Assoc. 1963;67:779-97.
3. Hatasaka HH. A radiographic study of roots in extraction sites. Angle Orthod. 1976;46(1):64-8.
4. Beyron H. Optimal occlusion. Dent Clin North Am. 1969;13(3):537-54.
5. Ingervall B. Functionally optimal occlusion: the goal of orthodontic treatment. Am J Orthod. 1976;70(1):81-90.
6. Mayoral G. Treatment results with light wires studied by panoramic radiography. Am J Orthod. 1982;81(6):489-97.
7. Williams R. Eliminating lower retention. J Clin Orthod. 1985;19(5):342-9.
8. Almeida-Pedrin RR, Pinzan A, Almeida RR, Ursi W, Almeida MR. Panoramic evaluation of mesiodistal axial inclinations of maxillary anterior teeth in orthodontically treated subjects. Am J Orthod Dentofacial Orthop. 2006;130(1):56-60.
9. Brandão AG. Estudo ortopantomográfico longitudinal das inclinações axiais mesiodistais em pacientes tratados ortodonticamente com extrações dos quatro primeiros pré-molares [dissertação]. Bauru (SP): Faculdade de Odontologia de Bauru; 2002.
10. Edwards JG. The prevention of relapse in extraction cases. Am J Orthod. 1971;60(2):128-44.
11. Jesuino FA, Costa LR, Valladares-Neto J. Mesiodistal root angulation of permanent teeth in children with mixed dentition and normal occlusion. J Appl Oral Sci. 2010;18(6):625-9.
12. Lucchesi MV, Wood RE, Nortje CJ. Suitability of the panoramic radiograph for assessment of mesiodistal angulation of teeth in the buccal segments of the mandible. Am J Orthod Dentofacial Orthop. 1988;94(4):303-10.
13. Ursi WJ, Almeida RR, Tavano O, Henriques JF. Assessment of mesiodistal axial inclination through panoramic radiography. J Clin Orthod. 1990;24(3):166-73.
14. Tavano O, Ursi WJS, Almeida RR, Henriques JFC. Determinação de linhas de referência para medições angulares em radiografias ortopantomográficas. Odontol Mod. 1989;16(9):22-5.
15. Akcam MO, Altiok T, Ozdiler E. Panoramic radiographs: a tool for investigating skeletal pattern. Am J Orthod Dentofacial Orthop. 2003;123(2):175-81.
16. McKee IW, Glover KE, Williamson PC, Lam EW, Heo G, Major PW. The effect of vertical and horizontal head positioning in panoramic radiography on mesiodistal tooth angulations. Angle Orthod. 2001;71(6):442-51.
17. McKee IW, Williamson PC, Lam EW, Heo G, Glover KE, Major PW. The accuracy of 4 panoramic units in the projection of mesiodistal tooth angulations. Am J Orthod Dentofacial Orthop. 2002;121(2):166-75.
18. Stramotas S, Geenty JP, Petocz P, Darendeliler MA. Accuracy of linear and angular measurements on panoramic radiographs taken at various positions in vitro. Eur J Orthod. 2002;24(1):43-52.
19. Larheim TA, Svanaes DB. Reproducibility of rotational panoramic radiography: mandibular linear dimensions and angles. Am J Orthod Dentofacial Orthop. 1986;90(1):45-51.
20. McDavid WD, Welander U, Brent Dove S, Tronjie G. Digital imaging in rotational panoramic radiography. Dentomaxillofac Radiol. 1995;24(2):68-75.
21. Bouwens DG, Cevidanes L, Ludlow JB, Phillips C. Comparison of mesiodistal root angulation with posttreatment panoramic radiographs and cone-beam computed tomography. Am J Orthod Dentofacial Orthop. 2011;139(1):126-32.
22. Van Elslande D, Heo G, Flores-Mir C, Carey J, Major PW. Accuracy of mesiodistal root angulation projected by cone-beam computed tomographic panoramic-like images. Am J Orthod Dentofacial Orthop. 2010;137(4 Suppl):S94-9.
23. Owens AM, Johal A. Near-end of treatment panoramic radiograph in the assessment of mesiodistal root angulation. Angle Orthod. 2008;78(3):475-81.
24. Strang RHW. Factors associated with successful orthodontic treatment. Am J Orthod. 1952;38(10):790-800.
25. Sella RC, Mendonça MR, Cuoghi OA. Avaliação ortopantomográfica das angulações mesiodistais de caninos, pré-molares e molares inferiores com e sem a presença dos terceiros molares. Rev Dental Press Ortod Ortop Facial. 2009;14(6):97-108.
26. Janson M. Ortodontia em adultos e tratamento interdisciplinar. 2a ed. Maringá: Dental Press; 2010.

16

Effect of saliva contamination on bond strength with a hydrophilic composite resin

Mauren Bitencourt Deprá[1], Josiane Xavier de Almeida[1], Taís de Morais Alves da Cunha[2],
Luis Filipe Siu Lon[2], Luciana Borges Retamoso[3], Orlando Motohiro Tanaka[4]

Objective: To evaluate the influence of saliva contamination on the bond strength of metallic brackets bonded to enamel with hydrophilic resin composite. **Methods:** Eighty premolars were randomly divided into 4 groups (n=20) according to bonding material and contamination: G1) bonded with Transbond XT with no saliva contamination, G2) bonded with Transbond XT with saliva contamination, G3) bonded with Transbond Plus Color Change with no saliva contamination and G4) bonded with Transbond Plus Color Change with saliva contamination. The results were statistically analyzed (ANOVA/Tukey). **Results:** The means and standard deviations (MPa) were: G1)10.15 ± 3.75; G2) 6.8 ± 2.54; G3) 9.3 ± 3.36; G4) 8.3 ± 2.95. The adhesive remnant index (ARI) ranged between 0 and 1 in G1 and G4. In G2 there was a prevalence of score 0 and similar ARI distribution in G3. **Conclusion:** Saliva contamination reduced bond strength when Transbond XT hydrophobic resin composite was used. However, the hydrophilic resin Transbond Plus Color Change was not affected by the contamination.
Keywords: Saliva. Orthodontic brackets. Bond strength. Adhesives.

[1] Graduate Student, School of Dentistry – PUCPR.
[2] MSc in Orthodontics, Orthodontic Department, School of Dentistry - PUCPR.
[3] PhD Student, Department of Dental Materials - PUCRS.
[4] Full professor - Orthodontics – PUCPR.

» The author reports no commercial, proprietary or financial interest in the products or companies described in this article.

Orlando Tanaka
Rua Imaculada Conceição, 1115 – CEP: 80.215-901 – Curitiba/PR
E-mail: tanakaom@gmail.com

INTRODUCTION

The adhesion to dental enamel started, in 1955, after discovery of acid conditioning by Buonocore. The application of an acid to enamel, demineralizes it selectively, making it appropriate to perform adhesive techniques.[10] This technique provides micromechanic bond between composite resins and enamel, facilitating the attachment of brackets, direct restorations, indirect restorations and adhesive prosthesis.[9] After enamel demineralization, the application of an adhesive system that penetrates into the microporosities and attaches the enamel to the composite resin is necessary. Basically, the function of enamel etching is the creation of an adhesive area by increasing enamel porosity and surface energy, resulting in better permeation of the adhesive. Thus, the micromechanic attachments of the resin in the porosities does not allow rupture of the enamel, providing greater longevity of bonding.[9,10] Some factors are capable of negatively influence the quality of adhesion, such as presence of saliva contamination, blood or remaining phosphoric acid.[8,14,15,20] The contamination by saliva is one of the most frequent defects in adhesion.[26] Rajagopal et al[14] and Sirirungrojying et al[21] reported that the enamel etching previous to the adhesive causes a reduction on the adhesive shear bond strength. On the other hand, the self-etching adhesives are considered hydrophilic and according to Trites et al[22] can be used in presence of humidity. However, the influence of saliva on the adhesive resistance of brackets bonded with self-etching adhesives still is controversial. Rajagopal et al[14] observed reduction on the bond strength when orthodontic brackets were bonded with self-etching adhesives in presence of saliva. These adhesive systems gathered the steps of acid conditioning and primer in one recipient making it self-etching, which would keep its properties even in humid environment. However, the use of these systems with conventional resins, hydrophobic, would reduce most of this capacity. In this way, the creation of a composite resin with the same hydrophilic characteristics, as Transbond Plus Color Change, would preserve this property. Thus, this work proposes to evaluate the bond strength of metallic brackets bonded to human enamel previously contaminated with saliva and analyze the area of adhesive defect after debonding.

MATERIAL AND METHODS

Eighty human premolars, donated by the tooth bank of the Catholic Pontifical University of Paraná (PUCPR), were selected, and had their roots sectioned with diamond burs (KG Sorensen) and discarded. The buccal surface of the teeth was positioned against a glass plate in order to allow most of the flat surface to be parallel to the ground. In this position, the crown was fixed, a PVC ring was positioned and the acrylic resin (Jet/Classic) shed over it (Fig 1A). Posteriorly, prophylaxis was performed, in low rotation, with rubber cups and pumice for 10 seconds. This was followed by rinsing and drying for 10 seconds each at a distance of 50 mm.

The 80 specimens were randomly divided in four groups (n = 20), according to Table 1:

» For G1, enamel etching was performed with 37% phosphoric acid for 15 seconds, rinsed for 10 seconds and dried for 10 seconds. It was followed by adhesive application (Transbond XT primer), insertion of Transbond XT on the bracket base, positioning on the central portion of the enamel under pressure of 400 KgF, measured by a tensiometer (ETM) (Fig 1B) and light cured for 40 seconds.

Table 1 - Division of experimental groups.

Group	Contamination	Adhesive system
G1	No	Transbond XT primer and Transbond XT
G2	Saliva	Transbond XT primer and Transbond XT
G3	No	Transbond self etching primer and Transbond Plus Color
G4	Saliva	Transbond self etching primer and Transbond Plus Color

» For G2, after enamel etching, rinsing and drying according to described in G1, non-stimulated saliva was applied on the surface. The saliva was collected directly from the researcher and applied on the bonding area with the help of a disposable microbrush.

» For G3, a self-etching primer (SEP, 3M/Unitek,USA) was used which was kept in contact with the enamel for 10 seconds. After that, the bracket was bonded using Transbond Plus Color Change (3M/Unitek, USA) in the central portion of the crown under pressure of 400 KgF and light cured for 40 seconds.

» For G4, after using a self-etching primer (SEP, 3M/Unitek, USA), non-stimulated saliva was applied on the enamel surface. The saliva was collected directly form the researcher and applied on bonding area with the help of a disposable microbrush. Premolars brackets (3M/Unitek, Monrovia, USA) were used in this study, with an area of 14.28 mm², measured by a digital caliper (Electron digital caliper 227 - Starret). After bracket bonding, the samples (Fig 1C) were stored in a closed recipient with distilled water at 37° C for 24 hours. After this period, the shear test was performed, with force applied in the occlusal gingival direction, in a universal testing machine (EMIC DL500R, São José dos Pinhais, PR, Brazil) at a speed of 0.5 mm/min. The testing machine was connected to a computer with the Mtest software® that registered the maximum debonding values (Figs 2A and B). After the shear test, the bonding defect was observed through a stereomicroscope with 40x of magnification and the adhesive remnant index (ARI) was analyzed according to Artun and Bergland:[2] Zero indicates no adhesive residue on the dental structure; 1, less than half of adhesive residue on the dental structure; 2, more than half of adhesive residue on the dental structure and 3, all the adhesive residue adhered to the bracket.

STATISTICAL ANALYSIS
Bond strength

The Kolmogorov-Smirnov and Levene's tests were used to verify the normality and homogeneity of variance, respectively. Normality and homogeneity obtained, the difference between groups was examined through the analysis of variance (ANOVA) and Tukey HSD multiple comparisons tests at a significance level of 5%.

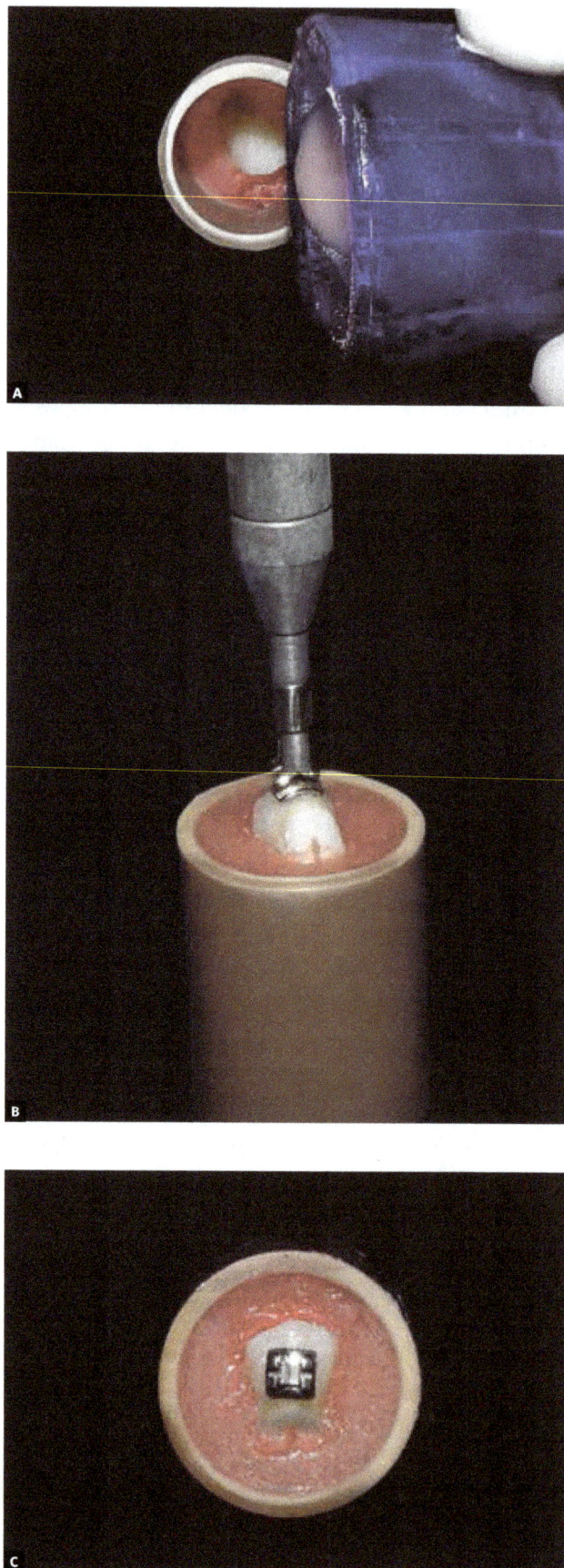

Figure 1 - Sequence of specimen confection. A) Tooth positioning, B) Pressure exerted on the bracket to standardize the thickness of the material, C) specimens finished.

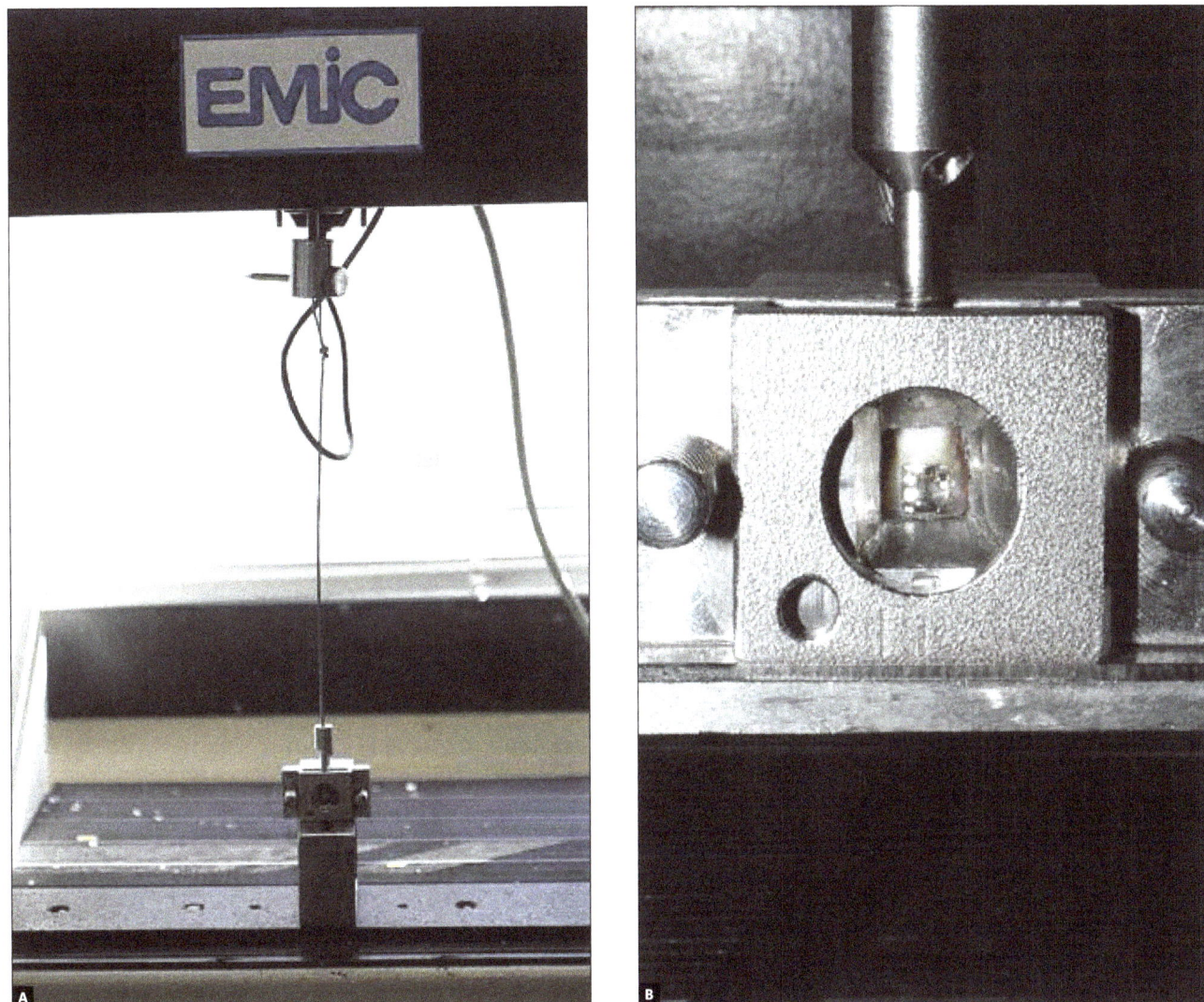

Figure 2 - Mechanical test: **A)** matrix used on the shear bond strength test, **B)** detail of the force applied in the occlusal gingival direction.

Table 2 - Descriptive statistic for bond strength.

Groups	n	Contamination	Resin	Mean	Standard-deviation
G1	20	No	Transbond XT	10.15^A	3.75
G2	20	Saliva	Transbond Plus	6.80^B	2.54
G3	20	No	Transbond XT	9.30^A	3.39
G4	20	Saliva	Transbond Plus	8.30^A	2.95

NOTE: different letters indicate significant difference by Tukey HSD ($p < 0.01$).

Table 3 - Descriptive statistic for adhesive remnant index (ARI).

Groups	n	Contamination	Resin	ARI scores (%)			
				0	1	2	3
G1	20	No	Transbond XT	40	30	10	20
G2	20	Saliva	Transbond Plus	90	10	0	0
G3	20	No	Transbond XT	25	30	25	20
G4	20	Saliva	Transbond Plus	40	40	20	0

Bond strength X Bond strength index

The correlation between bond strength and bond strength indication was obtained through application of the Spearman correlation test.

RESULTS

Bond strength

The Tukey HSD multiple comparison test identified significant statistical difference between the G1 and G2 (p<0.01), indicating that the contamination by saliva reduces shear bond strength when the hydrophobic resin Transbond XT is used (Table 2).

Adhesive Remnant Index (ARI)

Most specimens from G1 and G2 presented BSI ranging from 0 to 1. On G2 there was predominance of ARI 0. The specimens from G3 presented balanced distribution of ARI (Table 3).

The coefficient of Spearman's linear correlation was of 0.26, which indicates a weak correlation between shear bond strength and ARI.

DISCUSSION

The bonding contamination is a problem commonly found on the direct bracket bonding technique, especially in posterior teeth surgically exposed.[14] Among the main contaminants, stand out saliva and blood contamination. There is divergence about the influence of saliva on the shear bond strength. According to some studies,[4,5,18] this contamination reduces bond strength. On the other hand, some reports[3,16,21,23] show no difference on bond strength. These differences might be explained by the adhesive system used. Most of the articles in which the bond strength does not show reduction after the contamination used self-etching adhesive systems. This can be explained by the hydrophilic characteristics of these adhesives.[22] The results of the *in vitro* researches can be influenced by the thickness of the resin and direction of the force applied described by Eliades and Brantley.[12] Aiming to eliminate these factors, a tensiometer was used to standardize the thickness of the composite and the force used during the bonding procedure. Besides, all the experiment was performed by only one operator, as recommended by Ajlouni et al[1] and Bishara et al.[6] The bonding strength of the self-etching adhesives is also controversial. Authors[5,25,27] reported

statistically significant bonding strength reduction when self-etching adhesives were used. However, in this research, the bond strength was similar to the adhesives with previous acid conditioning. It is suggested that the hydrophilic characteristic was kept using a resin with the same property. But yet, there are no reports that evaluated the bonding strength of the hydrophilic resin Transbond Plus Color Change. Thus, studies are recommended to confirm this result. This way, during the choice of the bonding material, some factors must be considered: resistance, longevity, sensibility and ease for removal without dental surface damage. These can be evaluated *in vitro* and transposed to private practice through the evaluation of the shear bond strength and the adhesive remnant index (ARI).[11,17] In relation to bracket debonding, Bishara et al.[4] mentioned that when the adhesive defect occurs on the enamel-adhesive interface there is great risk of enamel fractured. Unlikely, the defect occurring on the adhesive/bracket interface or on the adhesive layer, the dental structure will normally be preserved[7,13,25]. Thus, the adhesives used in this research did not represent risk, for most of the bonding defects occurred on the adhesive layer (score 1 and 2 - ARI), reducing significantly the chances of fracture on the enamel. Only G2 presented high frequency of score 0. Regarding longevity of the bonding procedure, there are evidences that show that the resistance of adhesives with previous acid conditioning reduces after thermocycling. Saito et al[19] theorized that this fact is explained by the hydrophilic property and presence of HEMA in these self-etching solutions. Before these described properties, we recommend that in situations of imminent saliva contamination, the brackets should be bonded with an adhesive system and composite with hydrophilic characteristics, increasing the adhesive resistance and, consequently, the longevity of the bonding procedure.

CONCLUSION

The saliva reduces shear bond strength when brackets are bonded with hydrophobic resin Transbond XT. However, bond strength is not affected by the contamination by saliva when brackets are bonded with adhesive system and resin with hydrophilic properties (Transbond Plus + Transbond Plus Color Change).

REFERENCES

1. Ajlouni R, Bishara SE, Oonsombat C, Denehy GE. Evaluation of modifying the bonding protocol of a new acid-etch primer on the shear bond strength of orthodontic brackets. Angle Orthod. 2004;74(3):410-3.

2. Artun J, Bergland S. Clinical trials with crystal growth conditioning as an alternative to acid-etch enamel pretreatment. Am J Orthod. 1984;85(4):333-40.

3. Bishara SE, Gordan VV, VonWald L, Olson ME. Effect of an acidic primer on shear bond strength of orthodontic brackets. Am J Orthod Dentofacial Orthop. 1998;114(3):243-7.

4. Bishara SE, Gordan VV, VonWald L, Jakobsen JR. Shear bond strength of composite, glass ionomer, and acid primer adhesive systems. Am J Orthod Dentofacial Orthop. 1999;115(1):24-8.

5. Bishara SE, VonWald L, Laffoon JF, Warren JJ. Effect of a self-etch primer/adhesive on the shear bond strength of orthodontic brackets. Am J Orthod Dentofacial Orthop. 2001;119(6):621-4.

6. Bishara SE, Oonsombat C, Ajlouni R, Laffoon JF. Comparison of the shear bond strength of 2 self-etch primer/adhesive systems. Am J Orthod Dentofacial Orthop. 2004;125(3):348-50.

7. Brown CR, Way DC. Enamel loss during orthodontic bonding and subsequent loss during removal of filled and unfilled adhesives. Am J Orthod. 1978;74(6):663-71.

8. Campoy MD, Vicente A, Bravo LA. Effect of saliva contamination on the shear bond strength of orthodontic brackets bonded with a self-etching primer. Angle Orthod. 2005;75(5):865-9.

9. Carvalho RM, Yoshiyama M, Pashley EL, Pashley DH. In vivo study of the dimensional changes of human dentin after demineralization. Arch Oral Biol. 1996;41(4):369-77.

10. Carvalho RM. Adesivos dentinários: fundamentos para aplicação clínica. Rev Dent Rest. 1998;1(2):62-95.

11. De Munck J, Van Landuyt K, Peumans M, Poitevin A, Lambrechts P, Braem M, Van Meerbeek B. A critical review of the durability of adhesion to tooth tissue: methods and results. J Dent Res. 2005;84(2):118-32.

12. Eliades T, Brantley WA. The inappropriateness of conventional orthodontic bond strength assessment protocols. Eur J Orthod. 2000;22(1):13-23.

13. Joseph VP, Rossouw PE. The shear bond strengths of stainless steel orthodontic brackets bonded to teeth with orthodontic composite resin and various fissure sealants. Am J Orthod Dentofacial Orthop. 1990;98(1):66-71.

14. Rajagopal R, Padmanabhan S, Gnanamani J. A comparison of shear bond strength and debonding characteristics of conventional, moisture-insensitive, and self-etching primers in vitro. Angle Orthod. 2004;74(2):264-8.

15. Reddy L, Marker VA, Ellis E 3rd. Bond strength for orthodontic brackets contaminated by blood: composite versus resin-modified glass ionomer cements. J Oral Maxillofac Surg. 2003;61(2):206-13.

16. Retamoso LB, Collares FM, Samuel SMW, Ferreir ES. Influência do sistema adesivo na resistência de união de "brackets": um estudo in vitro. Rev Facul Odontol Porto Alegre. 2006; 47(3):17-22.

17. Retamoso LB, Onofre NML, Marchioro EM. Avaliação de diferentes fontes de polimerização na resistência de união de braquetes. Rev Clín Ortod Dental Press. 2008;7(2):74-8.

18. Romano FL, Tavares SW, Nouer DF, Consani S, Borges, AMMB. Shear bond strength of metallic orthodontic brackets bonded to enamel prepared with self-etching primer. Angle Orthod. 2005;75(5):849-53.

19. Saito K, Sirirungrojying S, Meguro D, Hayakawa T, Kasai K. Bonding durability of using self-etching primer with 4-META/ MMA-TBB resin cement to bond orthodontic brackets. Angle Orthod. 2005 Mar;75(2):260-5.

20. Schaneveldt S, Foley TF. Bond strength comparison of moisture-insensitive primers. Am J Orthod Dentofacial Orthop. 2002;122(3):267-73.

21. Sirirungrojying S, Saito K, Hayakawa T, Kasai K. Efficacy of using self-etching primer with a 4-META/MMA-TBB resin cement in bonding orthodontic brackets to human enamel and effect of saliva contamination on shear bond strength. Angle Orthod. 2004;74(2):251-8.

22. Trites B, Foley TF, Banting D. Bond strength comparison of 2 self-etching primers over a 3-month storage period. Am J Orthod Dentofacial Orthop. 2004;126(6):709-16.

23. Vicente A, Bravo LA, Romero M, Ortiz AJ, Canteras M. Shear bond strength of orthodontic brackets bonded with self-etching primers. Am J Dent. 2005;18(4):256-60.

24. Webster MJ, Nanda RS, Duncanson MG Jr, Khajotia SS, Sinha PK. The effect of saliva on shear bond strengths of hydrophilic bonding systems. Am J Orthod Dentofacial Orthop. 2001;119(1):54-8.

25. Yamada R, Hayakawa T, Kasai K. Effect of using self-etching primer for bonding orthodontic brackets. Angle Orthod. 2002;72(6):558-64.

26. Zachrisson BJ. A posttreatment evaluation of direct bonding in orthodontics. Am J Orthod. 1977;71(2):173-89.

27. Zeppieri IL, Chung CH, Mante FK. Effect of saliva on shear bond strength of an orthodontic adhesive used with moisture-insensitive and self-etching primers. Am J Orthod Dentofacial Orthop. 2003;124(4):414-9.

17

Cephalometric evaluation of the predictability of bimaxillary surgical-orthodontic treatment outcomes in long face pattern patients

Carla Maria Melleiro Gimenez[1], Francisco Antonio Bertoz[2], Marisa Aparecida Cabrini Gabrielli[3], Oswaldo Magro Filho[3], Idelmo Garcia[3], Valfrido Antonio Pereira Filho[3]

Objective: The aim of this study was to compare by means of McNamara as well as Legan and Burstone's cephalometric analyses, both manual and digitized (by Dentofacial Planner Plus and Dolphin Image software) prediction tracings to post-surgical results. **Methods:** Pre and post-surgical teleradiographs (6 months) of 25 long face patients subjected to combined orthognathic surgery were selected. Manual and computerized prediction tracings of each patient were performed and cephalometrically compared to post-surgical outcomes. This protocol was repeated in order to evaluate the method error and statistical evaluation was conducted by means of analysis of variance and Tukey's test. **Results:** A higher frequency of cephalometric variables, which were not statistically different from the actual post-surgical results for the manual method, was observed. It was followed by DFPlus and Dolphin software; in which similar cephalometric values for most variables were observed. **Conclusion:** It was concluded that the manual method seemed more reliable, although the predictability of the evaluated methods (computerized and manual) proved to be reasonably satisfactory and similar.

Keywords: Corrective orthodontics. Predictive value of tests. Oral surgery. Face.

» The authors report no commercial, proprietary or financial interest in the products or companies described in this article.

[1] PhD in Orthodontics, FOA-UNESP.
[2] Head Professor, Department of Pediatric Dentistry, FOA-UNESP.
[3] Assistant Professor, Oral and Maxillofacial Surgery, FOA-UNESP.

Carla Maria Melleiro Gimenez
Rua Padre Duarte 989, Ap. 24, Centro, Araraquara/SP – Brazil
CEP: 14801-310 – E-mail: carlamg@yahoo.com

INTRODUCTION

Accurate diagnosis of both structures involved in malocclusions and the severity of occlusal conditions, facial and functional, leads to the decision of surgical-orthodontic treatment. It is extremely important to carry out an individualized plan in order to obtain successful and consistent results. Initially, preparatory orthodontic procedures are performed prior to orthognathic surgery, aiming to position the teeth in their bone bases. At the latest stage of ideal arch placement, molding is performed in order to articulate the upper and lower models in Class I relationship. Should this relationship be suitable in sagittal, transverse and vertical dimensions, the patient is conducted to the oral and maxillofacial surgeon who will perform the surgical planning in all its particularities.[1]

The prediction tracings show the inclination of the incisors and anticipate all necessary surgical movements, providing visualization of potential results from the tangent to the soft tissue as well as from the tangent to the skeletal tissue. Based on these data, model surgery is performed in semi-adjustable articulator, in which the information concerning the prediction tracing is transferred. This phase will accurately determine both the magnitude and the direction of surgical movements performed to obtain proper occlusion. Afterwards, surgery is performed, followed by orthodontic finishing, removal of orthodontic appliance, placing of retention and post-retention monitoring phases.

This paper focuses on the phase of prediction tracings which is important for carrying out proper surgical planning as well as for guiding the patient and establishing communication with him. Reliability of the proposed result is a constant concern. These tracings create a situation in which it is possible to describe in detail all surgical alterations, leading to an optimized conduct of the case.[13] Conventionally, these tracings are manually carried out, however, there are computer software that perform the prediction of results based on the digitization of cephalometric teleradiographs landmarks, for instance: Dentofacial Planner, OPAL, Quick Ceph Image, COGsoft, TIOPS, Dolphin.[4,16] These software are able to simulate the effect of incisor decompensation and the resultant movements of bony bases, translating them into illustrations and providing a silhouette of post-surgical skeletal and soft tissue profiles. However, it is worth noting that the prediction of these profile changes is difficult due to

the variability of soft tissue behavior and differences in their translation accompanying skeletal changes promoted by orthognathic surgery.[17]

The present study is set within this context, with the purpose of comparing, through cephalometry, the accuracy of manual prediction tracings as well as those performed by both Dentofacial Planner Plus and Dolphin Image software, in relation to post-surgical results of long face patients subjected to bimaxillary orthognathic surgery.

MATERIAL AND METHODS

This study was approved by UNESP/Araçatuba Institutional Review Board, and analyzed pre and post-surgical lateral teleradiographs (6 months) of a sample comprised of 25 adult, long face patients, Angle's Class II, who were subjected to combined orthognathic surgery. These teleradiographs were obtained from the Center for Research and Treatment of Buccofacial Deformities (CEDEFACE – Araraquara/SP) and from the Oral and Maxillofacial Surgery and Traumatology course, given at UNESP College of Dentistry — Araraquara.

The inclusion criteria were:

1) Leucoderm, Brazilian, dentate and adult patients of both sexes.
2) Hyperdivergent patients.
3) Class II dental relationship, showing no open bite.
4) Bimaxillary surgical-orthodontic treatment performed in a minimum period of 6 months before the research, as this period assures sufficient regression of edema caused by surgery.
5) Radiographic documentation of initial periods, immediate preoperative phase, and well-performed post-surgical phase.
6) Absence of pathologies, fissures, facial anomalies or asymmetries.
7) Conventional Edgewise orthodontic technique was used for orthodontic preparation.
8) Absence of any other cosmetic and reconstructive surgeries performed on the patient's face during or after surgical-orthodontic treatment.

The sample comprised 22 (88%) females and 3 (12%) males with a mean age of 32.24 years (17 to 45 years).

Each teleradiography was traced three times (alternately and at weekly intervals in order to avoid memorization of traces), at an environment with controlled lighting (dark room). Seventy one landmarks were marked as they are necessary for the digitalization process performed with the Dentofacial Planner Plus software. The last trace of each patient, regarding pre and post-surgical teleradiographs (6 months), was used as a guide for an organized and sequential scan of these cephalometric landmarks. A scan of each trace was repeated twice in order to evaluate the method reproducibility (Intraexaminer Method Error).

Dentofacial ShowCase 2.0 for Microsoft Windows 95 and for Microsoft Windows NT 4.0 was used to scan the preoperative tracing, the prediction tracing obtained from this software as well as manual prediction tracing and post-surgical tracing. Dolphin Imaging 10.5 software (in the case of prediction tracings performed by this program) was used for the cephalometric evaluation, in which a single examiner was calibrated for tracing and digitizing the cephalograms.

Prediction tracings were built manually as well as with the use of Dentofacial Planner Plus (DFPlus) and Dolphin Imaging 10.5 (Dolphin) software. This process was based on data obtained from the surgery that was performed (clinical records in file folders of patients). The following sequence of tracings was obtained for each patient: manual prediction, DFPlus prediction, Dolphin prediction and post-surgical tracing (actual result). This sequence of tracings was subjected to McNamara's[12] as well as Legan and Burstone's[9] analyses for cephalometric evaluation.

The results (linear and angular measures obtained from the cephalometric analyses) were tabulated into Excel. A cephalometric analysis on the results obtained from manual and computerized prediction tracings as well as post-surgical tracings was carried out in order to check prediction error. This comparison was developed in three steps:

1) Evaluation carried out with Student's t test (paired) to determine whether or not there was prediction error statistically different from zero (for each cephalometric analysis measure cited for all prediction methods). The prediction error was given by subtracting post-surgical actual result from the value of cephalometric prediction.

2) Analysis of variance for comparison between post-surgical tracings and manual and computerized prediction tracings.

3) Tukey's test.

RESULTS
Method error

The method error analysis was indicated due to the importance of carrying out critical evaluation to verify the possibility of reproducibility as well as the effectiveness of the methodology used.[11] It should be noted that the data was read twice and that there was mutual agreement between readings, which proves the procedures to be reliable.

Table 1 - Means (M) and standard deviation (SD) of McNamara's cephalometric post-surgical measures and prediction errors means (M.E.) with their standard deviation (SD), according to the prediction methodology used.

Cephalometric measurement	Post-surgical		DFPlus		Dolphin		Manual	
	M	S.D.	E.M.	S.D.	E.M.	S.D.	E.M.	S.D.
A-Nperp	6.5	4.8	-6.6	3.9b*	<u>-4.7</u>	2.9a*	-6.7	3.9b*
Co-Gn	124.3	6.5	<u>-2.3</u>	4.4a*	-3.4	7.0a*	-8.3	6.5b*
CO-A	96.1	6.7	-7.4	4.5a*	<u>-7.3</u>	5.7a*	<u>-7.3</u>	5.9a*
Dif. Mx-Md	28.3	4.2	5.2	5.1b*	3.8	5.2b*	**-0.9**	5.4a
AIFH	77.7	5.5	2.1	3.9a*	2.4	5.4a*	1.6	4.3a
Pg-Nperp	0.1	6.3	<u>-4.0</u>	4.8a*	-5.3	5.8a*	-7.8	6.0b*
1-A perp	2.5	3.3	2.8	3.4b*	2.5	3.1b*	0.9	3.4a
1-A-Pg	1.8	3.1	3.5	2.0b*	4.0	2.6b*	<u>2.5</u>	2.5a*
FMA	30.6	5.0	-1.8	3.6a*	-0.7	3.8a	0.0	4.4a
Facial Axis	87.3	4.1	**-1.1**	3.6a	7.6	3.0c*	-3.9	4.1b*
Nasolabial Ang.	100.7	12.2	**0.7**	13.3a	11.0	10.4b*	**2.3**	13.9a

Means with the same letters in a row are not significantly different for Tukey's test at 5%.
* Means significantly different from zero for Student's t test at 5%.
» Bold: Measures of which prediction error was statistically equal to zero (actual result similar to the prediction).
» Underline: Measures with lower prediction error among the three evaluated methods.

Table 2 - Means (M) and standard deviation (SD) of Legan Burstone's cephalometric post-surgical measures, linear (mm) and angular (degrees), and prediction error means (E.M.) with their standard deviation, according to the prediction methodology used.

Cephalometric measurement	Post-surgical		DFPlus		Dolphin		Manual	
	M	S.D.	E.M.	S.D.	E.M.	S.D.	E.M.	S.D.
Sn-G Vert	10.7	4.9	<u>-4.0</u>	2.6ᵃ*	-5.3	4.4ᵃ*	-4.9	4.5ᵃ*
Pg-G Vert	4.0	7.1	<u>-4.7</u>	5.4ᵃ*	-8.7	7.8ᵇ*	-5.9	7.1ab*
Middle third	67.7	5.6	**0.9**	3.8ᵃ			-1.2	5.7ᵇ
Lower third	74.4	6.0	-1.1	2.9ᵇ*			0.9	5.1ᵃ
Upper Lip Protrusion	5.2	2.3	-1.1	1.8ᵇ*	-1.1	1.6ᵇ*	**0.5**	1.9ᵃ
Lower Lip Protrusion	3.2	3.4	**-0.3**	3.5ᵃ	2.9	3.4ᶜ*	0.9	2.8ᵇ
Upper Incisor Exposure	3.5	2.4	**-0.6**	2.2ᵃ	**-0.9**	2.2ᵃ	2.2	2.4ᵇ*
Interlabial Space	3.6	3.7	-2.7	2.7ᵇ*	**1.0**	3.1ᵃ	3.7	3.1ᶜ*
Facial Convexity	15.4	5.3	-2.7	4.5ab*	**-1.1**	4.9ᵃ	-3.2	5.5ᵇ*
Cervico-mental angle	75.4	9.6	**-2.0**	10.2ᵃ	-10.1	11.5ᵇ*	-13.8	13.8ᵇ*
Nasolabial angle	100.7	12.2	**0.7**	13.3ᵃ	11.0	10.4ᵇ*	2.3	13.9ᵃ
Mentolabial sulcus	5.4	1.4	-1.6	1.9ᵇ*	-12.2	2.0ᶜ*	<u>1.1</u>	2.1ᵃ*
Medium / inf.%	91.5	9.4	2.8	6.7ᵃ*	7.7	9.2ᶜ*	**-2.4**	8.5ᵇ

Means with the same letters in a row are not significantly different for Tukey's test at 5%.
* Means significantly different from zero for Student's t test at 5%.
» Bold: Measures of which prediction error was statistically equal to zero (actual result similar to the prediction)
» Underline: Measures with lower prediction error among the three evaluated methods.
NOTE: The averages of the middle and lower facial thirds are not provided by Dolphin Imaging 10.5 software.

DISCUSSION

Each measure regarding the selected analyses was systematically evaluated from a cephalometric point of view[9,12] in order to relate the prediction error: the difference between the actual post-surgical measure and the prediction measure of each method (Dentofacial Planner Plus, Dolphin Imaging, manual prediction tracing). If the difference was zero, it would mean that the prediction would have been identical to the actual post-surgical results, indicating an excellent degree of accuracy concerning predictability. Therefore, the closer the cephalometric measures are to zero, the more accurate the method of predictability. Moreover, positive or negative prediction error indicate that the predicted value is, respectively, higher or lower than the actual value.

In accordance with Student's t test, the results shown in Table 1 (McNamara Jr Cephalometric Analysis,[12]) demonstrate that only 8 out of 33 evaluated means were not significantly different from zero; i.e., only eight presented a prediction result that did not differ statistically from the actual final result. These measures were: Maxillomandibular difference (manual method), AIFH (manual method), 1-Aperp (manual method), FMA (manual method and Dolphin), Facial axis (DFPlus), nasolabial angle (manual method and DFPlus). Therefore, the predictions which did not differ statistically from the actual post-surgical result were more frequent when using the manual method (5 cephalometric variables), followed by the DFPlus computerized method (2 cephalometric variables) and Dolphin (only one cephalometric variable).

Analyses of variance were used to compare the three methods concerning the prediction error. When such analyses indicated significant difference between methods, Tukey's test was used for multiple comparisons of means.

Despite presenting statistically significant differences, the following measures were close to the actual result: 1-APg (manual method), Pg-Nperp (DFPlus), CO-A (manual method and Dolphin), CO-Gen (DFPlus), A-Nperp (Dolphin). In this case, the three methods (Manual method, DFPlus and Dolphin) presented the same frequency (2 cephalometric variables for each method).

Results also demonstrated that some cephalometric measures showed very close values between two methods: A-Nperp (manual method and DFPlus), CO-A (manual method, DFPlus, Dolphin), AIFH (DFPlus and Dolphin), 1-A perp (DFPlus and Dolphin), FMA (Dolphin, DFPlus). In this case, Dolphin Imaging and DFPlus computerized methods proved to have a higher frequency of agreement.

The results displayed in Table 2 refer to the cephalometric measures established by Legan and Burstone.[9] From a total of 37 cephalometric means evaluated by Student's t test, 14 were not significantly different from zero, i.e., not statistically different from the actual post-surgical result, which indicates a good level of prediction. These cephalometric references are: middle third of the face (DFPlus and manual method), lower third of the face (manual method), upper lip protrusion (manual method), lower lip protrusion (DFPlus and manual method), upper incisor exposure (Dolphin and DFPlus), interlabial space (Dolphin), facial convexity (Dolphin), cervico-mental angle (DFPlus), nasolabial angle (DFPlus and manual method) proportion of the facial thirds - Medium/Inf.% (manual method). The manual method had the highest number of cephalometric variables (6) with no statistically significant difference concerning the actual post-surgical result; followed by DFPlus (5) and Dolphin (3).

Except for the last two cephalometric measures, the means which significantly differ from zero, regarding a single measure, present equal signs: positive or negative, thus, demonstrating the same behavior towards cephalometric prediction. Analyses of variance were used to compare the three methods concerning the prediction error. Such analyses were complemented by Tukey's test.

Despite presenting statistically significant differences, the following measures were close to the actual result: Sn-G Vert (DFPlus), Pg-G Vert (DFPlus), mentolabial sulcus (manual method). In this regard, the prediction of DFPlus software (2 cephalometric variables) was more often closer to the actual result.

Results also demonstrate that some cephalometric measures showed very close values between two methods: Sn-G Vert (manual method and DFPlus), upper incisor exposure (DFPlus and Dolphin), facial convexity (DFPlus and Dolphin), cervico-mental angle (manual method and Dolphin), nasolabial angle (DFPlus and manual method), Medium / inf.% (DFPlus and manual method). Therefore, manual and DFPlus methods proved to have a higher frequency of agreement, followed by DFPlus and Dolphin. The study of Power et al[16] corroborates the findings of the present study. These authors compared the accuracy of prediction using Dolphin Imaging Software (Version 8.0) and the traditional manual technique; in comparison with actual post-surgical results. Manual tracings proved to be more predictable. The comparison of actual results to the predictions of the software demonstrated clinically significant differences for all measures.

Similarly, in the study carried out by Chunmaneechote and Friede,[3] prediction proves to be higher in the manual method. The authors concluded that conventional prediction tracings were significantly closer to post-surgical results than the pre-programmed proportions ($p < 0.05$).

Smith, Thomas and Proffit[18] evaluated five software (Dentofacial Planner Plus, Dolphin Imaging, Orthoplan, Quick Ceph Image and Vistadent) and their differences in the ability to simulate results in orthognathic surgery. Dentofacial Planner Plus software was considered the best simulator. The results showed that the differences in the ability to simulate results depend on several factors, such as: software performance, easy to use, cost, compatibility, image quality and practical application of available resources. In the present study, the frequency of cephalometric variables that were closer to post-surgical results proved to be higher when using DFPlus software in comparison to Dolphing Imaging software, corroborating the aforementioned authors.

Furthermore, Schultes et al[17] also claim that the prediction of DFPlus software is appropriate. The authors found that the software was frequently in accordance with the real situation regarding the nasal and labial areas, while the highest margins of errors were seen in the submental region. In general, predictability was greater than 80 %, which ensures accurate planning.

Csaszar, Bruker-Csaszar and Niederllmann[5] also evaluated the accuracy of prediction of DFPlus software and concluded that this proves to be satisfactory, although the profile of the labial region presents difficulties of predictability, which indicates the need for further development of this software.

In the study carried out by Gosset et al,[7] which compared the traditional prediction tracings (manual method) and the Dolphin Imaging software tracings with actual post-surgical results, it was shown that seven out of the sixteen measures showed statistically significant differences for the conventional method, while nine measures were statistically significant different for Dolphin Imaging software. Based on these data, the authors concluded that both methods seem to demonstrate reasonable predictability, thus, being similarly accurate. This statement corroborates the findings of this study, since the evaluated methods also demonstrated reasonable predictability, the differences between them were slight and the degree of accuracy observed was similar.

Claiming that it is necessary to have common sense when using any system regarding prediction of results, Lu et al,[10] emphasized that although computerized imaging systems are valuable for establishing communication with patients as well as giving explanations to them, further efforts are needed to improve their accuracy, including considerations related to the stress of soft tissue and quality of muscle tissue. Therefore one must consider that the prediction obtained by imaging systems must be carefully interpreted.

Facing the possibility of high individual variability, Cousley et al[4] compared post-surgical results with prediction tracings and noted that the predictions of some cephalometric variables were reasonably accurate in terms of mean values. However, there was high individual variation for most measures, with the presence of systematic error. In particular, there was a tendency toward orthognathic surgery "overprediction", inducing backward mandibular rotation.

Pektas et al[15] evaluated the accuracy of predictability of tegumentar tissue response resulting from surgical-orthodontic treatment and observed that in the sagittal plane,

the tip of the nose was the most accurate area, while the upper lip area presented the highest level of difference. In the vertical plane, the subnasal area was the most accurate, while the lower lip area was the least precise. The authors suggested that the predictions in sagittal plane were superior to those in the vertical plane.

Several authors suggest that variability factors related to the soft tissue (such as thickness, soft tissue tonicity, shape, functional application, and free functional space) be carefully considered when interpreting the predictability within the context of surgical-orthodontic treatment.[6,8,14]

Statistical analysis of the method error proved that the methodology used for marking cephalometric landmarks as well as angular, linear and proportion measures, was reliable and reproducible, which confirms the considerations of Buschang et al,[2] Martins[11] and Trajano et al.[19]

CONCLUSION

The experimental conditions of this study show that:

• The manual method proved to be closer to the cephalometric variables evaluated in relation to the actual post-surgical results, followed by DFPlus and Dolphin.

REFERENCES

1. Araújo CU, Tamaki T. Posição labial em repouso e sorriso e a sua relação com os incisivos centrais superiores. Rev Odontol Univ São Paulo. 1987;1(2):28-34.

2. Buschang PH, Tanguay R, Demirjian A. Cephalometric reliability: a full ANOVA model for the estimation of true and error variance. Angle Orthod. 1987;57(2):168-75.

3. Chunmaneechote P, Friede H. Mandibular setback osteotomy: facial soft tissue behavior and possibility to improve the accuracy of the soft tissue profile prediction with the use of a computerized cephalometric program: Quick Ceph Image Pro: v. 2,5. Clin Orthod Res. 1999;2(2):85-98.

4. Cousley RR, Grant E, Kindelan JD. The validity of computerized orthognathic predictions. J Orthod. 2003;30(2):149-54; discussion 128.

5. Csaszar GR, Brüker-Csaszar B, Niederdellmann H. Prediction of soft tissue profiles in orthodontic surgery with the Dentofacial Planner. Int J Adult Orthodon Orthognath Surg. 1999;14(4):285-90.

6. Gabrielli MFR. Alterações de posição dos tecidos moles da face após osteotomias Le Fort I: um estudo retrospectivo [tese]. Araraquara (SP): Universidade Estadual Paulista; 1990.

7. Gossett CB, Preston CB, Dunford R, Lampasso J. Prediction accuracy of computer-assisted surgical visual treatment objectives as compared with conventional visual treatment objectives. J Oral Maxillofac Surg. 2005;63(5):609-17.

8. Kuyl MH, Verbeeck RM, Dermaut LR. The integumental profile: a reflection of the underlying skeletal configuration? Am J Orthod Dentofacial Orthop. 1994;106(6):597-604.

9. Legan HL, Burstone CJ. Soft tissue cephalometric analysis for orthognathic surgery. J Oral Surg. 1980;38(10):744-51.

10. Lu CH, Ko EW, Huang CS. The accuracy of video imaging prediction in soft tissue outcome after bimaxillary orthognathic surgery. J Oral Maxillofac Surg. 2003;61(3):333-42.

11. Martins LP. Erro de reprodutibilidade das medidas das análises cefalométricas de Steiner e Ricketts pelos métodos convencional e computadorizado [tese]. Araraquara (SP): Universidade Estadual Paulista; 1993.

12. McNamara JA Jr. A method of cephalometric evaluation. Am J Orthod. 1984;86(6):449-69.

13. Omura T, Glickman RS, Super S. Method to verify the accuracy of model surgery and prediction tracing. Int J Adult Orthodon Orthognath Surg. 1996;11(3):265-70.

14. Park YC, Burstone CJ. Soft tissue profile: fallacies of hard tissue standards in treatment planning. Am J Orthod Dentofacial Orthop. 1986;90(1):52-62.

15. Pektas ZO, Kircelli BH, Cilasun U, Uckan S. The accuracy of computer-assisted surgical planning in soft tissue prediction following orthognathic surgery. Int J Med Robot. 2007;3:64-71.

16. Power G, Breckon J, Sherriff M, McDonald F. Dolphin Imaging Software: an analysis of the accuracy of cephalometric digitization and orthognathic prediction. Int J Oral Maxillofac Surg. 2005;34(6):619-26.

17. Schultes G, Gaggl A, Kärcher H. Accuracy of cephalometric and video imaging program Dentofacial Planner Plus in orthognathic surgical planning. Comput Aided Surg. 1998;3(3):108-14.

18. Smith JD, Thomas PM, Proffit WR. A comparison of current prediction imaging programs. Am J Orthod Dentofacial Orthop. 2004;125(5):527-36.

19. Trajano FS, Pinto AS, Ferreira AC, Katu CMB, Cunha RB, Viana FM. Estudo comparativo entre os métodos de análise cefalométrica manual e computadorizada. Rev Dental Press Ortod Ortop Facial. 2000;5(6):57-62.

18

Comparative analysis of the anterior and posterior length and deflection angle of the cranial base, in individuals with facial Pattern I, II and III

Guilherme Thiesen[1], Guilherme Pletsch[2], Michella Dinah Zastrow[3], Caio Vinicius Martins do Valle[4], Karyna Martins do Valle-Corotti[5], Mayara Paim Patel[6], Paulo Cesar Rodrigues Conti[7]

Objective: This study evaluated the variations in the anterior cranial base (S-N), posterior cranial base (S-Ba) and deflection of the cranial base (SNBa) among three different facial patterns (Pattern I, II and III). **Method:** A sample of 60 lateral cephalometric radiographs of Brazilian Caucasian patients, both genders, between 8 and 17 years of age was selected. The sample was divided into 3 groups (Pattern I, II and III) of 20 individuals each. The inclusion criteria for each group were the ANB angle, Wits appraisal and the facial profile angle (G'.Sn.Pg'). To compare the mean values obtained from (SNBa, S-N, S-Ba) each group measures, the ANOVA test and Scheffé's Post-Hoc test were applied. **Results and Conclusions:** There was no statistically significant difference for the deflection angle of the cranial base among the different facial patterns (Patterns I, II and III). There was no significant difference for the measures of the anterior and posterior cranial base between the facial Patterns I and II. The mean values for S-Ba were lower in facial Pattern III with statistically significant difference. The mean values of S-N in the facial Pattern III were also reduced, but without showing statistically significant difference. This trend of lower values in the cranial base measurements would explain the maxillary deficiency and/or mandibular prognathism features that characterize the facial Pattern III. **Keywords:** Cranial base. Orthodontics. Maxillofacial development. Face.

[1] MSc in Orthodontics and Facial Orthopedics, PUCRS. Professor of Orthodontics, UNISUL and UNIASSELVI.

[2] Specialist in Orthodontics, UNISUL.

[3] MSc in Radiology, UFSC. Professor of Radiology and Stomatology, UNISUL.

[4] MSc in Orthodontics, Bauru School of Dentistry – São Paulo University (FOB-USP). Coordinator of the Specialization Course in Orthodontics, UNIASSELVI. PhD Student in Oral Rehabilitation, FOB-USP.

[5] MSc and PhD in Orthodontics, FOB-USP. Associate Professor, Department of Orthodontics, São Paulo City University (UNICID). Professor of the MSc Program in Orthodontics, UNICID.

[6] MSc and PhD in Orthodontics, FOB-USP. Professor of the Specialization Course in Orthodontics, Dentistry and Health Catarinense Institute.

[7] Head Professor of the Prosthesis Department, FOB-USP. Honorary member of the Ibero Latin American Academy of Craniomandibular Dysfunction and Orofacial Pain.

» The author reports no commercial, proprietary or financial interest in the products or companies described in this article.

Guilherme Thiesen
Av. Madre Benvenuta, 1285, Santa Mônica
CEP: 88.035-001 – Florianópolis / SC – Brazil
E-mail: guilherme.thiesen@unisul.br

INTRODUCTION

The cranial base has been the subject of numerous studies.[1,4] It is a special interest region in orthodontics, once its growth and development are interrelated to the face, directly influencing the growth of the maxilla and mandible and, consequently, the establishment of their anteroposterior relationship.

The cranial base is composed of different bones (sphenoid, ethmoid, frontal, parietal, temporal, and occipital) interconnected by synchondrosis.[11] It can also be divided into anterior base (S-N) and posterior base (S-Ba or S-Ar).[29]

Initially, during intrauterine life, the cranial base is practically flat. But gradually it suffers deflection, increasing its angulation, due to the growth of the brain.[9] According to Björk,[4] the cranial base develops mainly from the chondrocranium, and its shape, during development, may vary considerably. There is a flattening tendency until birth, which changes during the first years of life, gradually flexing until approximately ten years old, when normally its final shape is reached. According to Bishara,[3] the cranial base reaches 87% of its adult size at two years of age, 90% at 5 years and 98% at 15 years. Also, according to Moore and Lavelle,[19] the cranial base reaches about 90% of its total size of about five years of age, and from this age on it can be considered stable. Therefore, its development is fast during the first years of life, followed by a decelerated growth. According to Moyers,[21] the growth of the cranial base is mainly in the anterior-inferior direction, influencing the growth of the maxilla and mandible, being its main growth sites the spheno-occipital, the sphenoethmoidal, the sphenoidal inter-and intraoccipital synchondrosis.

Brodie[5] emphasized the importance of understanding the growth of the cranial base for orthodontists, since the successful treatment of malocclusions depends, largely, of the entire craniofacial growth. Therefore, orthodontists were gradually understanding that the facial skeleton, in which the teeth and alveolar process are inserted, is closely related with the cranial base, with the nasomaxillary portion connected to its anterior region, and the jaw, to its posterior region. For this reason, any changes that occur between the anterior and posterior cranial base (e.g., changes in the length and angle between them) may generate significant results in the relationships of the facial parts.[15]

Ricketts[23] stated that the cranial base has an important influence over the total facial prognathism and the establishment of the jaws anteroposterior relationship. Moyers[21] reported that the growth of the cranial base has a direct effect on the positioning of the mandible and the middle region of the face, and as this base is the most stable of all parts of the craniofacial skeleton, it is less affected by external influences (orthodontic treatment, for example). In 1993, Enlow[9] mentioned the cranial base as the template over which the face develops. So what happens in the cranial base directly affects the structure, the angles, the size and positioning of the various parts of the face. According to Enlow,[9] the opening of the cranial base angle causes a retrusive effect on the mandible, and its closure, a protrusive effect.

Therefore, the deflection angle and the size of the cranial base have been considered as potential causes of skeletal Class II malocclusions, where an increased length of the anterior cranial base would be associated with an anterior displacement of the maxilla[24] and a increased cranial base angle would be correlated with a higher degree of mandibular retrusion. However, when Ngan, Byczek and Scheick[22] and Varella[28] studied the early morphological characteristics of the Class II malocclusion, they found a normal configuration and bending of the cranial base.

Guyer et al[13] compared cephalometric radiographs of Class III patients with Class I patients. They found a shorter posterior cranial base in subjects with Class III, and no significant difference for the angle of the cranial base. On the other hand, Marquez[18] using cephalometric radiographs of 30 patients with mandibular prognathism and comparing them with a control group, observed that the anterior portion and the deflection angle of the cranial base are smaller in Class III patients. Sanborn[25] compared 42 Class III subjects with a control group (35 individuals), and observed a lower S-N value in the Class III group. The author also found statistically significant correlation between the slope of cranial base and the Class I, II and III malocclusions, being that the SNBa angle is sharper in Class III malocclusion.

Mouakeh,[20] when analyzing the morphological characteristics of the craniofacial complex in children with Class III malocclusion, reported that the anterior and posterior cranial base were significantly lower than the control group. However, in a retrospective cephalometric study performed by Dhopatkar et al.[8] the results showed that the deflection of cranial base have no fundamental importance in determining the malocclusion, since the mandibular size was significantly different in the different malocclusions.

According to Moyers,[21] a pattern is a set of restraining rules acting to preserve the integration of the parts under various conditions. In this way, it was suggested that the face morphogenetic patterns and the maxillomandibular growth should be considered with the same connotation. In 1907, Angle[2] said that the orthodontist would be able to classify malocclusion by facial evaluation only. According to Capelozza Filho,[6] a facial pattern is the "management of facial configuration throughout time", and once the facial morphology is defined, the individual is diagnosed as having particular facial pattern with all its relevant features, therefore allowing the understanding of the malocclusion and its prognosis. One must understand that the study of some variables is not enough to determine the morphological facial pattern of the individual. However, these may be aggregated to the characteristics pertinent to a specific facial pattern. Therefore, the objective of this study was to compare the angular (SNBa) and linear (S-N and S-Ba) measurements of the cranial base in subjects with different facial patterns (Pattern I, II and III).

MATERIAL AND METHODS

For this study, sixty cephalometric radiographs from Brazilian individuals aged between 8 and 17 years, of both genders, were selected., All subjects were or have been under orthodontic treatment at the Clinic of Orthodontics, University of Southern Santa Catarina - UNISUL. The sample was subdivided into three groups (Pattern I group; Pattern II group and Pattern III group), each group being composed of twenty (20) cephalometric radiographs.

The selection criterion for the age group ranging from 8 to 17 years of age was based on the age at which the cranial base has already reached the growth peak and also its final morphology. From this age on it continues to grow, but in reduced proportions and without changing its configuration. On the other hand, during this same period, the different facial patterns characteristics are developed and confirmed. The sample's mean age was 12 years and 4 months, and for each group as follows.

» Pattern I – 12 years and 10 months.
» Pattern II – 13 years and 1 month.
» Pattern III – 11 years and 2 months.

The lateral cephalometric radiographs, part of the initial orthodontic records of each individual, were previously obtained at the same radiological service, pertaining to UNISUL. Kodak® radiographic films, size 18 x 24 cm were used. The radiographs were processed by the radiological service using an Imaging Corp® (All-Pro), model All-Pro in a proper darkroom, using a total processing time of 2 minutes. No correction was performed for the linear magnification of the radiographic images (approximately 7% compared to the median plane). All cephalometric tracings were manually performed by the same previously calibrated investigator, using black pencil 0.3 mm HB. The comparative analysis between groups was performed by means of angular and linear measurements obtained from the cephalometric radiographs, with scale of 0.50 degrees and 0.5 mm. These measurements allowed the assessment of the cranial base morphology and also its relations with the maxilla and the mandible. The cephalometric points, planes and angles used in this study were the following:

» S (sella): Situated at the midsagittal region of the sphenoid bone center. The point should be marked at the sella turcica's geometric center.
» Ba (basion): Located at the most inferior point on the anterior margin of the foramen magnum, in the sagittal plane.
» N (nasion): Located in the most anterior region of the frontonasal suture (suture between the frontal and nasal bone).
» A-point (subspinale): Located in deepest region of the premaxilla's anterior curvature.
» B-point (supramentale): Located at the deepest point of the anterior curvature of the alveolar process of the mandible.
» G' (soft tissue glabella): Located at the soft tissue glabella.
» Sn (subnasale).
» Pg' (soft tissue pogonion).
» S-Ba (posterior cranial base).
» S-N (anterior cranial base).
» SNBa: Expresses the degree of deflection of the cranial base.
» ANB: Expresses the maxillomandibular relation to the cranial base.

» G'.Sn.Pg' (angle of facial convexity): Expresses the maxilla-mandibular anteroposterior relationship in soft tissue profile.

» Wits: Expresses linearly, the anteroposterior relationship between the maxilla and the mandible.

The Figure 1 shows a standard cephalogram used in this study.

For examiner calibration, twenty radiographs of the sample were selected masked (to avoid any biased analysis) and analyzed for a second time, respecting a 10 days interval. From these measurements, the Kappa test was applied. To calculate the random error, Dahlberg's formula was used.

To determine the inclusion of individuals in their respective group each facial pattern characteristics (Pattern I, II or III) was taken into account, as recommended by Capelozza Filho[6] as well as the facial convexity angle (G'.Sn.Pg') according to Suguino et al.[27] In addition, each individual's ANB angle and Wits appraisal were analyzed. The mean values for ANB, Wits and G'.Sn.Pg' of each group were as follows (Table 1):

» Pattern I group: ANB = 3.25°, Wits = 0.82 mm and G'.Sn.Pg' = 166.8°.

» Pattern II group: ANB = 8.53°, Wits = 5.26 mm and G'.Sn.Pg' = 158.27°.

» Pattern III group: ANB = - 1.5°, Wits = - 6.2 mm and G'.Sn.Pg' = 174.3°.

Once the groups were delimited, the measurements of the cranial base (SNBa, S-N and S-Ba) were assessed for the whole sample. The study data were then presented as mean and standard deviation for the three groups. To assess if there was difference in the SNBa, S-N and S-Ba analyses between different facial patterns, we used the one-way analysis of variance (ANOVA) followed by Scheffé post-hoc tests.

RESULTS

From the analysis, Kappa test and percent agreement were applied (Table 2), observing that the examiner was able to conduct all analyses of this research. For the random error, no significant value was found for representative of error for angular and linear measurements, with the greatest measurement difference found being of 0.5 ° and 0.5 mm, respectively.

The mean value found for the cranial base deflection angle (SNBa) for Pattern I individuals was 131.7°, with a

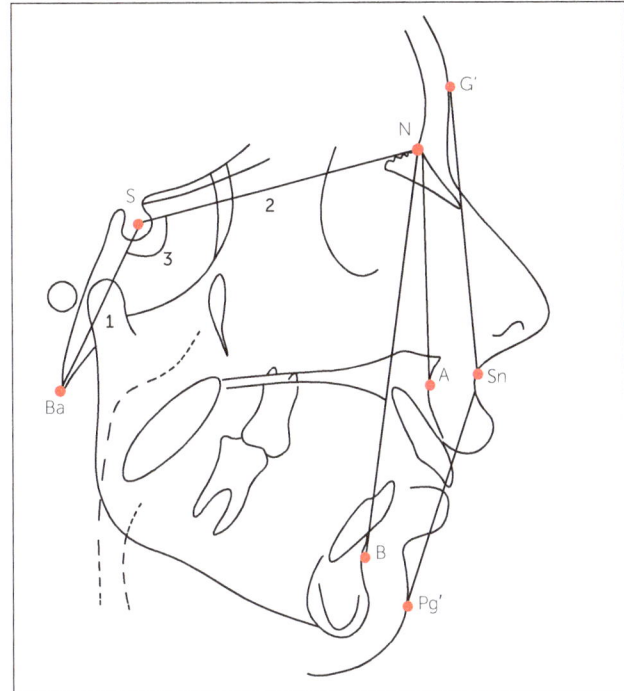

Figure 1 - Standard cephalogram used in the study. 1) posterior cranial base; 2) anterior cranial base; 3) cranial base angle.

standard deviation of 4.5°. In Pattern II group, the average value of SNBa was 132.8°, with a standard deviation of 4.9°. For Pattern III group, the average value of SNBa was 132.5°, with a standard deviation of 3.2°. There was no statistically significant difference for the SNBa value in the different facial patterns assessed, using the one-way analysis of variance (ANOVA) (Table 2).

In the evaluation of the anterior cranial base (S-N, the mean value found for Pattern I group was 69.4 mm, with a standard deviation of 2.3 mm. In Pattern II group, the mean value of S-N was slightly higher, presenting with 70.4 mm and a standard deviation of 4.7 mm. Although there was no statistically significant difference, the Pattern III group had the lowest mean value for the anterior cranial base, which was 67.1 mm (SD = 4.1 mm) (Table 3).

The posterior cranial base (S-Ba) mean value for Pattern I group was 46.0 mm, with a standard deviation of 2.7 mm. For the Pattern II group, showed a 46.8 mm mean, with a standard deviation of 2.9 mm. In Pattern III group the mean value was once again reduced and showed statistically significant difference, being 42.5 mm, with a standard deviation of 3.0 mm (Table 3).

Table 1 - Mean values for ANB, Wits and G'.Sn.Pg' for the three studied facial patterns.

Group	Pattern I	Pattern II	Pattern III
ANB	3.25°	8.53°	-1.5°
Wits	0.82 mm	5.26 mm	- 6.2 mm
G'.Sn.Pg'	166.8°	158.27°	174.3°

Table 2 - Kappa test and percentage agreement values for intraexaminer calibration.

Analysis	Kappa Values	P	Percent agreement
SNBa	1.000	<0.0001*	100%
G'.Sn.Pg'	0.928	<0.0001*	95%
S-Ba	0.935	<0.0001*	95%
S-N	1.000	<0.0001*	100%
Wits	1.000	<0.0001*	100%
ANB	1.000	<0.0001*	100%

* Statistically significant.

Table 3 - Mean and standard deviation values for the different measurements performed in the three studied facial patterns.

Group	Pattern I	Pattern II	Pattern III
SNBa	131.7 ± 4.5	132.8 ± 4.9	132.5 ± 3.2
S-Ba	46.0 ± 2.7	46.8 ± 2.9	42.5 ± 3.0
S-N	69.4 ± 2.3	70.4 ± 4.7	67.1 ± 4.1

Table 4 - ANOVA (F) results and respective significance probability performed for the different facial patterns.

Analysis	Test result (F)	P
SNBa	0.257	0.774
S-Ba	9.626	<0.0001*
S-N	2.828	0.070

* Statistically significant.

After performing the ANOVA test, it was found statistically significant difference between of the groups only for the posterior cranial base (S-Ba) mean values (Table 4). Post-hoc Scheffé tests were conducted to locate the significant differences between the different patterns. Differences were detected to the value of S-Ba between Pattern III and Pattern I groups (P = 0.007), and between Pattern III and Pattern II groups (P = 0.001).

DISCUSSION

The human skull, especially its base, has always aroused the interest of many scientists, such as anthropologists and orthodontists. Current orthodontics is no longer restricted to dental arches and their occlusion. Its constant evolution has enabled a better understanding of the craniofacial growth and development, thus obtaining an integrated view of the cranium, face, TMJ and dental occlusion.

Coben[7] analyzing the integration of the craniofacial skeleton variants, emphasized that, when evaluating individual craniofacial skeletal patterns, a greater perspective on the etiology of malocclusions is found. This is because not all Class II and III malocclusions can be explained based on the mandibular and/or maxillary size. When considering the relationship of the cranial base with the dentofacial complex, one concludes that the factors combination is complex, with a great array of adjustments, and the integration of these factors determines the facial harmony or disharmony.

In this study, the size of the posterior cranial base, in Pattern III, showed a statistically significant difference (reduced when compared to Pattern I and II). This may help explain the prognathism that occurs in this facial type. A reduced posterior cranial base generates a more anterior position of the glenoid fossa of the temporal bone, where the mandibular condyles are articulated with the cranial base.[9] Being this joint in a more anterior position, the ramus and, consequently, the entire jaw, will also be more anteriorly positioned, leading to mandibular prognathism.[4] Enlow,[9] in one of his papers on the relationship between the cranial base and the jaws, states that individuals with a cranial base of reduced size have a tendency to a more brachycephalic head shape. As a result on the face, it is found a relatively retrusive nasomaxillary complex and a more anterior positioned jaw, resulting in a greater tendency for a prognathic profile. However, Enlow[9] himself states that most individuals presents structural characteristics that compensate these morphogenetic trends of facial pattern (in this case, a smaller jaw or a larger maxilla, for example). Thus, these features can compensate in a greater or lesser degree, a structural disharmony presents in cranial base, where the individual can present at least reasonable facial proportions. However, if these compensatory characteristics do not occur, or if it is insufficient, the cranial base intrinsic morphogenetic tendencies will be expressed with great severity and gravity on the face of the individual.

Comparative analysis of the anterior and posterior length and deflection angle of the cranial base, in individuals...

133

In this study, Pattern III also presented difference when compared to Pattern I and II, for the mean values of the anterior cranial base length. Although there was no statistically significant difference, this value was reduced in Pattern III group. This result, like the reduced posterior base, can help explain the concave facial profile in Pattern III. This is because the nasomaxillary complex develops over this region.[5,7,9,21] Thus, a reduced length of anterior cranial base can result a retrusive positioning of the whole nasomaxillary complex. In the facial profile, this is expressed as a tendency to poor middle-third of the face. Björk,[4] when studying the human prognathism, stated that a shortening of the anterior cranial base is accompanied by an increase of facial prognathism if the other structures involved remain unchanged. This is consistent with the results of this study. However, the shortening of the cranial base is not the prime factor for a facial Pattern III, since it can present other important etiologic factors. Nevertheless this shortening is usually present in Pattern III, contributing in a greater or lesser degree, to the characteristic profile of this group.

According to Weidenreich,[30] a sharper SNBa angle is usually related to a more brachycephalic skull and greater mandibular prognathism. Enlow[9] found a sharper SNBa angle, a short middle-third of the face and mandibular ramus with a more anterior orientation in subjects with Angle's Class III malocclusion, when compared to a control group. The same authors found, in subjects with Class II malocclusion, a less sharp SNBa angle, with a base of greater length when compared to a control group (Class I).

According to Björk,[4] a reduced SNBa angle and shortening of the cranial base, would some of the facial prognathism causes. He also asserts that the opposite is true, where an increase in the angle of the cranial base, as well as a greater length base, would be responsible for a more retrognathic facial pattern. However, the difference between the anteroposterior positioning of the maxilla and mandible is partly due to variation in the size of the jaws, and partly due to variation in the length and flexure angle of the cranial base, which are associated with the both jaws.

The angle of the cranial base (SNBa) did not differ between the different groups. This result is consistent with what Freitas[12] found on his studies. There were also no statistically significant differences between the

linear dimensions of the cranial base (S-N and S-Ba) between Pattern I and Pattern II. But these results do not confirm what part of the literature describes about the subject.[1,4,8,9,12,15]

This study investigated the differences in the deflection angle of the cranial base, as well as in the length of its anterior (S-N) and posterior (S-Ba) portions in different facial patterns (Pattern I, II and III). However, it is important to keep in mind that the morphogenetic facial pattern is formed by a series of specific characteristics of each face type. And each of these characteristics alone does not define a facial pattern. It also possible to have compensations in maxillomandibular structures. These compensations can act minimizing an abnormal morphological pattern of the cranial base.

The fact that these values (SNBa for the three groups and S-N and S-Ba for Pattern I and II) did not show significant differences can be explained by such morphological compensation existing in the studied subjects. For example, when comparing Pattern I and II individuals, they can present values for SNBa, S-N and S-Ba, within the normal range. The difference in these facial patterns may have been caused by a smaller mandible and / or a larger maxilla in the Pattern II individual.

Therefore, it would be interesting to conduct further studies on the topic, including larger specificities between different facial patterns (separating the Pattern III caused by maxillary deficiency from the Pattern III caused by mandibular excess; separating the Pattern II caused by maxillary excess from the Pattern II caused by mandibular deficiency, for example), thus distinguishing the main etiological factor for each facial pattern.

Current orthodontics does not accept absolute normal values anymore. Facial harmony is expressed by a combination of floating norms of the angles and proportions, especially in a population with high racial miscegenation as the Brazilian population. Each person has a unique facial architecture. Therefore, the study of one variable, alone, is not sufficient to understand the characteristics of a facial type. However, the orthodontist should not forget that in some cases the causative morphological factor of a disharmonic facial pattern, such as Patterns II and III, can also result from alterations present in the cranial base, and not only from a linear disproportion between the structures of the jaws. This "missing link" often ends up being neglected by the professionals in the patients' craniofacial evaluation. We must know the role of each variable within a whole, and thus successfully diagnose the main etiology of a certain disease.

CONCLUSIONS

In the studied sample, there was no difference between the mean values for the deflection angle of the cranial base (SNBa) in different facial patterns (I, II, III).

There was statistically significant difference for the mean values of the posterior cranial base (S–Ba) for the Pattern III group. In this group, the posterior cranial base was reduced when compared with Pattern I and II groups.

Although without statistical difference, the anterior cranial base (S–N) in the Pattern III group was reduced when compared to Pattern I and II.

REFERENCES

1. Anderson D, Popovich F. Relation of cranial base flexure to cranial form and mandibular position. Am J Phys Anthropol. 1983;61(2):181-7.
2. Angle EH. Treatment of malocclusion of the teeth. Philadelphia: The S. S. With Dental Manufacturing; 1907.
3. Bishara SE. Ortodontia. São Paulo: Ed. Santos; 2004.
4. Björk A. Cranial base development. Am J Orthod. 1955;41(3):198-225.
5. Brodie AG Jr. The behavior of the cranial base and its components as revealed by serial cephalometric roentgenograms. Angle Orthod. 1955;25(3):148-160.
6. Capelozza Filho L. Diagnóstico em Ortodontia. Maringá: Dental Press; 2004.
7. Coben SE. The integration of facial skeletal variants. Am J Orthod. 1955;41(6):407-34.
8. Dhopatkar A, Bhatia S, Rock P. An investigation into the relationship between the cranial base angle and malocclusion. Angle Orthod. 2002;72(5):456-63.
9. Enlow DH. Crescimento facial. 3ª ed. São Paulo: Artes Médicas; 1993.
10. Faltin Jr. K. A individualização do diagnóstico e conseqüentes opções de tratamento. In: Grupo brasileiro de Professores de Ortodontia e Odontopediatria. São Paulo; 1997. p. 166-72.
11. Ferner AG, Staubesand RT. Sobotta Atlas de Anatomia Humana. Rio de Janeiro: Guanabara Koogan; 1983.
12. Freitas JC. Influência da base craniana nas más oclusões [dissertação]. Rio de Janeiro (RJ): Universidade Federal do Rio de Janeiro; 1983.
13. Guyer EC, Ellis EE 3rd, McNamara JA Jr, Behrents RG. Components of Class III malocclusion in juveniles and adolescents. Angle Orthod. 1986;56(1):7-30.
14. Jacobson A, Evans WG, Preston CB, Sadowsky PL. Mandibular prognathism. Am J Orthod. 1974; 66(2):140-71.
15. Kasai K, Moro T, Kanazawa E, Iwasawa T. Relationship between cranial base and maxilofacial morphology. Eur J Orthod. 1995;17(5):403-10.
16. Klocke A, Nanda RS, Kahl-Nieke B. Skeletal Class II paterns in the primary dentition. Am J Orthod Dentofacial Orthop. 2002;121(6):596-601.
17. Lanza P, Santos Pinto A, Bolini PDA. Estudo cefalométrico do crescimento e flexão da base do crânio humano do nascimento aos seis meses de idade. Rev Dental Press Ortod Ortop Facial. 2003;7(2):33-9.
18. Marquez IM. Avaliação do padrão facial, preparo ortodôntico e capacidade do tratamento cirúrgico em pacientes Classe III com prognatismo mandibular [tese]. Bauru (SP): Faculdade de Odontologia de Bauru; 1993.
19. Moore WJ, Lavelle CLB. Growth of the facial skeleton in the hominoidea. New York: Academic; 1974.
20. Mouakeh M. Cephalometric evaluation of craniofacial pattern of Syrian children with Class III malocclusion. Am J Orthod Dentofacial Orthop. 2001;119(6):640-9.
21. Moyers RE. Ortodontia. 4ª ed. Rio de Janeiro: Guanabara Koogan; 1991.
22. Ngan PW, Byczek E, Scheick J. Longitudinal evaluation of growth changes in Class II division 1 subjects. Semin Orthod. 1997;3(4):222-31.
23. Ricketts RM. Planning treatment on the basis of the facial pattern and an estimative os its growth. Angle Orthod. 1957;27(1):14-37.
24. Rothstein T, Yoon-Tarlie C. Dental and facial skeletal characteristics and growth of males and females with Class II, division 1 malocclusion between the ages of 10 and 14 (revisited) – Part I: characteristics of size, form, and position. Am J Orthod Dentofacial Orthop. 2000;117(3):320-32.
25. Sandborn RT. Differences between the facial skeletal patterns of Class III malocclusion and normal occlusion. Angle Orthod. 1955;25(4):208-22.
26. Scott JH. Dentofacial development and growth. Oxford: Pergamon; 1967.
27. Suguino R, Ramos AL, Terada HH, Furquim LZ, Maeda L, Silva OG Filho. Análise Facial. Rev Dental Press Ortod Ortop Maxilar. 1996;1(1):86-107.
28. Varrela J. Early developmental traits in Class II malocclusion. Acta Odontol Scand. 1998;56(6):375-7.
29. Vion PE. Anatomia cefalométrica. São Paulo: Ed. Santos; 1994.
30. Weidenreich F. Some particulars of skull and brain of early hominids and their bearing on the problem of the relationship between man and anthropoids. Am J Phys Anthropol. 1947;5(4):387-427.

19

Sterilizing elastomeric chains without losing mechanical properties

Matheus Melo Pithon[1], Caio Souza Ferraz[2], Francine Cristina Silva Rosa[3], Luciano Pereira Rosa[4]

Objective: To investigate the effects of different sterilization/disinfection methods on the mechanical properties of orthodontic elastomeric chains. **Methods:** Segments of elastomeric chains with 5 links each were sent for sterilization by cobalt 60 (Co60) (20 KGy) gamma ray technology. After the procedure, the elastomeric chains were contaminated with clinical samples of *Streptococcus mutans*. Subsequently, the elastomeric chains were submitted to sterilization/disinfection tests carried out by means of different methods, forming six study groups, as follows: Group 1 (control - without contamination), Group 2 (70°GL alcohol), Group 3 (autoclave), Group 4 (ultraviolet), Group 5 (peracetic acid) and Group 6 (glutaraldehyde). After sterilization/disinfection, the effectiveness of these methods, by Colony forming units per mL (CFU/mL), and the mechanical properties of the material were assessed. Student's t-test was used to assess the number of CFUs while ANOVA and Tukey's test were used to assess elastic strength. **Results:** Ultraviolet treatment was not completely effective for sterilization. No loss of mechanical properties occurred with the use of the different sterilization methods (p > 0.05). **Conclusion:** Biological control of elastomeric chains does not affect their mechanical properties.

Keywords: Orthodontics. Disinfection. Elastomers.

[1] Professor of Orthodontics, Universidade Estadual do Sudoeste da Bahia (UESB), Jequié, Bahia, Brazil.
[2] Undergraduate student in Dentistry, Universidade Estadual do Sudoeste da Bahia (UESB), Jequié, Bahia, Brazil.
[3] Professor of Microbiology, Universidade Federal da Bahia (UFBA), Vitória da Conquista, Bahia, Brazil.
[4] Professor of Radiology, Universidade Federal da Bahia (UFBA), Vitória da Conquista, Bahia, Brazil.

Matheus Melo Pithon
Av. Otávio Santos, 395, sala 705, Centro Odontomédico Dr. Altamirando da Costa Lima, Bairro Recreio, CEP 45020-750 - Vitória da Conquista - Bahia - Brazil - E-mail: matheuspithon@gmail.com

» The authors report no commercial, proprietary or financial interest in the products or companies described in this article.

INTRODUCTION

Fighting infections in dental offices has been a daunting challenge to dentists, researchers and immunologists. Most of times, germs have been able to dodge contemporary safety measures, thereby exposing professionals and patients to risk. On the other hand, lack of care by some professionals with regard to biosafety has favored the intensification of infection.[1,2]

Of the dental specialties, Orthodontics is outstanding among those with a higher number of predisposing factors for cross-infection.[3,4] Orthodontics is characterized by a high turnover of patients and multiplicity of vehicles for disease transmission (equipment, instruments, operators' hands, etc.), thus exposing clinicians, assistants and patients to serious risks of infection.[5,6]

In Orthodontics, elastomeric chains are among the different types of material that highly favor the occurrence of cross-infection, given that this type of material is commercially presented in reels ranging from 1 to 4.5 meters, which hinders its individual use.[7,8]

Despite wide acceptance and use of elastomeric chains, doubt is cast on their mechanical and biological properties after they have been submitted to sterilization procedures.[9] Considering that elastics and elastomeric chains are amorphous polymers made of polyurethane material, presenting characteristics of both rubber and plastic, their characteristics may be altered in contact with physical and or chemical agents.[10]

Thus, the present study aimed at assessing which method would be most indicated to sterilize elastomeric chains without causing them to lose their mechanical properties.

MATERIAL AND METHODS

Elastomeric chains (Morelli, Sorocaba, Brazil) of the short spacing type were carefully removed from the reel without being elongated/stretched, and cut into segments with 5 links each. Subsequently, they were wrapped in surgical grade paper (n = 15) and sent to sterilization by gamma radiation with cobalt 60 (20 KGy) (Empresa Brasileira de Radiação - EMBRARAD, Cotia-SP, Brazil) without alterations in their physical properties.

Assessing effectiveness of different methods

After specimens were sterilized, they were contaminated in test tubes containing 10 mL of TODD liquid culture medium with 100 microliters of standardized suspension for assessment by spectrophotometry (optical density = 0.620; wavelength = 398) of 1×10^6 cells/mL of ten different randomly selected clinical samples of *Streptococcus mutans*. Specimens were then incubated at 37 °C for 48 h.

After the incubation period and *Streptococcus mutans* monospecies biofilm formation adherent to the specimens, the latter were introduced into polypropylene tubes, containing 2 mL of sterile saline solution (0.85% NaCl), for 10 seconds, so as to remove excess biofilm. Specimens were then introduced into appropriate and sterile receptacles so as to be subjected to sterilization tests, as follows:

» Group 1: Elastomeric chains which were not submitted to any sterilization method (control group).

» Group 2: Elastomeric chains immersed in polypropylene tubes containing 2 mL of 70° GL alcohol for 1 minute.

» Group 3: Elastomeric chains autoclaved for a cycle of 15 minutes.

» Group 4: Elastomeric chains sterilized in ultraviolet light (SPLabor, Presidente Prudente, São Paulo, Brazil) for 30 minutes, divided by 15 minutes on each side of the elastic.

» Group 5: Elastomeric chains immersed in polypropylene tubes containing 2 mL of peracetic acid for 30 minutes.

» Group 6: Elastomeric chains immersed in polypropylene tubes containing 2 mL of 2% glutaraldehyde solution for 30 minutes.

After sterilization/disinfection procedures were carried out by the different methods, the specimens were removed in a sterile environment inside a laminar flow chamber and introduced into polypropylene tubes containing 2 mL of sterile saline solution (0.85% NaCl), agitated in a vortex appliance for 1 minute. From the suspension obtained, decimal dilutions of 10^{-1}, 10^{-2} were made. Aliquots of 100 microliters of initial suspension and the other dilutions were seeded on Petri dishes containing Todd Hewitt broth at 37 °C for 48 h.

Subsequently, each dish was examined by a single previously calibrated investigator to determine the number of colony forming units per mL (CFU/mL) with the aid of a colony counter (CP602, Phoenix, Araraquara, São Paulo, Brazil).

Table 1 - Methods with description of respective groups.

	Sterilization method	Time	Pressure	Volume	Temperature
Group 1	-	-	-	-	-
Group 2	70° GL alcohol	1 min	-	1 mL	Room
Group 3	Autoclave	15 min	1 atm	-	121 °C
Group 4	Ultraviolet	15 min p/surface	-	-	Room
Group 5	Peracetic acid	30 min	-	2 mL	Room
Group 6	Glutaraldehyde	30 min	-	2 mL	Room

Assessing mechanical properties

After being submitted to different biological control methods, the strength generated by the elastomeric chains was measured (n = 15)according to the previously established sequence of groups.

Elastomeric chains were taken to a digital dynamometer (Instrutherm DD-300, São Paulo, Brazil) mounted on a platform specifically set up for this investigation. Elastomeric chains were distended for 23.5 cm.

Statistical analysis

After assessing the number of colonies formed and the maximum values obtained by the elastomeric chains, statistical analyses were carried out. To this end, SPSS 13.0 software (SPSS Inc., Chicago, Illinois, USA) was used. Descriptive statistical analysis including mean and standard deviation was carried out for all groups. The values referring to the number of colonies formed were submitted to Student's t-test with a significance level set at 5%. The values referring to the amount of strength released were submitted to analysis of variance (ANOVA) so as to determine whether there were statistical differences among groups. Tukey's test was later performed.

RESULTS

Results referring to the mean number of colony forming units (CFU/mL) reveal that the control group obtained the highest mean of around 220,000 CFU/mL, whereas the group in which ultraviolet light (UV) was used as the method for microorganism control obtained an approximate mean of 80,000 CFU/mL.

When UV was compared to the other biological control methods, it proved to be the least effective in reducing microorganisms (p = 0.010) (Table 1). There were statistical differences between the control group and the other groups (p < 0.05) (Fig 1 and Table 2).

Table 2 - Mean, standard deviation and statistical analysis of the number of colony forming units for the different groups evaluated.

Group	Biological control methods	Mean (SD)	Statistics
1	Control	220133.2 (53911.093)	-2/p = 0.000*
			-3/p = 0.000*
			-4/p = 0.000
			-5/p = 0.000
			-6/p = 0.000
2	70° GL alcohol	0.00 (0)	-3/p = 1.000
			-4/p = 0.010*
			-5/p = 1.000
			-6/p = 1.000
3	Autoclave	0.00 (0)	-4/p = 0.010*
			-5/p = 1.000
			-6/p = 1.000
4	Ultraviolet	75956 (83643)	-5/p = 0.010*
			-6/p = 0.010*
5	Peracetic acid	0.00 (0)	-6/p = 1.010
6	Glutaraldehyde	0.00 (0)	

SD = standard deviation;
*= statistical differences (p < 0.05).

With regard to the percentage of decontamination of elastomeric chains, the UV group obtained the lowest percentage of around 65%, whereas the other methods obtained 100%.

In terms of mechanical properties, no differences were found among the different sterilization methods (p > 0.005) (Table 3).

DISCUSSION

When manipulating orthodontic elastomeric chains at the time of inserting them into patient's oral cavity, the orthodontist indirectly contaminates the reel that contains the material which may trigger a cross-infection.

Table 3 - Statistics of different biological control methods in terms of evaluation of the mechanical properties of elastomeric chains.

Groups	Methods of sterilization	Mean (SD)	p value
1	Control	6.36 (0.79)	-2/p = 0.571
			-3/p = 1.000
			-4/p = 0.478
			-5/p = 0.810
			-6/p = 0.997
2	70° GL alcohol	5.74 (0.84)	-3/p = 0.370
			-4/p = 0.012
			-5/p = 0.999
			-6/p = 0.292
3	Autoclave	6.48 (0.85)	-4/p = 0.686
			-5/p = 0.618
			-6/p = 1.000
4	Ultraviolet	7.02 (1.03)	-5/p = 0.036
			-6/p = 0.771
5	Peracetic acid	5.89 (1.21)	-6/p = 0.524
6	Glutaraldehyde	6.53 (1.11)	

SD = standard deviation.
*= statistical differences (p < 0.05).

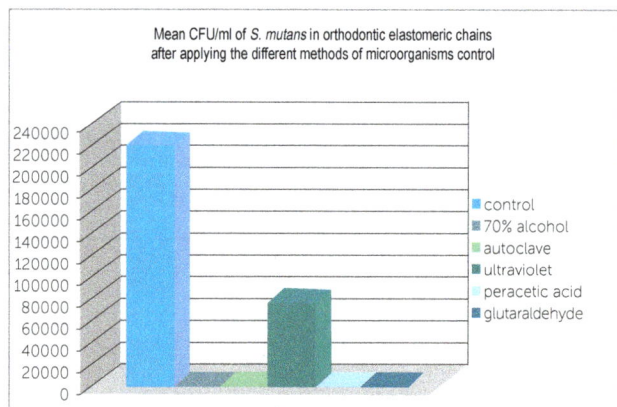

Figure 1 - Mean CFU/mL of *S. Mutans* on orthodontic elastomeric chains after applying the different methods of microorganisms control.

Cross-infection is defined as the transmission of infectious agents among patients and health personnel within a clinical environment. Transmission occurs from person to person or by contact with contaminated objects. Transmission may occur through blood, saliva droplets, or instruments contaminated with blood, saliva and tissue debris. Transmission pathway is either by contact, inhalation or inoculation.[1]

According to Silva et al,[11] there is a high incidence of cross-infection in the dental office. Thus, the use of decontaminating agents is relevant in clinical practice. A number of methods is used in the dental office with a view to dodging cross-infection, namely: autoclave, alcohol, glutaraldehyde, peracetic acid and ultraviolet radiation.

According to Berger,[12] ultraviolet radiation (UV) is used in Dentistry as a disinfectant agent for toothbrush surfaces; however, its effectiveness is greatly related to the time of exposure. In the present study, ultraviolet radiation obtained the lowest percentage (65%) in the reduction of colony forming units (CFU/mL) in comparison to the other groups in which disinfectant agents were used. The latter reduced CFUs/mL in 100%. When the mechanical properties of elastomeric chains were compared, UV obtained the best mean, around 7.02; however, without significant differences among groups.

In the present study, glutaraldehyde proved an efficient disinfectant agent, in addition to not affecting the mechanical properties of elastomeric chains, given that there was no significant difference between this group (6.53) and the control group (6.36). These data corroborate the findings by Suprono et al[13] who reported that glutaraldehyde does not cause deterioration of the elastomeric chain surface.

Peracetic acid has been used in food and water industries, sewage treatment companies and for decontamination and sterilization of heat-sensitive medical-hospital devices and equipment.[14-17] Peracetic-acid proved an efficient decontaminating agent and completely reduced the number of colony forming units (CFU/mL). Furthermore, peracetic acid does not leave residues and does not produce harmful products, as its mechanism of action involves the release of free oxygen and hydroxyl radicals in decomposition in water, oxygen and acetic acid.[14-17] This was proved in the present study, since all elastomeric chains evaluated kept their mechanical properties, in addition to being completely sterilized.

The method most used for sterilization of medical and dental instruments worldwide is damp steam sterilization (autoclave).[18] It proved efficient in reducing the number of colony forming units (CFU/mL), thereby completely reducing the existent bacteria. Moreover, it yielded surprising results in terms of the mechanical properties of elastomeric chains, since even in contact with heat, the mechanical properties remained the same, without statistical differences in comparison to the control group.

Based on the results obtained in this study, the simplest method of promoting sterilization/disinfection of orthodontic elastomeric chains was alcohol. After 1 minute, it was possible to eliminate the microorganisms adhered to the elastics without losing their mechanical characteristics. Nevertheless, the fact that only *S. Mutans* was used in the experiment must be considered. In spite of being the most prevalent and most important infectious agent in the oral cavity, this bacterium is not the most resistant; therefore, further studies are warranted to investigate other microorganisms.

Importantly, orthodontic clinic success not only involves mastery of corrective techniques to achieve the ideal dental occlusion, but also requires the application of biosafety rules and concerns about the local and systemic consequences of dental material used for this purpose.

CONCLUSION

Based on the results of this study it is reasonable to conclude that except for the ultraviolet method, all other methods promoted sterilization of elastomeric chains; no sterilization methods led to loss of elastomeric chains mechanical properties.

REFERENCES

1. Barghout N, Habashneh RA, Ryalat ST, Asa'ad FA, Marashdeh M. Patients' perception of cross-infection prevention in dentistry in Jordan. Oral Health Prev Dent. 2012;10(1):9-16.

2. Sofola OO, Uti OG, Onigbinde OO. Public perception of cross-infection control in dentistry in Nigeria. Int Dent J. 2005;55(6):383-7.

3. Davies C. Orthodontic products update. Cross infection control and elastomeric module delivery systems. Br J Orthod. 1998;25(4):301-3.

4. Shcherbakov AS, Ivanova SB, Nikonorov VI. [The organizational problems of preventing cross infection in orthodontic departments and offices]. Stomatologiia (Mosk). 1996;Spec No:94-5.

5. Casaccia GR, Gomes JC, Alviano DS, Ruellas ACO, Sant'Anna EF. Microbiological evaluation of elastomeric chains. Angle Orthod. 2007;77(5):890-3.

6. Tebbett PM. Gloves: a recommended aid in cross infection control in orthodontics. A comparison of gloves available from UK supply houses. Br J Orthod. 1993;20:367-371.

7. Dittmer MP, Demling AP, Borchers L, Stiesch M, Kohorst P, Schwestka-Polly R. The influence of simulated aging on the mechanical properties of orthodontic elastomeric chains without an intermodular link. J Orofac Orthop. 2012;73(4):289-97.

8. Takla GS, Cunningham SJ, Horrocks EN, Wilson M. The effectiveness of an elastomeric module dispenser in cross-infection control. J Clin Orthod. 1998;32(12):721-6.

9. Jeffries CL, von Fraunhofer JA. The effects of 2% alkaline gluteraldehyde solution on the elastic properties of elastomeric chain. Angle Orthod. 1991;61(1):25-30.

10. Josell SD, Leiss JB, Rekow D. Force degradation in elastomeric chain. Semin Orthod. 1997;3(3):189-97.

11. Silva FC, Kimpara ET, Mancini MN, Balducci I, Jorge AO, Koga-Ito CY. Effectiveness of six different disinfectants on removing five microbial species and effects on the topographic characteristics of acrylic resin. J Prosthodont 2008;17(8):627-33.

12. Berger JR, Drukartz MJ, Tenenbaum MD. The efficacy of two UV toothbrush sanitization devices. A pilot study. NY State Dent J. 2008;74(1):50-2.

13. Suprono MS, Kattadiyil MT, Goodacre CJ, Winer MS. Effect of disinfection on irreversible hydrocolloid and alternative impression materials and the resultant gypsum casts. J Prosthet Dent. 2012;108(4):250-8.

14. Kauppinen A, Ikonen J, Pursiainen A, Pitkanen T, Miettinen IT. Decontamination of a drinking water pipeline system contaminated with adenovirus and Escherichia coli utilizing peracetic acid and chlorine. J Water Health. 2012;10(3):406-18.

15. Sagsen B, Ustun Y, Aslan T, Canakci BC. The effect of peracetic acid on removing calcium hydroxide from the root canals. J Endod. 2012;38(9):1197-201.

16. Gonzalez A, Gehr R, Vaca M, Lopez R. Disinfection of an advanced primary effluent with peracetic acid and ultraviolet combined treatment: a continuous-flow pilot plant study. Water Environ Res. 2012;84(3):247-53.

17. Fernandes FH, Orsi IA, Villabona CA. Effects of the peracetic acid and sodium hypochlorite on the colour stability and surface roughness of the denture base acrylic resins polymerised by microwave and water bath methods. Gerodontology. 2013;30(1):18-25.

18. Jabbari H, Alikhah H, Sahebkaram Alamdari N, Naghavi Behzad M, Mehrabi E, Borzui L, et al. Developing the use of quality indicators in sterilization practices. Iranian. J Publ Health. 2012;41:64-9.

20

Orthodontic post-adjustment pain control with acupuncture

Daniela de Cassia Faglioni Boleta-Ceranto[1], Ricardo Sampaio de Souza[2], Sandra Silverio-Lopes[3], Nathalie Canola Moura[4]

Objective: This study aimed to evaluate the analgesic efficacy of systemic acupuncture therapy on the pain caused after orthodontic adjustments. **Methods:** An initial sample of 30 orthodontic patients with fixed appliances monthly adjusted was selected; however, only 11 participants completed the study. For this reason, final sample comprised these patients' data only. Initially, average pain levels were assessed at different periods by means of an analogue visual scale (VAS) for three months without acupuncture. In the following three months, the volunteers were submitted to systemic acupuncture sessions on Hegu (LI4) and Jiache (St6) points,before orthodontic adjustments were carried out. **Results:** Results revealed statistically significant reduction in pain level indexes both for men (P = 0.030) and women (P = 0.028) when acupuncture therapy was performed prior to orthodontic adjustment. Patients did not present any side effects. **Conclusion:** Acupuncture is a safe and effective method in reducing orthodontic post-adjustment pain.

Keywords: Orthodontics. Acupuncture analgesia. Pain.

[1] Full professor, Paranaense University (UNIPAR).

[2] Full professor, Department of Orthodontics, UNIPAR.

[3] Professor, Graduate program, Brazilian Institute of Therapy and Education (IBRATE).

[4] Specialist in Orthodontics, UNIPAR.

» The authors report no commercial, proprietary or financial interest in the products or companies described in this article.

Daniela de Cassia Faglioni Boleta Ceranto
Rua Carlos Bartolomeu Canceli, 950 – sobrado 42 – Bairro Canceli
Cascavel/PR – Brazil – CEP 85.811-280 – E-mail: dcboleta@unipar.br

INTRODUCTION

Dental therapy in general, including orthodontic treatment, usually causes pain or distress. Pain is considered a very subjective symptom, for this reason, it is best defined as: "An uncomfortable sensory and emotional experience associated with real or potential injuries or described in terms of such injuries".[1] Individual's past experiences, emotional state, cultural background, age and sex[2,3] are among the facts that influence pain level, all of which may pose difficulties in measuring symptoms.

The literature shows that all orthodontic procedures, such as separator placement, fixed orthodontic appliances installation and activation, and orthopedic force application, cause pain. Additionally, fixed appliances tend to cause more pain than removable or functional ones, and the correlation between applied forces and pain is small.[4]

There are two major forms of distress caused by fixed orthodontic appliances: traumatic ulcers and pain during orthodontic movement.

In case of traumatic ulcers, orthodontic appliance functions as a traumatic factor that lesions the mucosa and causes epithelial tissue loss, thereby exposing subjacent conjunctive tissue and causing pain by local nociceptors stimulation.

As for orthodontic movement, there are no doubts that pain perception is part of the inflammatory reaction caused by blood flow alterations after orthodontic forces are applied. As a result, many chemical mediators are released as follows: Substance P, histamine, encephalin, dopamine, serotonin, glycine, glutamate, gamma-aminobutyric acid (GABA), prostaglandin, leucotriene, cytokine; thereby causing local hyperalgesia.[4,5] Bergius et al[3] analyzed 203 orthodontic patients, and demonstrated that 91% of them reported pain caused by orthodontic appliance, whereas 39% reported pain in every orthodontic appointment while adjustment was carried out. Studies show that nearly 95% of patients under orthodontic treatment present different levels of discomfort,[6,7] especially within the first 24 hours after orthodontic adjustment. Pain caused by fixed orthodontic treatment gradually increases 4 hours after appliance adjustment, returning to normality on the seventh day.[2,7,8,10]

Studies reveal that the first 48 hours of pain after orthodontic adjustment cause as much disturbance as to interfere in patient's sleep and induce the need for medication. Krishnan[4] conducted a literature review and found that nearly all orthodontic patients report moderate to extreme difficulty in chewing and swallowing solid food because of pain, proving that orthodontic pain can also interfere in patient's diet, thus raising another major concern for patients and professionals.

Erdinç and Dinçer[11] reported that nearly 50% of their patients suffered pain within 6 hours to two days after orthodontic adjustment, which interfered in their daily activities. The authors also reported a reduction in pain intensity and the number of patients with pain from the third day on.

Considering the high rate of patients complaining about pain suffered during orthodontic treatment, different methods have been tested for its control, namely: low-level laser (LEDs) application, transcutaneous electrical nerve stimulation (TENS), neural stimulation, vibration to stimulate periodontal ligament, among others resulting in pain control.[5]

In addition to conventional techniques, researchers have sought new procedures for pain control. As a result, Dentistry is trying alternative methods to aid professionals bring more comfort to their patients. Nevertheless, new methods do not include the development of new ultra-modern equipments and/or last generation drugs, only. Researches show that ancient techniques are scientifically efficient in pain control, and acupuncture is among the most effective ones.

The present study assessed the analgesic efficacy of systemic acupuncture therapy on pain caused after orthodontic adjustments. The tested hypotheses were whether acupuncture was efficient or not in reducing pain caused by orthodontic adjustment.

MATERIAL AND METHODS

This research was approved by the Ethics Committee on Human Research under protocol 00080375000-08. All volunteers filled an informed consent form.

This research was conducted as a blind study. The researcher responsible for acupuncture was aware of the treatment modality each patient would be submitted to. However, results were analyzed by a statistician unaware of the treatment to which each volunteer was subjected to.

Patients under fixed orthodontic treatment at the Graduate Program Orthodontic Clinic participated in this research. First, research volunteers were selected. To be included in the group, the patient had to be complaining of pain after orthodontic adjustment and accept acupuncture treatment. Thirty patients volunteered, although, only 11 (7 women and 4 man) concluded the study. Patients' mean age was of 16.2 years (Table 1). The volunteers were monthly assessed during 6 months by means of a visual analogue scale (VAS) for pain. Each scale corresponds to a 10-cm horizontal line with two points meaning "no pain" and "the worst pain possible". Participants were instructed to mark a transversal trace on the line, representing the equivalence of pain intensity they felt.[3]

VAS allowed pain to be quantified during different periods (before orthodontic adjustment, right after adjustment, 4, 8, 24 and 72 hours after adjustment). Each participant received 7 scales every month in accordance with previously described periods. In the following appointments, the scales were filled and collected for analysis which measured each scale with a millimetric ruler so as to obtain numerical data.[3]

Within the first 3 months, the volunteers were instructed to fill out VAS after orthodontic adjustment so as to obtain an average of participant's pain without acupuncture treatment. In the following 3 months, antisepsis of the areas of needle insertion was done with cotton and 70% alcohol 5 minutes prior to each orthodontic adjustment. Subsequently, systemic needles were inserted at Hegu (LI4) and Jiache (St6) points on both sides. The needles remained in place for twenty minutes.[12] Dragon® Sterile stainless steel needles (0.20 x 25 mm) were used.

New VASs were filled out during the same periods previously described. Results were used to calculate the average pain described by each patient during the three orthodontic adjustment appointments after acupuncture therapy. Therefore, volunteers performed self-analyses.

Patients were instructed not to take any other analgesic medication while the effect of acupuncture therapy was being analyzed. Should pain be too intense so as to require analgesic medication, the instruction was to record the date, time, type and doses of medication.

Analysis of results of the 11 volunteers was carried out with Sigma-Stat statistic program. Data was first submitted to analysis of variance (ANOVA) ($P \leq 0.05$). Should ANOVA yield significant values, Tukey test was used to identify significant differences between the average pain level obtained through VAS.

RESULTS

Since significant statistic differences were found in pain perception between male and female patients, results were separately assessed according to that variable.

Variation of pain perception according to time

Results reveal a gradual increase in volunteers' pain level right after orthodontic adjustments and within the first 24 hours with gradual reduction during the following periods. Table 2 and Figure 1 show the averages between female and male patients.

General pain level average of male and female volunteers with and without acupuncture therapy

Analysis of variance (ANOVA) followed by Tukey test at a 5% significance level was conducted between male and female patients and showed a statistically significant difference in pain level after orthodontic activation with or without previous acupuncture therapy. Results are shown in Table 3 and Figure 2.

Average pain level of female volunteers during different periods with and without acupuncture

Averages obtained with or without acupuncture treatment at different studied periods submitted to analysis of variance (ANOVA) at 5% significance level between male and female patients showed that although there was a reduction in pain level during all periods when acupuncture was performed before orthodontic adjustments, it was only statistically significant during the pre-orthodontic adjustment period. Results are shown in Table 4 and Figure 3A.

Table 1 - Volunteers' age and sex.

Sex	Mean ± SD
Female	15.33 ± 3.933
Male	17.4 ± 3.43
Total	16.2 ± 3.68

Table 2 - Average pain level alterations over time.

	Before*	After**	4 h	8 h	24 h	48 h	72 h
Without acupuncture	1.08	3.76	4.09	3.96	3.965	3.2	2
With acupuncture	0.104	2.2504	2.711	1.71	2.4	1.6	1.29

* Before orthodontic adjustment.
** Right after orthodontic adjustment.

Table 3 - Average values of pain level after orthodontic adjustment with or without previous acupuncture therapy in male and female volunteers. Data expressed as mean ± standard deviation.

Treatment	Mean ± SD
Without acupuncture male	2.61 ± 1.263
With acupuncture male	1.27 ± 0.677
Without acupuncture female	3.72 ± 1.129
With acupuncture female	2.22 ± 1.113

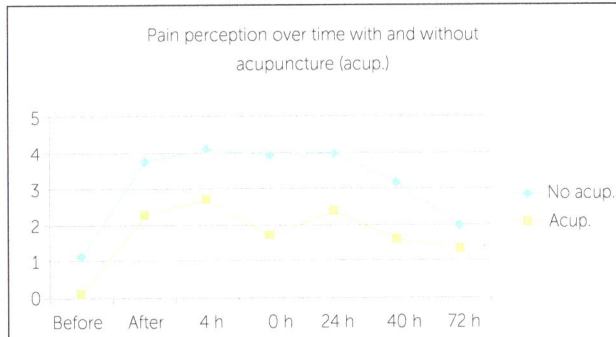

Figure 1 - Average pain perception alteration over time, with and without previous acupuncture therapy.

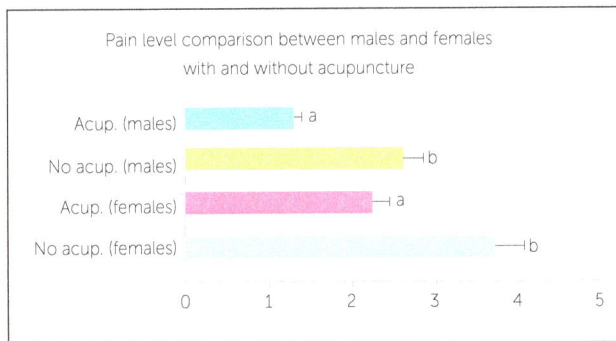

Figure 2 - Average (and standard deviation) of male and female volunteers' pain level after orthodontic adjustment with or without previous acupuncture therapy. The comparison using distinct letters through Tukey test statistically distinguishes the averages among themselves.

Average pain level of male volunteers during different periods with and without acupuncture

Analysis of variance (ANOVA) was performed at 5% significance level among male participants during different periods with and without acupuncture and revealed a statistically significant difference in pain level 8 hours after orthodontic adjustment, only. Nevertheless, there was a visual reduction in the levels of pain perception recorded during all periods. Results are shown in Table 4 and Figure 3B.

DISCUSSION

Even if analgesic and anesthetic medications are used, dental therapy, including orthodontic treatment, is acknowledged by most people to cause pain or even a light distress. The literature shows that all orthodontic procedures, such as separator placement, bracket installation and activation, and the application and activation of orthopedic forces, cause pain. Additionally, fixed appliances cause more pain than removable or functional ones and the correlation among applied forces and pain felt by patients is small.[4]

Table 4 - Average values of pain levels in different periods with or without previous acupuncture (acup.) treatment in female and male volunteers. Data expressed as mean ± standard deviation.

	Before	After	4 h	8 h	24 h	48 h	72 h
No acup. (female)	1.77 ± 1.68	4.21 ± 2.69	4.36 ± 2.39	4.63 ± 1.84	4.3 ± 2.22	4.31 ± 1.88	2.43 ± 1.90
Acup. (female)	*0.02 ± 0.03	2.92 ± 2.34	3.34 ± 2.11	2.50 ± 2.49	2.90 ± 2.64	2.20 ± 1.94	1.64 ± 2.03
No acup. (male)	0.4 ± 0.62	3.32 ± 1.77	3.83 ± 1.67	3.3 ± 1.64	3.63 ± 1.96	2.22 ± 1.52	1.6 ± 2.38
Acup. (male)	0.18 ± 0.29	1.59 ± 2.10	2.08 ± 2.17	*0.93 ± 0.39	2.03 ± 0.88	1.18 ± 2.39	0.95 ± 1.54

* $p < 0.05$.

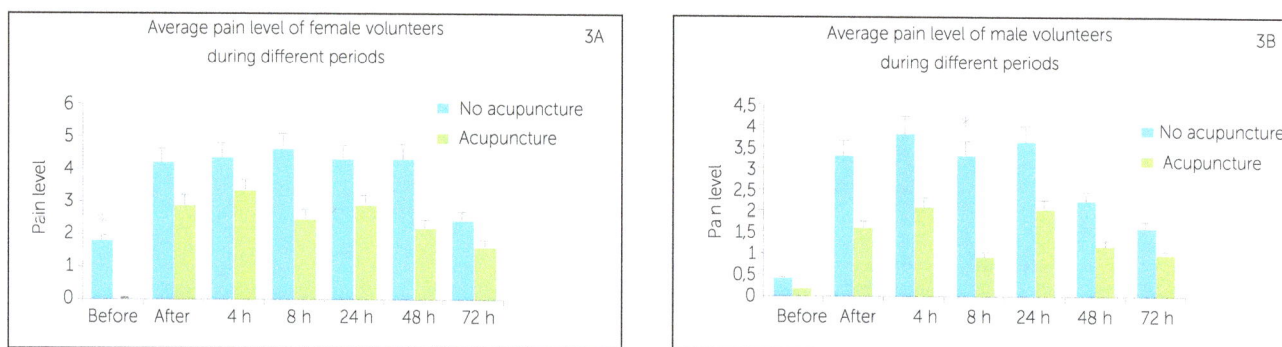

Figure 3 - Average pain level (and standard deviation) of female (**A**) and male (**B**) volunteers during different periods of orthodontic adjustment with and without previous acupuncture treatment. * $p < 0.05$.

Among the facts that influence pain level are: former experiences, emotional state, cultural background, age and sex,[2,3,18] all of which may pose difficulties in measuring the symptom. Except for patient's age and sex, which can be easily be assessed, all other factors are quite personal and can be considered as limitations of the present study, since they were not considered as variants that influence pain levels and could interfere in the results.[3] Participants' motivation and expectations towards the acupuncture analgesic effect also seem not to influence the results. Since the average values were monthly collected, participants had no access to former analyses and could hardly compare the records in a way that allowed them to forge final results. This could be considered a limitation of this study. Ideally, Sham acupuncture (needle applications at non-analgesic points) should have also been used; however, once a great number of participants quit, it was impossible to divide the group due to the limited number of volunteers comprising the sample. Further studies will be able to correct this fact.

Considering the high rate of patients complaining about pain suffered during orthodontic treatment, different methods have been tested for its control, namely: Low-power laser (LEDs) application, transcutaneous electrical nerve stimulation (TENS), neural stimulation, vibration to stimulate periodontal ligament, among others resulting in pain control.[5] In addition to conventional techniques to control pain, Dentistry has introduced alternative methods to aid professionals bring more comfort to their patients. Those alternative techniques have been acknowledged and approved by the Federal Council of Dentistry (Resolution 82, July, 2008), and can be applied to reduce pain in dental patients. Acupuncture is one of the most effective techniques.

The aim of the present study was to assess the analgesic efficiency of systemic acupuncture performed before orthodontic adjustment to treat orthodontic post-adjustment pain. The research started with 30 patients gathered from an Orthodontic Graduate Program, but only 11 participants concluded it. Some degree of desistance is expected during human research. No volunteers declined to participate in this study due to its methodology. A great number of absences during orthodontic adjustment appointments were observed, thereby eliminating some participants. In some cases, the orthodontist responsible for the orthodontic adjustment was absent, which also hindered patient's particiation on the research. All volunteers had their pain level analyzed by Visual Analogical Scales (VAS).

VAS was chosen due to being greatly used to measure pain and having some advantages among verbal scales, such as the facility children have in filling it out.[13] Patients were asked to register the intensity of pain they felt on the line representing the estimate variable.[13] A numerical value was assigned by the researcher using a millimetric ruler. Consequently, precise values were not possible.[14] No volunteers had difficulties in filling out the scales, reinforcing their easiness.

Bergius et al[3] assert that pain caused by orthodontic adjustment can be immediate or delayed. Immediate pain occurs after the archwire is attached and periodontal ligament is compressed. The latter starts a few hours later when hyperalgesia of periodontal ligament generates allodynia through the release of chemical active substances (as prostaglandin, histamine and substance P), thereby causing partial depolarization of afferent fibers, neural facilitation and peripheral sensitization. When an orthodontic force is applied to a tooth, an initial distress and/or pain phase of 1 or two days usually occur.[10] The intensity of pain generally increases within 4 to 24 hours and then reduces to normal levels within a 7-day period.[3] There is generally a circadian variation in pain intensity, with an increase of pain between late afternoon and night, although that does not intensely interfere in sleep.[8] Our results confirm the fact that pain begins after orthodontic adjustment, its apex occurs within 8 to 24 hours and gradually reduces over time, even with previous acupuncture treatment. However, the present work shows that intense decrease occurs when acupuncture treatment is previously performed.

Scheurer[7] also showed that general pain intensity perception, analgesic taking, pain during feeding and distress influence on daily life were significantly greater in women than men. Women are more sensitive to experimental painful stimuli than men, with clinical pain of greater frequency and severity lasting for a longer period of time and in a larger range of body locations.[15,16] In the present study, we also observed greater feminine pain sensitiveness, with or without previous acupuncture treatment. This fact could be related to women's great hormonal variability, mainly in female teenagers voluntaries. For both males and females, acupuncture treatment significantly reduced pain after orthodontic adjustments, thus proving its efficiency.

Even when results showed a reduction in pain levels after acupuncture treatment during all studied periods (both for men and women), it was only statistically significant during two periods. Before orthodontic adjustment in female patients, which is justified by their hormonal alterations — a limitation for the study since their menstrual period was not assessed. For men, within 8 hours after adjustment, corresponding, according to the literature, to the time of pain apex.[3]

Pain reduction observed in the present study probably occurred due to acupuncture action mechanism, activating descending pain inhibition and antinociceptive substances release, such as β-endorphin (analgesics), cortisol (anti-inflammatory) and serotonin (antidepressant) in the blood flow and cephalorachidian liquid.[17]

Data obtained in the present study confirm the efficiency of acupuncture as a complementary treatment in Orthodontics. It is important since nearly all orthodontic patients, as described in many studies, report moderate to extreme difficulty in chewing and swallowing solid food because of pain, proving that orthodontic pain can also interfere on patient's diet, a major concern for patients and professionals.[4] Also, Erdinç and Dinçer[11] reported that nearly 50% of their patients suffered from pain that interfered on their daily activities within 6 hours to two days after orthodontic adjustments, which could be diminished by stimulation of analgesic points through acupuncture, as shown in the present study.

The literature highlights many analgesic acupoints. Microsystems of acupuncture such as ear acupuncture, hand acupuncture and scalp acupuncture points are another treatment option, instead of systemic acupuncture. Hegu (LI4) and Jiache (St6) points were used for its location and professional easy access.

Acknowledgment and approval of acupuncture practice as a complement to dental treatment, issued by the Federal Council of Dentistry in July 2008, will certainly bring progress in this matter, since national researches using acupuncture for dental treatment are few and, for this reason, narrow the benefits of the method for both patients and professionals. Acupuncture does not produce side effects and can be safely practiced by a qualified professional. In this study, a total of 33 acupuncture sessions were done (3 on each one of the 11 volunteers), and no patients presented side effects related to needle insertion.

The fact that it is not an onerous technique is important and must also be observed, particularly considering the present social-economic situation in Brazil.

CONCLUSION

Within the limitations and conditions of this experiment, it is reasonable to conclude that systemic acupuncture treatment performed before orthodontic therapy can reduce pain level in both men and women. Additionally, acupuncture proves to be a safe technique employed for this purpose.

REFERENCES

1. Mersky YH. Classification of chronic pain. Descriptions of chronic pain syndromes and definitions of pain terms. Prepared by the International Association for the Study of Pain, Subcommittee on Taxonomy. Pain Suppl. 1986;3:S1-S226.

2. Okeson JP. Tratamento das desordens temporomandibulares e oclusão. 4a ed. São Paulo: Artes Médicas; 2000.

3. Bergius M, Kiliaridis S, Berggren U. Pain in orthodontics. A review and discussion of the literature. J Orofac Orthop. 2000;61(2):125-37.

4. Krishnan, V. Orthodontic pain: from causes to management: a review. Eur J Orthod. 2007;29(2):170-9.

5. Polat O, Karaman AI. Pain control during fixed orthodontic appliance therapy. Angle Orthod. 2005;75(2):214-9.

6. Kvam E, Bondevik O, Gjerdet NR. Traumatic ulcers and pain during orthodontic treatment. Community Dent Oral Epidemiol. 1989;17(3):154-7.

7. Scheurer P, Firestone A, Bürgin W. Perception of pain as a result of orthodontic treatment with fixed appliances. Eur J Orthod. 1996;18(1):349-57.

8. Jones M, Chan C. The pain and discomfort experienced during orthodontic treatment. A randomized controlled trial of two aligning archwires. Am J Orthod Dentofacial Orthop. 1992;102(4):373-81.

9. Okeson JP. Bell's orofacial pain. 5th ed. Carol Stream, Ill: Quintessence; 1995.

10. Fernandes LM, Øgaard B, Skoglund L. Pain and discomfort experienced after placement of a conventional or a superelastic NiTi aligning archwire. J Orofac Orthop. 1998;59(6):331-9.

11. Erdinç AM, Dinçer B. Perception of pain during orthodontic treatment with fixed appliances. Eur J Orthod. 2004;26(1):79-85.

12. Vachiramon A, Wang WC. Acupuncture and acupressure techniques for reducing orthodontic post-adjustment pain. J Contemp Dent Pract. 2005;6(1):163-7.

13. Seymour R, Simpson J, Chariton J, Phillips M. An evaluation of length and end-phrase of visual analogue scales in dental pain. Pain. 1985;21(2):177-85.

14. Ferreira-Bacci, AV. Comparação da Escala CR10 de Borg com a Escala Analógica Visual na avaliação da dor em pacientes com Desordens Temporomandibulares [dissertação]. Ribeirão Preto (SP): Universidade de São Paulo; 2002.

15. Unruh AM. Gender variations in clinical pain experience. Pain. 1996;65(2-3):123-67.

16. Wise EA, Price DD, Myers CD, Heft MW, Robinson ME. Gender role expectations of pain: relationship to experimental pain perception. Pain. 2002;96(3):335-42.

17. Rosted P. Introduction to acupuncture in dentistry. Br Dent J. 2000;189(3):136-40.

21

Long-term stability of maxillary anterior alignment in non-extraction cases

Luiz Filiphe Gonçalves Canuto[1], Marcos Roberto de Freitas[2], Karina Maria Salvatore de Freitas[3], Rodrigo Hermont Cançado[4], Leniana Santos Neves[5]

Objective: The purpose of this retrospective study was to evaluate long-term stability of maxillary incisors alignment in cases submitted to non-extraction orthodontic treatment. **Methods:** The sample comprised 23 patients (13 female; 10 male) at a mean initial age of 13.36 years (SD = 1.81 years), treated with fixed appliances. Dental cast measurements were obtained at three different time points (T_1 – pretreatment, T_2 – posttreatment and T_3 – long-term posttreatment). Variables assessed in maxillary arch were Little Irregularity Index, intercanine, interpremolar and intermolar widths, arch length and perimeter. The statistical analysis was performed by one-way ANOVA and Tukey tests when necessary. Pearson' correlation coefficients were used to investigate possible associations between the evaluated variables. **Results:** There was no significant change in most arch dimension measurements during and after treatment, however, during the long-term posttreatment period, it was observed a significant maxillary incisors crowding relapse. **Conclusion:** The maxillary incisors irregularity increased significantly (1.52 mm) during long-term posttreatment. None of the studied clinical factors demonstrated to be predictive of the maxillary crowding relapse.
Keywords: Relapse. Corrective orthodontics. Malocclusion.

[1] Post-Doctor in Orthodontics, FOB-USP. Professor, Specialization Course in Orthodontics, ABO-PE and FACSETE.
[2] Professor, Orthodontics, FOB-USP.
[3] PhD in Orthodontics, FOB-USP. Post-Doctor in Orthodontics, Toronto Dentistry University.
[4] Adjunct Professor, Uningá. Professor, Specialization Course in Orthodontics, UFVJM.
[5] Professor, Specialization Course in Orthodontics, UFVJM.

» The authors report no commercial, proprietary or financial interest in the products or companies described in this article.

Luiz Filiphe Gonçalves Canuto
Alameda Octávio Pinheiro Brisolla, 9-75
CEP: 17.012-901 – Bauru/SP – Brazil
E-mail: luizfiliphecanuto@yahoo.com.br

INTRODUCTION

The primary purpose of orthodontic treatments is malocclusion correction; however, treatment stability shows considerable variability during post-retention phase. Despite the literature consensus that some occlusal changes will inevitably occur after orthodontic treatment,[15,19,28] it is noted that long-term stability of the aligned teeth is highly variable and unpredictable.[17]

Greater research emphasis has been placed on relapse of mandibular anterior crowding and little emphasis has been given to investigating the maxillary crowding relapse and parameters that may be helpful in predicting its long-term stability.[2,3,9,12,18,23,25]

Alignment stability of mandibular incisors is less than that of the maxillary anterior teeth.[8,10,22,26,29,30] Factors such as pretreatment crowding severity[25] and gingival fibers traction[5,6,7] are considered risk factors for maxillary incisors crowding relapse. However, there is an association between a prolonged period of retention and greater stability of maxillary teeth alignment.[23] Maxillary incisors tend to rotate in the direction of their initial positions,[25,26] despite buccolingual relapse being unpredictable.[25] Furthermore, palatal contacts between maxillary and mandibular incisors preclude lingual movement of the maxillary teeth and any vestibular movement is probably determined by the lips position and function.[12]

Accordingly to Little,[14] evidence of progressive instability is often first noted by progressive crowding of mandibular incisors following removal of retaining devices. Whatever the multiplicity of causes for relapse, mandibular incisor irregularity is often the precursor of maxillary crowding, deepening of the overbite, and generalized deterioration of orthodontic treated cases.

Kahl-Nieke, Fischbach and Schwarze,[13] evaluated pretreatment, posttreatment, and post-retention models of 226 cases with all types of anomaly. Findings indicated that relapse of incisors crowding occurred in approximately half of the sample and that post-retention crowding increased more frequently in mandible than in the maxilla. Pretreatment variables such as severe crowding and incisors irregularity, arch length deficiency, arch constriction and increased overbite were found to be associated factors in the process of post-retention increase of crowding and incisors irregularity. Premolars extraction treatment exhibited greater maxillary and mandibular crowding relapse than non-extraction protocol.

In a longitudinal study, Moussa, O'Reilly and Close,[18] evaluated 55 non-extraction orthodontic patients that were previously submitted to rapid palatal expansion (RPE). The authors[18] observed that maxillary incisors irregularity increased 0.60 mm during post-retention. They suggested that RPE procedure may be helpful in long-term stability; however, due to the absence of a control group there was no clear evidence about a possible influence of RPE procedure on the crowding relapse. However, Canuto et al,[3] compared the long-term stability of maxillary incisor alignment in patients treated with and without rapid maxillary expansion. They concluded that RME did not influence long-term maxillary anterior alignment stability.

Vaden, Harris and Gardner,[30] concluded that most (96%) of the maxillary incisor irregularity correction was maintained after 15 years of treatment. At the post-retention recall, the maxillary irregularity index increased only 0.30 mm. Surbeck et al[25] evaluated whether pretreatment misalignment of the maxillary anterior teeth are of significance for post-retention relapse of alignment. The results suggested that anatomic contact point displacement of the maxillary anterior teeth and maxillary incisor rotation relative to the dental arch are significant risk factors for post-retention relapse of alignment and that the pattern of rotational displacement relative to the dental arch has a strong tendency to repeat itself.

Taner et al[27] evaluated the effects of fiberotomy in alleviating dental relapse of incisors after orthodontic treatment. The authors described that there was significant increase of irregularity index in the control group, for both maxillary and mandibular anterior segments. Meanwhile, in the group where circumferential supracrestal fiberotomy was performed, no significant increase of the irregularity index was noted. One year later, Huang and Artun,[12] evaluated whether post-retention relapse of maxillary and mandibular incisor alignment were associated. The authors suggested[12] that the occlusal contacts with the mandibular anterior teeth represent lingual boundaries for the maxillary incisor movement, and any labial movement is likely to be determined by the position and function of the lips. In addition, also suggested that the post-retention movement of the mandibular incisors may be influenced by the position of the maxillary incisors and vice versa and indicated that an association between the post-retention misalignment of the incisors in the 2 arches might exist.

Ferris et al[9] investigated the long-term post-retention stability of RPE-lip bumper therapy followed by full fixed appliances. The sample comprised 20 patients at the late mixed dentition that were recalled to obtain post-retention records. The subjects were out of retention for an average of 7.9 years. The majority of treatment increases in maxillary and mandibular arch dimensions were maintained during post-retention phase. Post-retention incisor irregularity increased 0.5 mm in the maxillary arch and 1.1 mm in the mandibular arch. The authors[9] concluded that use of RPE–lip bumper therapy in the late mixed dentition followed by full fixed appliances is an effective form of treatment for patients with up to moderate tooth size-arch length discrepancies.

Erdinc, Nanda and Isiksal,[8] evaluated long-term stability of incisor crowding in orthodontic patients treated with and without premolar extractions. Minimal incisor crowding relapse occurred (0.19 mm and 0.12 mm for extraction and non-extraction groups, respectively). Maxillary incisor irregularity relapse was smaller than mandibular incisor relapse for both groups. Intercanine width expanded during treatment. Incisor positions in both groups tended to return to pretreatment values. Clinically acceptable stability was obtained.[8]

Because of insufficient studies on maxillary anterior tooth alignment and parameters that may be helpful in predicting its long-term stability, this study aimed to evaluate the long-term maxillary incisors crowding relapse and possible factors that may influence tooth alignment stability.

MATERIAL AND METHODS
Material

The sample was obtained from the files of Bauru Dental School, University of São Paulo, Bauru, São Paulo, Brazil, and consisted of Class I and II malocclusion patients treated orthodontically without extractions.

The criteria for sample selection included the presence of all permanent teeth at treatment beginning (at least first permanent molars) and the absence of shape and/or number dental anomalies. All patients had complete orthodontic records, including study models of the initial phase (T_1), end of treatment (T_2) and post-retention (T_3). None of the subjects underwent rapid maxillary expansion.

Sample comprised 69 dental casts of 23 subjects (13 girls and 10 boys; initial mean age: 13.36 years; SD = 1.81 years) who received full maxillary and mandibular fixed edgewise appliances. These patients underwent orthodontic treatment for a mean period of 2.18 years (SD = 0.93) and were satisfactorily finished at a mean age of 15.54 years (SD = 1.86). The post-retention study models were taken after a mean period of 4.92 years (SD = 1.11).

Regarding initial malocclusion, ten patients had Class I, 8 had quarter-cusp Class II, and 5 had half Class II anteroposterior molar relationships. None of the patients exhibited posterior crossbite at T_1.

After active treatment, all patients wore a full time Hawley retainer in the maxillary arch for 12 months. A lingual canine-to-canine mandibular bonded retainer was placed and left for a mean period of 3 years.

Methods
Dental cast measurements

The T_1, T_2 and T_3 maxillary dental casts were used. All dental cast measurements were made with a centesimal precision digital caliper (Mitutoyo America, Aurora, Ill, São Paulo, Brazil).

All were linear measurements, in millimeters, described as follows:

A) Maxillary incisor irregularity[14] (LITTLE) (Fig 1).
B) Intercanine width (A; INTERC): The linear distance between the cusp tips of the maxillary canines. When there was a facet, the cusp tip was estimated (Fig 2).
C) Inter-premolar widths (INTERPB and INTERPB'): The linear distance between left and right central fossae of the maxillary first (B) and second (B') premolars (Fig 2).
D) Intermolar width (C; INTERMOL): The linear distance between the mesiobuccal cusps tips of the maxillary first molars. When there was a facet, the cusp tip was estimated (Fig 2).
E) Arch length (D + E; LENGTH): The linear distance along the midline from the interincisal midline to the mesial contact of the first molars (Fig 2).

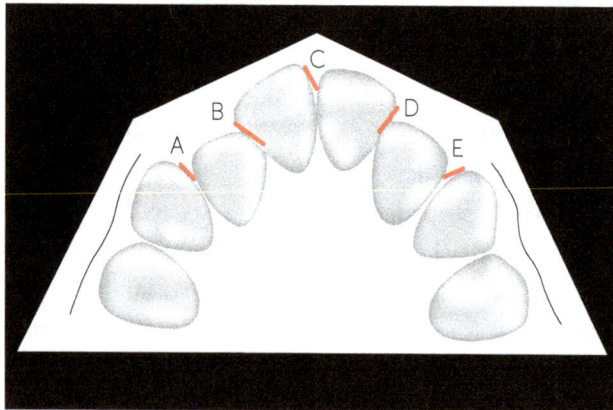

Figure 1 - Little Irregularity Index (modified for the upper arch) = A+B+C+D+E.

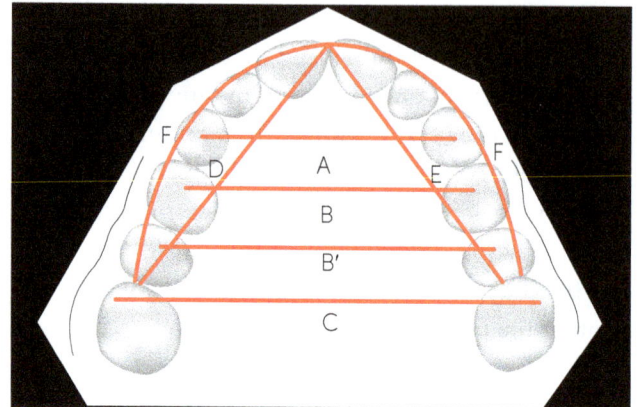

Figure 2 - Variables studied on dental casts: A, intercanine width; B, inter-first-premolar width; B', inter-second-premolar width; C, intermolar width; D + E, arch length; F, arch perimeter.

F) Arch perimeter (F; PERIM): The distance in millimeters from the mesial dental contact of the left first molars to the mesial dental contact of the right first molars to (Fig 2).

Statistical analysis
Method error

Within a month interval from the first measurement, ten dental casts from T_1, T_2 and T_3 phases were randomly selected and remeasured. The casual error was calculated according to Dahlberg's formula ($Se^2 = \Sigma d^2/2n$).[4] The systematic error was calculated with dependent t tests, according to Houston.[11]

Statistical method

One-way dependent ANOVA and Tukey tests were used to evaluate the behavior of the measured variables during the three phases (Initial – T_1; Post-treatment – T_2; Post-retention – T_3).

The Pearson correlation coefficient was calculated by using the whole sample to investigate a significant correlation between maxillary incisors crowding relapse and the pretreatment irregularity or the amount of crowding correction.

Pearson correlation coefficient was also calculated to investigate a association between maxillary incisors crowding relapse and the relapse of intercanine, interpremolar or intermolar widths, arch length and perimeter.

The results were considered statistically significant at $p < 0.05$. All statistical analyses were performed with the software Statistica for Windows, version 6.0, Statsoft, Tulsa, Okla, USA.

RESULTS

Dahlberg's formula and Paired t tests showed no significant casual and systematic errors.

The Table 1 exhibits results of one-way analysis of variance (ANOVA) with the post-hoc Tukey test (different letters means a statistically significant difference between variables) that were used to determine whether there was a significant difference between the measured variables during T_1, T_2 and T_3. The results showed that the incisors irregularity had significant changes not only during treatment but also at posttreatment. Maxillary crowding relapse occurred in most patients with a mean percentage of 30.64% of the treatment correction. However, no significant differences were detected to the dimensional variables evaluated during the 3 phases, except for the inter-first-premolar width (INTERPB), that exhibited a statistically significant increase from pretreatment (T_1) to posttreatment (T_2).

Results of the Pearson correlation tests are in the Tables 2 and 3. There was a significant and negative correlation between maxillary incisors crowding relapse and the relapse of the intercanine and inter-first-premolar widths.

DISCUSSION

Although incisors alignment relapse in maxillary arch is less prevalent than in mandibular arch, the evaluation of possible factors that may influence maxillary tooth alignment stability has validity. Relapse of crowding in this region may also results in esthetic and functional occlusal deficiencies. Mainly due to its

Table 1 - Results of one-way analysis of variance (ANOVA) with the post-hoc Tukey test (different letters means a statistically significant difference between variables) for the variables measured on dental casts (N = 23), at the three stages studied (T_1, T_2 and T_3).

Variable	Initial (T_1) Mean ± SD	Posttreatment (T_2) Mean ± SD	Post-retention (T_3) Mean ± SD	p
LITTLE	6.56 ± 2.83[A]	1.59 ± 0.73[B]	3.11 ± 1.41[C]	0.000*
INTERC	34.07 ± 3.79[A]	34.65 ± 1.44[A]	34.53 ± 1.87[A]	0.653
INTERPB	34.71 ± 1.86[A]	36.34 ± 1.81[B]	35.76 ± 1.81[B]	0.012*
INTERPB'	40.20 ± 2.31[A]	41.35 ± 2.15[A]	41.09 ± 2.16[A]	0.186
INTERMOL	51.13 ± 2.62[A]	51.52 ± 2.50[A]	51.94 ± 2.51[A]	0.560
LENGTH	72.09 ± 4.08[A]	73.76 ± 2.49[A]	72.07 ± 2.58[A]	0.118
PERIM	75.18 ± 3.77[A]	76.52 ± 2.66[A]	75.32 ± 2.55[A]	0.269
LITTLE	6.56 ± 2.83[A]	1.59 ± 0.73[B]	3.11 ± 1.41[C]	0.000*

Table 2 - Results of the Pearson correlation test.

Variable	r	p
LITTLE1 x LITTLE3	0.252	0.071
LITTLE1 x LITTLE3-2	0.241	0.084
LITTLE2-1 x LITTLE3-2	-0.264	0.055

Table 3 - Results of the Pearson correlation test.

Variable	r	p
LITTLE3-2 x INTERC3-2	-0.459	0.000*
LITTLE3-2 x INTERPB3-2	-0.419	0.001*
LITTLE3-2 x INTERPB'3-2	-0.269	0.053
LITTLE3-2 x INTERMOL3-2	-0.064	-0.649
LITTLE3-2 x LENGTH3-2	0.028	0.842
LITTLE3-2 x PERIM3-2	-0.012	0.930

*Statistically significant at p < 0.05.

location, maxillary incisors crowding relapse tends to become more visible and therefore promote greater esthetic impacts than mandibular irregularity.

Results for one-way analysis of variance (ANOVA) with the post-hoc Tukey test (Table 1) showed that occurred statistically significant changes in the Little irregularity index during the three phases studied. It was observed a significant maxillary crowding reduction during treatment. However, there was a significant relapse of the incisors irregularity after treatment. Regarding changes in maxillary arch dimensions during treatment, there was only a significant change in the variable INTERPB (Inter-first-premolar width), suggesting that most maxillary arch dimensions were maintained during treatment, and remained stable during post-retention. Sadowsky et al[23] evaluating stability in maxillary and mandibular dental arches of patients treated without extractions and Edgewise mechanics, observed no significant changes in the intercanine and inter-premolars widths, five years post-retention. Erdinc, Nanda and Isiksal,[8] evaluated stability of the orthodontic treatment, with and without extractions. Similarly to the present study, it was

observed significant decreases in maxillary incisors irregularity during treatment. Patients treated without extractions exhibited significant increases of the intercanine and inter-premolars widths during treatment. The maxillary arch dimensional measurements showed no significant changes after treatment, however, relapse of maxillary crowding was significant. These studies[8,23] and the present suggests a favorable prognosis regarding maxillary arch long-term dimensional stability of orthodontic cases treated without premolars extractions.

In the present study, mean post-retention crowding relapse was 1.52 mm. Sadowsky et al,[23] assessing stability of subjects treated non-extraction, reported a relatively similar amount of relapse (1.1 mm), 5 years post-retention. However, Moussa, O'Reilly and Close[18] observed more favorable results regarding crowding relapse, 8 to 10 years post-retention, in a sample comprising 18 subjects treated with rapid maxillary expansion and fixed appliances. It was observed a mean maxillary crowding relapse of 0.6 mm (SD = 1.30). Vaden, Harris and Gardner,[30] noted that 96% of the maxillary crowding correction remained stable 15 years after treatment. The amount of crowding increased from 1.5 mm at posttreatment to 1.8 mm at post-retention. Ferris et al[9] also evaluated the maxillary crowding relapse in non-extraction cases. It was observed only 0.47 (SD = 1.19) of maxillary irregularity increase during the post-retention (7.9 years). The increased stability observed in these studies may be explained by the prolonged retention protocol after orthodontic treatment.[23] In the Sadowsky et al[23] study, retainers were placed and left for a mean period of 8.4 years. Moussa, O'Reilly and Close,[18] described a mean period of 6.6 years of retention for the mandibular arch and full time Hawley retainer in the maxillary arch for 2 years. The study conducted by Vaden, Harris and Gardner,[30] reports that patients used these retainers in the maxillary and mandibular arches or these retainers in the maxillary arch and a lingual canine-to-canine mandibular bonded retainer. The first posttreatment control was carried out only after six years. The study by Ferris et al[9] described a retention protocol that included the use of Hawley in the maxillary for 3 years (full time during one year) and lingual bonded retainer or Hawley plates in the mandibular arch for a mean period of 3 years. In the present study, all subjects wore a full time Hawley retainer in the maxillary arch for 12 months. A lingual canine-to-canine mandibular bonded retainer was placed and left for a mean period of 3 years.

Erdinc, Nanda and Isiksal[8] described an increase in maxillary incisors irregularity of 0.19 mm and 0.12 mm for patients treated with or without extractions, respectively, 4 years and 11 months after treatment. The extraction group showed 4.4 mm of pretreatment crowding. However, the non-extraction group exhibited only 1.94 mm of initial irregularity. The initial crowding was significantly less severe than that observed in our sample (6.56 mm). Maxillary and mandibular retainers were removed at least two years before the post-retention measurements. The exceptional stability of this study may be related to the amount of initial crowding and due to a short interval between retainer removal and the post-retention evaluation.

Although the results indicate a posttreatment maxillary crowding relapse greater than that reported in previous studies,[8,9,18,23,30] the mean irregularity index at posttreatment (3.12 mm) is considered clinically acceptable according to Little.[14]

Results of the Pearson correlation tests showed no significant correlations to most variables evaluated (Tables 2 and 3). It was observed that the amount of initial crowding had no effect on relapse, as described in previous studies.[1,17] Surbeck et al,[25] in contrast, reported a positive correlation between the amount of maxillary incisors irregularity and the amount of incisors crowding relapse. The authors reported[25] that the tendency to maxillary crowding relapse increases 2.3 times for each 0.2 mm of incisors contact point displacement in relation to the dental arch. Furthermore, each 4° of tooth rotation at pretreatment has increased by 2.7 times the probability of irregularity relapse. The authors[25] also pointed out that partially aligned tooth exhibits significant risk of relapse. They suggested the use of individualized retention protocols and that patients should be aware about the possibility of relapse accordingly to the initial irregularity.[25] However, a positive correlation between the amount maxillary incisors crowding at pretreatment and the crowding relapse after treatment seems unlikely when analyzing our results and previous studies. For example, ours results indicated that the experimental group exhibited 6.56 mm of initial irregularity and had a mean post-retention relapse of 1.52 mm. The mean crowding relapse observed in the present study was higher than that reported by Ferris et al,[9] Sadowsky et al[23] and Vaden, Harris and Gardner,[30] with samples that exhibited more maxillary incisors irregularity at pretreatment (10.45 mm, 8.0 mm and 7.9 mm, respectively). Despite more initial crowding, these studies reported less posttreatment irregularity relapse (0.47 mm, 1.1 mm, 0.3 mm, respectively).

The amount of maxillary crowding relapse (LITTLE3-2) showed a statistically significant and negative correlation ($p < 0.05$) with the post-retention changes in intercanine (INTERC3-2) and inter-first-premolars (INTERPB3-2) widths (Table 3). These results suggest that the higher the post-retention decreases of intercanine and inter-first-premolars widths the higher the maxillary crowding relapse. However, although these correlations have statistical significance, the coefficients values observed implicate in a weak correlation (r values of -0.459 and -0.419, respectively). Therefore, it can be argued that the observed correlation between relapse of the maxillary crowding and the reduction of these dimensional measurements has poor clinical significance.

Moreover, it seems obvious that the reduction of these measurements tends to be consequence of maxillary arch constriction in the anterior region. Therefore, it is expected a space availability decrease and an increase in the amount of tooth crowding.

Despite numerous studies that evaluated a possible relationship between changes in intercanine width and mandibular incisors crowding relapse, the correlation between maxillary crowding relapse and maxillary intercanine width changes were only investigated by Surbeck et al,[25] and Erdinc, Nanda and Isiksal.[8] Surbeck et al[25] found a significant association (p < 0.001) between intercanine width decreases and maxillary incisors crowding relapse, however, the correlation test result also revealed a weak association (r < 0.70). Erdinc, Nanda and Isiksal,[8] found no correlation between post-retention changes in incisors irregularity and changes in intercanine width.

Clinical implications

Maxillary anterior alignment shows better prognosis regarding stability when compared to the same region in the mandibular arch, this fact may explain the scarce studies in literature about this issue. Despite the greater stability, maxillary crowding relapse can compromise orthodontic results after retention appliances removal. The post-retention relapse observed in this study (1.52 mm), although statistically significant, may be considered clinically acceptable.[14] Otherwise, this minimal amount of crowding relapse can lead to patient dissatisfaction.

Maxillary incisors crowding relapse shows some etiological factors as retention time, initial crowding severity; relapse of teeth in the opposite side, changes in arch dimensions, rotated teeth at pretreatment and lack of complete correction of rotated teeth resulting in absence of adequate interdental contacts. Thus, it becomes clear that more stable results can be obtained with a prolonged retention protocol and an adequate alignment of maxillary incisors during treatment.

CONCLUSION

The maxillary incisors irregularity increased significantly (1.52 mm) five years posttreatment.

None of the clinical factors studied in the dental casts demonstrated to be predictive of the maxillary crowding relapse.

The results suggest that more attention regarding maxillary arch retention protocol should be taken by the clinician. Although alignment stability of mandibular incisors is less than that of the maxillary anterior teeth, maxillary crowding relapse can be significant.

REFERENCES

1. Artun J, Garol JD, Little RM. Long-term stability of mandibular incisors following successful treatment of Class II, Division 1, malocclusions. Angle Orthod. 1996;66(3):229-38.

2. Busdrang PH, Horton-Reuland SJ, Legler L, Nevant C. Non-extraction approach to tooth size arch length discrepancies with the Alexander discipline. Semin Orthod. 2001;7(2):117-31.

3. Canuto LF, Freitas MR, Janson G, Freitas KM, Martins PP. Influence of rapid palatal expansion on maxillary incisors alignment stability. Am J Orthod Dentofacial Orthop. 2010;137(2):164.e1-6.

4. Dahlberg G. Statistical methods for medical and biological students. New York: Interscience; 1940.

5. Edwards JG. A study of the periodontium during orthodontic rotation of teeth. Am J Orthod. 1968;54(6):441-61.

6. Edwards JG. A surgical procedure to eliminate rotational relapse. Am J Orthod. 1970;57(1):35-46.

7. Edwards JG. A long-term prospective evaluation of the circumferential supracrestal fiberotomy in alleviating orthodontic relapse. Am J Orthod Dentofacial Orthop. 1988;93(5):380-7.

8. Erdinc AE, Nanda RS, Işiksal E. Relapse of anterior crowding in patients treated with extraction and non-extraction of premolars. Am J Orthod Dentofacial Orthop. 2006;129(6):775-84.

9. Ferris T, Alexander RG, Boley J, Buschang PH. Long-term stability of combined rapid palatal expansion-lip bumper therapy followed by full fixed appliances. Am J Orthod Dentofacial Orthop. 2005;128(3):310-25.

10. Heiser W, Niederwanger A, Bancher B, Bittermann G, Neunteufel N, Kulmer S. Three-dimensional dental arch and palatal form changes after extraction and non-extraction treatment. Part 1. Arch length and area. Am J Orthod Dentofacial Orthop. 2004;126(1):82-90.

11. Houston WJ. The analysis of errors in orthodontic measurements. Am J Orthod. 1983;83(5):382-90.

12. Huang L, Artun J. Is the post-retention relapse of maxillary and mandibular incisor alignment related? Am J Orthod Dentofacial Orthop. 2001;120(1):9-19.

13. Kahl-Nieke B, Fischbach H, Schwarze CW. Post-retention crowding and incisor irregularity: a long-term follow-up evaluation of stability and relapse. Br J Orthod. 1995;22(3):249-57.

14. Little RM. The irregularity index: a quantitative score of mandibular anterior alignment. Am J Orthod. 1975;68(5):554-63.

15. Little RM. Stability and relapse of dental arch alignment. Br J Orthod. 1990;17(3):235-41.

16. Little RM, Riedel RA, Artun J. An evaluation of changes in mandibular anterior alignment from 10 to 20 years post-retention. Am J Orthod Dentofacial Orthop. 1988;93(5):423-8.

17. Little RM, Wallen TR, Riedel RA. Stability and relapse of mandibular anterior alignment – first premolar extraction cases treated by traditional edgewise orthodontics. Am J Orthod. 1981;80(4):349-65.

18. Moussa R, O'Reilly MT, Close JM. Long-term stability of rapid palatal expander treatment and edgewise mechanotherapy. Am J Orthod Dentofacial Orthop. 1995;108(5):478-88.

19. Parker WS. Retention: retainers may be forever. Am J Orthod Dentofacial Orthop. 1989;95(6):505-13.

20. Richardson ME. A review of changes in lower arch alignment from seven to fifty years. Semin Orthod. 1999;5(3):151-9.

21. Rossouw PE, Preston CB, Lombard CJ, Truter JW. A longitudinal evaluation of the anterior border of the dentition. Am J Orthod Dentofacial Orthop. 1993;104(2):146-52.

22. Sadowsky C, Sakols EI. Long-term assessment of orthodontic relapse. Am J Orthod. 1982;82(6):456-63.

23. Sadowsky C, Schneider BJ, BeGole EA, Tahir E. Long-term stability after orthodontic treatment: non-extraction with prolonged retention. Am J Orthod Dentofacial Orthop. 1994;106(3):243-9.

24. Sinclair PM, Little RM. Maturation of untreated normal occlusions. Am J Orthod. 1983;83(2):114-23.

25. Surbeck BT, Artun J, Hawkins NR, Leroux B. Associations between initial, posttreatment, and post-retention alignment of maxillary anterior teeth. Am J Orthod Dentofacial Orthop. 1998;113(2):186-95.

26. Swanson WD, Riedel RA, Danna JA. Post-retention study: incidence and stability of rotated teeth in humans. Angle Orthod. 1975;45(3):198-203.

27. Taner TU, Haydar B, Kavuklu I, Korkmaz A. Short-term effects of fiberotomy on relapse of anterior crowding. Am J Orthod Dentofacial Orthop. 2000;118(6):617-23.

28. Thilander B. Orthodontic relapse versus natural development. Am J Orthod Dentofacial Orthop. 2000;117(5):562-3.

29. Uhde MD, Sadowsky C, BeGole EA. Long-term stability of dental relationships after orthodontic treatment. Angle Orthod. 1983;53(3):240-52.

30. Vaden JL, Harris EF, Gardner RL. Relapse revisited. Am J Orthod Dentofacial Orthop. 1997;111(5):543-53.

22

Finishing procedures in Orthodontics: dental dimensions and proportions (microesthetics)

Roberto Carlos Bodart Brandão[1], Larissa Bustamente Capucho Brandão[2]

Objective: The objective of the present article is to describe procedures that can be performed to achieve excellence in orthodontic treatment finishing. The content is limited to microesthetics, which comprises the concept of ideal dental dimensions and proportions (white esthetics) and its correlation with the periodontium (pink esthetics). Standards of normality are described both in their real dimensions (dental height and width), and in those effectively perceived by the observer, the virtual dimensions. **Methods:** The best scientific evidence was sought in the literature to support the clinical procedures that must guide the professional to obtain maximum esthetic quality on their treatments. Therefore, it is necessary to investigate what the other specialties in Dentistry expect from Orthodontics and, specially, what they have to offer. Clinical cases will be used to illustrate the dental movement that might maximize treatment outcome and to confront the ideal standards with the current state of the art. **Conclusion:** Treatment quality is directly related to the amount of procedures implemented by the orthodontist, associated with concepts and resources from Periodontics and Dental Prosthesis. Microesthetics cannot be seen in isolation, but rather as the key to establish a pleasant smile (miniesthetics) in addition to a harmonious face (macroesthetics) and a human being with high self-esteem (hyper-esthetics).

Keywords: Orthodontics. Dentistry. Dental esthetics. Smile.

» The authors report no commercial, proprietary or financial interest in the products or companies described in this article.

Roberto Carlos Bodart Brandão
Av. Américo Buaiz, 501/1007 – Torre Norte – Enseada do Suá
CEP: 29.050-911 – Vitória/ES — Brazil
E-mail: consultorio@ortobrandao.com.br

[1] Adjunct professor of Orthodontics, Federal University of Espírito Santo (UFES).
[2] Specialist in Orthodontics, Fluminense Federal University (UFF).

INTRODUCTION

The subject of orthodontic finishing is instigating and extensive. After all, it is all about achieving the objectives of orthodontic treatment, seeking excellence of results, justifying the patient's financial investment and, consequently, prior professional referral, so that new treatments can be initiated. Adequately finishing the cases means investing in professional longevity, remaining in our work place with approval of the society — colleagues and patients, in an increasingly competitive market, as a private pension in its true meaning, which is: to prepare the future.

For being quite a large subject, orthodontic treatment finishing must be discussed in four different and, at the same time, complementary, topics:

1) Fundamental principles.
2) Esthetic orthodontic procedures.
3) Transdisciplinary approaches.
4) Occlusal adjustment.

We began to discuss orthodontic finishing in a reverse order when the article *Occlusal adjust in Orthodontics: why, when and how* was published.[8] This reverse order was purposeful. If the orthodontist intends to perform a quick and stable treatment, he must begin backwards, i.e., establish the best molar intercuspation as soon as possible, then premolars, enabling the perfect canine occlusion. Thus, a stable and reproducible occlusion, with no premature contacts, is established first. This is the foundation for the success in orthodontic finishing; the esthetic procedures will only be complete and durable if there is stability in dental occlusion.[8]

We also had the opportunity to approach the fundamental principles that guide orthodontic finishing in an interview,[9] in which it was asserted that finishing begins even before the appliance is placed, paradoxical as it may seem. Most often, we are concerned about the finishing phase during the last months of orthodontic treatment, specially when the rectangular arches are placed. When this occurs, there is a waste of time and opportunities that could shorten and optimize orthodontic finishing. A solid planning and an individualized appliance placement define a better finishing. And it is worth remembering that treatment onset is when there is greater patient collaboration. When this collaboration is demanded at the final moments of treatment, what we have is a tired and, often, unmotivated patient.[9]

An interesting division of esthetics in Orthodontics is that presented by Sarver and Ackerman,[48] who divided it into three sections: 1) Microesthetics, which includes the dental aspect, considering the arrangement of teeth on the arches, their color, shape, dimensions and proportions; 2) Miniesthetics, which includes smile esthetics, how teeth are exposed and perceived in smile dynamics, specially its relation with the lips; 3) Macroesthetics, which refers to the face, its harmony and proportions, and the esthetic impact of the several structures in its composition (Fig 1).

In this article, the Microesthetics approach, specially the dental dimensions and proportions, with its variations, will be discussed within the topic *Esthetic orthodontic procedures*.

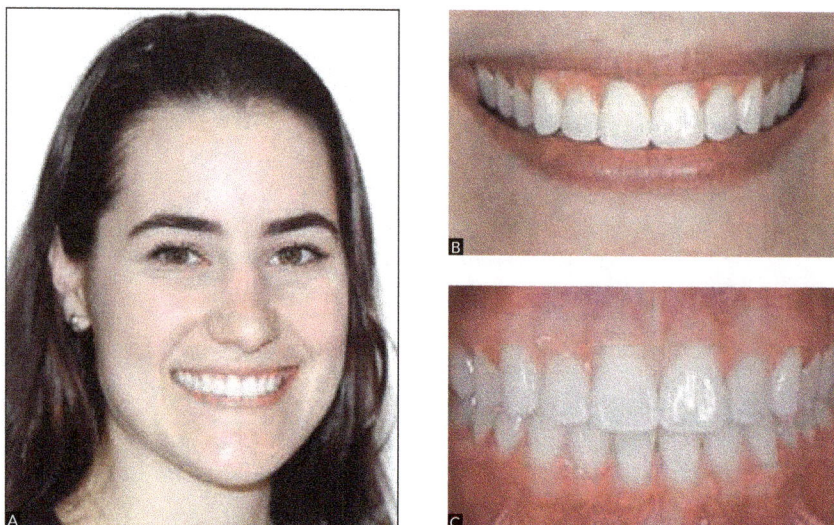

Figure 1 - Esthetical approaches according to Sarver and Ackerman[48]: **A)** Macroesthetics, seeks the harmony of facial structures; **B)** Miniesthetics, evaluated by the oral structures that comprise the smile; **C)** Microesthetics, related to the teeth and to the periodontium.

ESTHETIC IMPACT OF DENTAL DIMENSIONS AND PROPORTIONS

The fact that the evaluation of facial beauty is essentially subjective cannot be forgotten. The artist Albrecht Dürer,[16] from the XVI century, wrote: " I don't know what beauty is, but I do know it affects many things in life", and considered that, although the concept of facial beauty is immersed in subjectivity, the evaluation of facial proportions could be objectively performed. The discussion is about how ideal patterns can be defined, within a theme that experiences important changes with the evolution of society.[44]

In a recent study, Orce-Romero et al.[45] investigated the common characteristics which influenced esthetical perception in different populations around the world. This study was based on the analysis of the smile of 500 celebrities exposed on Time magazine. They found that upper lip vertical height, smile width, upper central incisors exposure, dental symmetry and intra-dental proportions are the most influential factors in defining a smile as pleasant, corroborating the findings of other authors who found an evolution on the esthetical criteria of professionals and laypeople.[3,25,25,52] Four of these factors are characteristics related to microesthetics and, if well managed by the orthodontist and his team of colleagues of related specialties, are determinant to achieve the esthetical excellence of the smile.

It is important to note that there is a wide range of combinations of smile characteristics that make it more or less pleasant, specially when the entire face of the patient is included in the observation. Kokich Jr, Kiyak and Shapiro[35] observed that people, when seeing a smiling face, look first and for a longer period of time to other areas of the face before they look at the teeth. For this reason, microesthetics must be considered within a context: other variables related to the smile (miniesthetics) and to the face (macroesthetics) must be in harmony with the proportions and dimensions in the dental arches.

WIDTH AND HEIGHT OF CROWNS

There is a variation on dental dimensions that can be considered as normal or desirable, specially when considering that there are individuals with different facial patterns. Some works show that the dimensions of anterior teeth can be defined within a limited range. The height of the central incisor varies from 10.4 to 11.2 mm while its width varies from 8.73 to 9.3 mm, and, usually,

these references are used in prosthetic reconstructions, when no other parameters are available.[37,54,55]

The most important is the correlation of these dimensions, i.e., the dental proportions.[4,20,50] Two proportions must be considered: the relation between height and width of each tooth, and the relation of height and width among the teeth. In these cases, we will always be referring to the real dimension of the teeth, i.e., the clinical crown dimensions of anterior teeth.

A classic study that investigated dental proportions was that by Gillen et al[20] who found the following proportions of width among the upper anterior teeth: a) lateral incisors have 78% of the width of the central incisor (lateral incisor = central incisor x 0.78); b) lateral incisor has 87% of the width of the canine (lateral incisor = canine x 0.87); c) canine has 90% of the width of the central incisor (canine = central incisor x 0.90), as shown in Figure 2.

The studies by Sterrett et al.[58] demonstrated that the relation between width and height of central and lateral incisors and canines is practically the same in both genders. Females tend to have slightly wider teeth in comparison to males, being: central incisors 86% and 85%, lateral incisors 79% and 76%, and canines 81% and 76%, respectively. The most recent research available found the proportion between height and width of upper anterior teeth ranging from 75 to 80% in central incisors, from 66 to 70% in lateral incisors, and from 80 to 85% in canines, without statistical difference between men and women.[45]

Most authors define the height/width ratio of 0.80 for the upper central incisor (which represents the key tooth to esthetical composition of the smile) as a standard to be used in Prosthesis, Periodontics and Orthodontics.[50,55,58] Therefore, on establishing ideal widths, based on intact teeth, it is suggested to use the proportion of 80 ± 5%

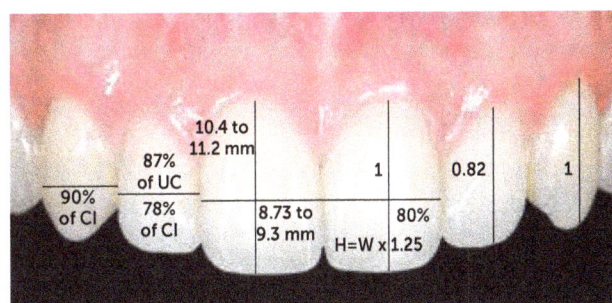

Figure 2 - Real proportions and dimensions of teeth with four approaches: variations on the dimensions of height and width of the central incisor (red), height/width proportion of the central incisor (black), relations of width between anterior teeth (green) and relations of height of anterior teeth (blue).

to define the ideal height, relating it to the facial pattern and to the individual's natural dental proportions (Fig 2).

The relation of proportion between the crown heights of anterior teeth proposed by Gillen et al.[20] is widely used. It suggests that the height of the clinical crown of the upper lateral incisor must be 82% of the height of the crowns of the central incisor and canine. Therefore, canines and upper central incisors would have the same anatomical crown height. (Fig 2). This study was used to justify the bonding of orthodontic brackets at the same height for canines and upper central incisors, during placement of the orthodontic appliance.

In the decision making process, these proportions must be considered in two clinical situations. The first one is when interproximal wear is used to obtain space in the dental arch, or to close black spaces when the contact point is brought closer to the alveolar bone crest, which shall be discussed in a specific topic later on. The second situation in which the height x width relation is essential occurs when the patient has loss of dental volume, compromising the height of the crown, when there is incisal wear by attrition or abrasion, or compromising the width of the crown due to cavities or unsatisfactory restorations. The recovery of these proportions must be defined during treatment planning, and it would be a priority for the definition of transverse and vertical corrections of the dental arches.[30,57] When loss of dimensions of the upper anterior teeth is detected, the first treatment step must be to provide spaces for these dimensions to be restored within the ideal proportionality, using extractions, distalizations or maxillary expansions, even when surgical assistance is necessary (Fig 3).

Another practical way to use dental proportions to establish the width of anterior teeth is by fixed measures, based on averages of tooth size.[14] In this case, database of tooth sizes of different populations are used, which generates formulas for the dental widths to relate to each other, specially for anterior teeth. Figure 4 shows a proposal of a mathematical formula used to define the size of a tooth based on the size of other teeth. In this case, the letter Y represents the width of the upper central incisor and the letter X, the width of the lower central incisor.[14,15] The width of the upper lateral incisor would be the width of the upper central incisor minus 2 mm, and the width of the upper canine would be the width of the central minus 1 mm. Based on the width of the lower central incisor, the width of the upper central incisor would be

defined by adding 3 mm, while the width of the lower central incisor would be defined by adding 0.5 mm, and the width of the lower canine by adding 1 mm.

Contrary to golden proportions and based on measures of dental dimensions and of harmonious proportions derived from observations on the population, as those previously described, Chu[14,15] developed an instrument to measure proportionality. This proportionality gauge (commercialized by Hu-Friedy®) does not need mathematical calculations and uses a formula that was predetermined by its creator, for dental proportions that are visually available in a color scale that must be considered by the professional. In other words, for each tooth width marked by the colors on the horizontal rod of the measurer, it would be necessary that the height of the crown were equivalent to the same color available on the vertical rod, this would define the best proportion (Fig 5).

CROWN VIRTUAL WIDTHS

Real width and height are data based on direct measurements carried out on the teeth (anthropometric measures), i.e., their absolute dimensions. It is recommended to consider the virtual dimensions which are, effectively, what is perceived by people – the esthetics that really matters.

The perception of dental dimension different from reality is a physical, better yet, optical phenomenon. When we take a shower with a green soap, we evidently do not become green, because there is no pigment in the soap, but rather an optical phenomenon, due to the arrangement of the crystals of the soap that reflect only part of the light spectrum, where the green color is. We only see what is reflected to our retina; the part of light that focuses an object and is deflected in another direction, or absorbed, escapes our visual perception. Therefore, the flat surfaces are completely perceived by the reflection of light that focuses in 90º on them — it is what we effectively clearly see, the virtual dimensions of the teeth. The shades represent the curved surfaces where the light is deviated in another direction, because it is deflected.[40]

The dimension of the virtual width of the teeth follows its position, the shape of the dental arch and the anatomy of each tooth. The central incisors, for being closer to the observer, at the front of the dental arch, are privileged by the parallax effect, attracting the perception of the human eye.[10] Starting with the concept of central incisor predominance, the perception of the other teeth in the anterior region begins to follow the golden proportion.

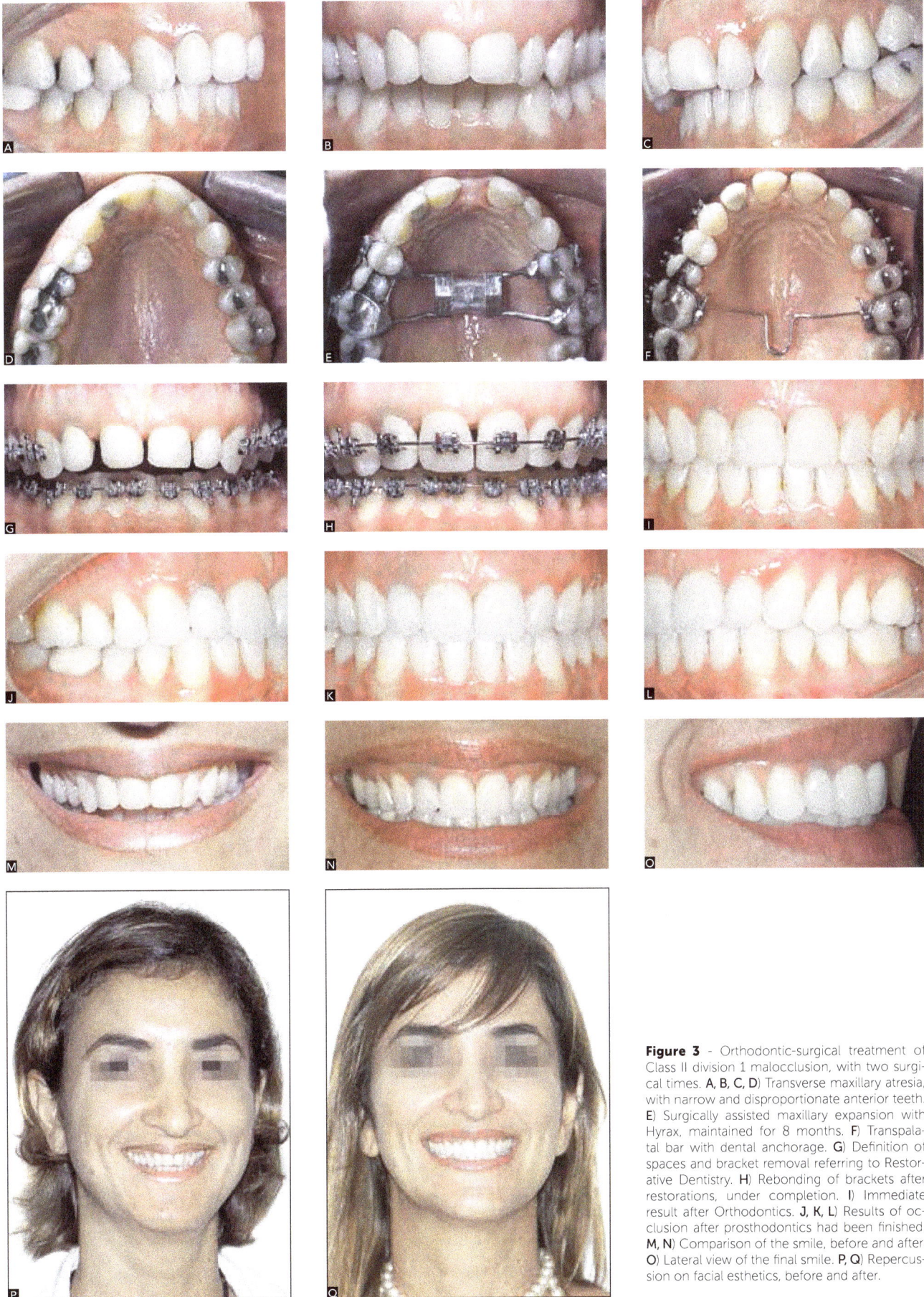

Figure 3 - Orthodontic-surgical treatment of Class II division 1 malocclusion, with two surgical times. **A, B, C, D)** Transverse maxillary atresia, with narrow and disproportionate anterior teeth. **E)** Surgically assisted maxillary expansion with Hyrax, maintained for 8 months. **F)** Transpalatal bar with dental anchorage. **G)** Definition of spaces and bracket removal referring to Restorative Dentistry. **H)** Rebonding of brackets after restorations, under completion. **I)** Immediate result after Orthodontics. **J, K, L)** Results of occlusion after prosthodontics had been finished. **M, N)** Comparison of the smile, before and after. **O)** Lateral view of the final smile. **P, Q)** Repercussion on facial esthetics, before and after.

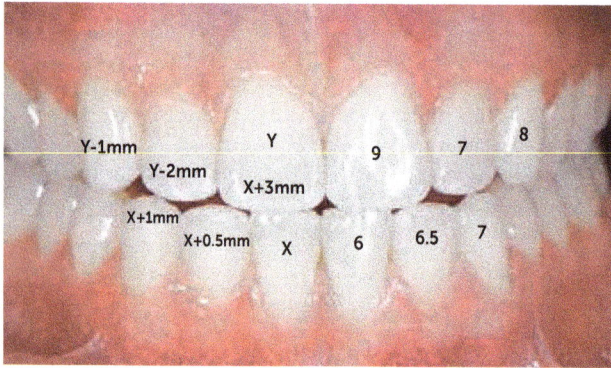

Figure 4 - Formulas to achieve the best relation between the widths of anterior teeth, emphasized by Chu,[14,15] enabling definition of the width of a tooth based on the dimension of another. In the left hemiarch, example of application of the formulas of correlation between the dental widths.

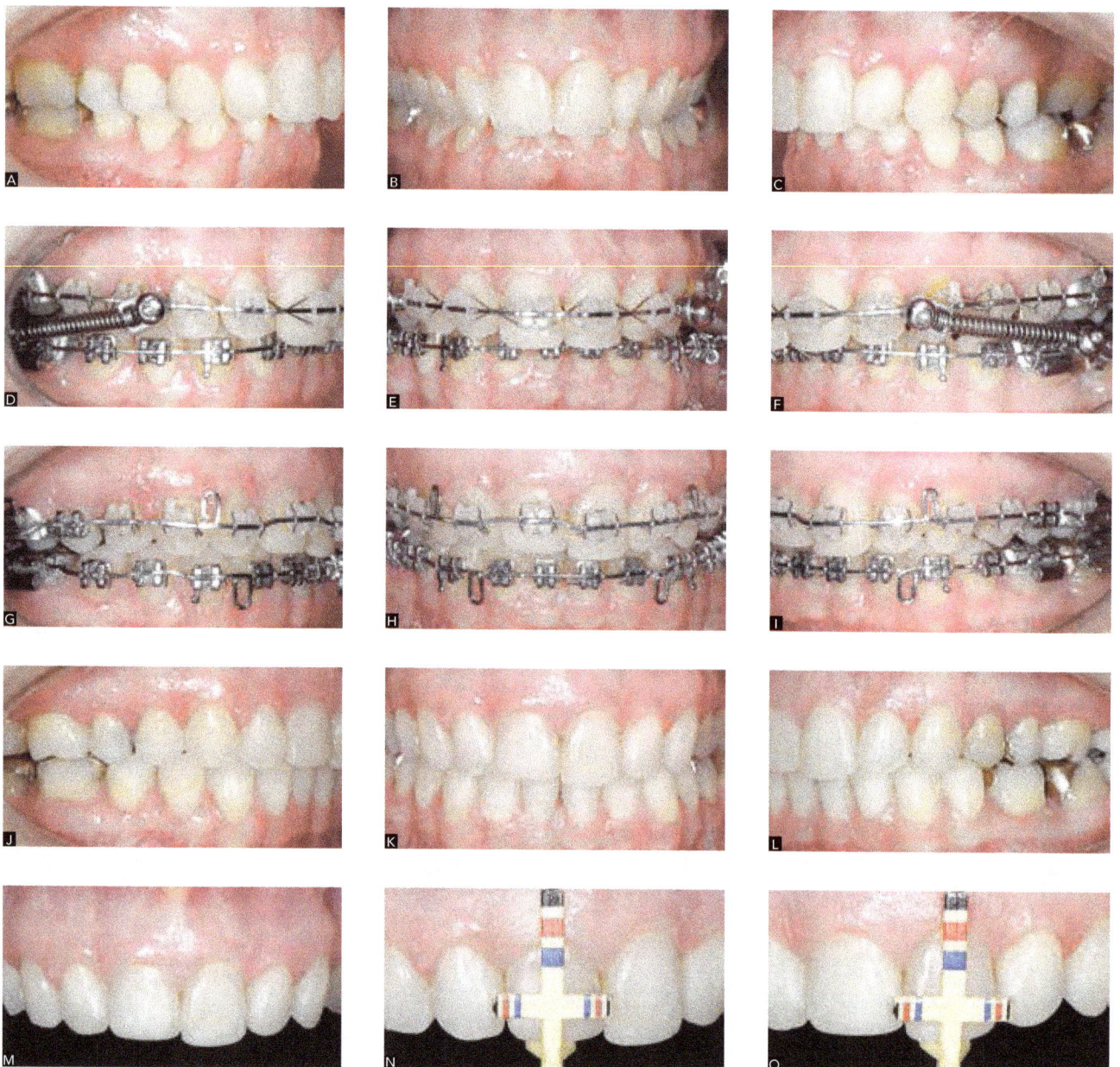

Figure 5 - Class II division 1 patient, right subdivision with excessive overbite. **A, B, C)** Initial case, upper arch with atresia and asymmetric extrusion of anterior teeth. **D, E, F)** Dynaflex® appliance, for action similar to the Class II intermaxillary rubber bands. **G, H, I)** Correction of gingival contour, intruding the right upper central incisor. **J, K, L)** Immediate result after Orthodontics, central incisors with asymmetric dimensions. **M, N, O)** Verification of height and width proportions with Chu's gauge,[15] showing that the teeth should be dimensioned by the red marking, as the left central incisor.

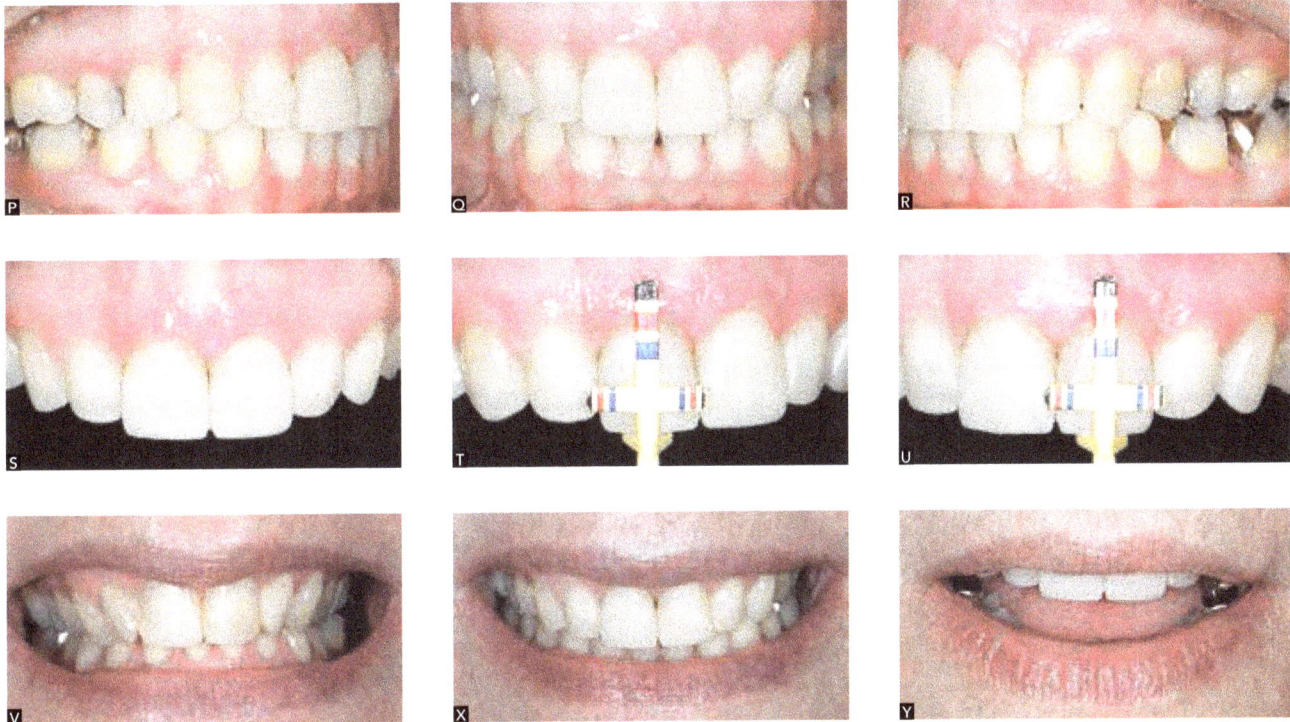

Figure 5 (continuation) - P, Q, R) Restorations in provisional resin, serving as mock-up for the patient to give his opinion and also guide the prosthodontist. S, T, U) Verification of the symmetry and proportions achieved. V) Smile before treatment, wide buccal corridor. X, Y) Smile and speech after Orthodontics and provisional restorations.

Also known as divine proportion, the golden proportion rises from an algebraic constant denoted by the greek letter φ (phi), with approximate value of 1.618, and it is used in arts, since Antiquity, by sculptors and painters. It defines the size proportion between structures or parts, directly related to harmony. This proportion was verified in human beings, related to the size of phalanges and to growth, and introduced in Dentistry by Lombardi,[36] when it began to be used as a parameter for the evaluation of smile amplitude measure and of the visible portion of the teeth. The distal reduction of the virtual width of the teeth must be similar to this constant. By this parameter, the lateral incisors must appear proportionally smaller (62%) in relation to the central incisors. Similarly, the proportion of canine appearance in relation to the lateral incisors must be 62% smaller and coincident with the appearance proportion of the premolar, and so on (Fig 6).

The upper central incisor and the canine have approximate real dimensions, but the virtual width of the canine, due to its convex anatomy and position on the dental arch curvature, represents only 33% of the virtual width of the central incisor. This tooth is privileged by its wide flat surface, reflecting most of the light that focuses on its clinical crown. A tool that is widely used by Dental Prosthesis is the generation of optical illusion,

for example, when the central and lateral incisors have approximate sizes: the professional builds different anatomical contours on the restoration or on the porcelain crown, totally flat on the central incisor, increasing its virtual width, and with marked curvature on the distal face of the lateral incisor, hiding its real dimension.[2,12,19,37]

The possibility of working with optics, modifying the virtual width of the teeth, can be verified in two situations. The first one is related to the torque effects on the posterior teeth, and influences on the buccal

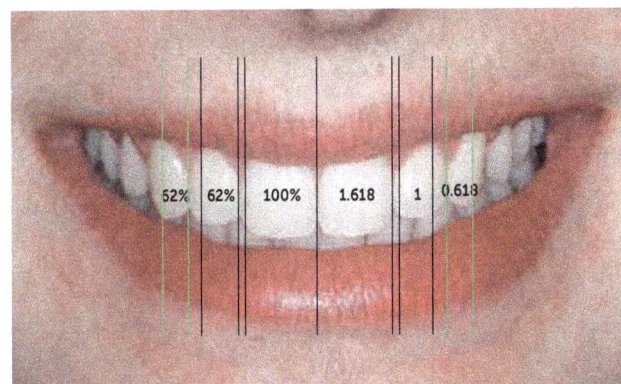

Figure 6 - Virtual width of the teeth, taking the golden proportion as parameter. There is a reduction in the perception of the size of teeth from the central incisors on due to the smaller flat area available to reflect light. The conformation of the arches, dental alignment and shape of the teeth define the amount of flat surface on which the light will focus and, thus, the beauty and naturality of the smile.

corridor and on the smile amplitude. In expanded arches, due to the buccal torque of the crowns of posterior teeth, the teeth seem to be larger or in greater amount in the oral cavity.[8] On the other hand, in contracted arches, due to the excessive lingual torque of the crowns of posterior teeth, the teeth seem to be smaller, with little expression in the smile, and wide and dark buccal corridors. In these cases, the contraction or expansion of the dental arches, at the expense of coronary movement, and the definition of the correct implantation of teeth on their bone base may significantly change the esthetical perception of size and number of teeth in the smile. It is clear that the best buccal corridor and the

best amplitude of the smile are established with adequate torques on canines and posterior teeth (Fig 7).[9,47]

The other way to work the virtual width to achieve the best esthetics is related to correct dental alignment, specially when the dental arch shape is respected, setting the teeth with well positioned contact points in the buccolingual direction, without rotations. Otherwise, mesially rotated teeth tend to expose more the clinical crown to the light, making the real width larger. This might generate the illusion of a lateral incisor or canine with dimensions that are larger than or equivalent to the central incisor. A distal rotation hides the buccal surface, creating the appearance of microdontia.

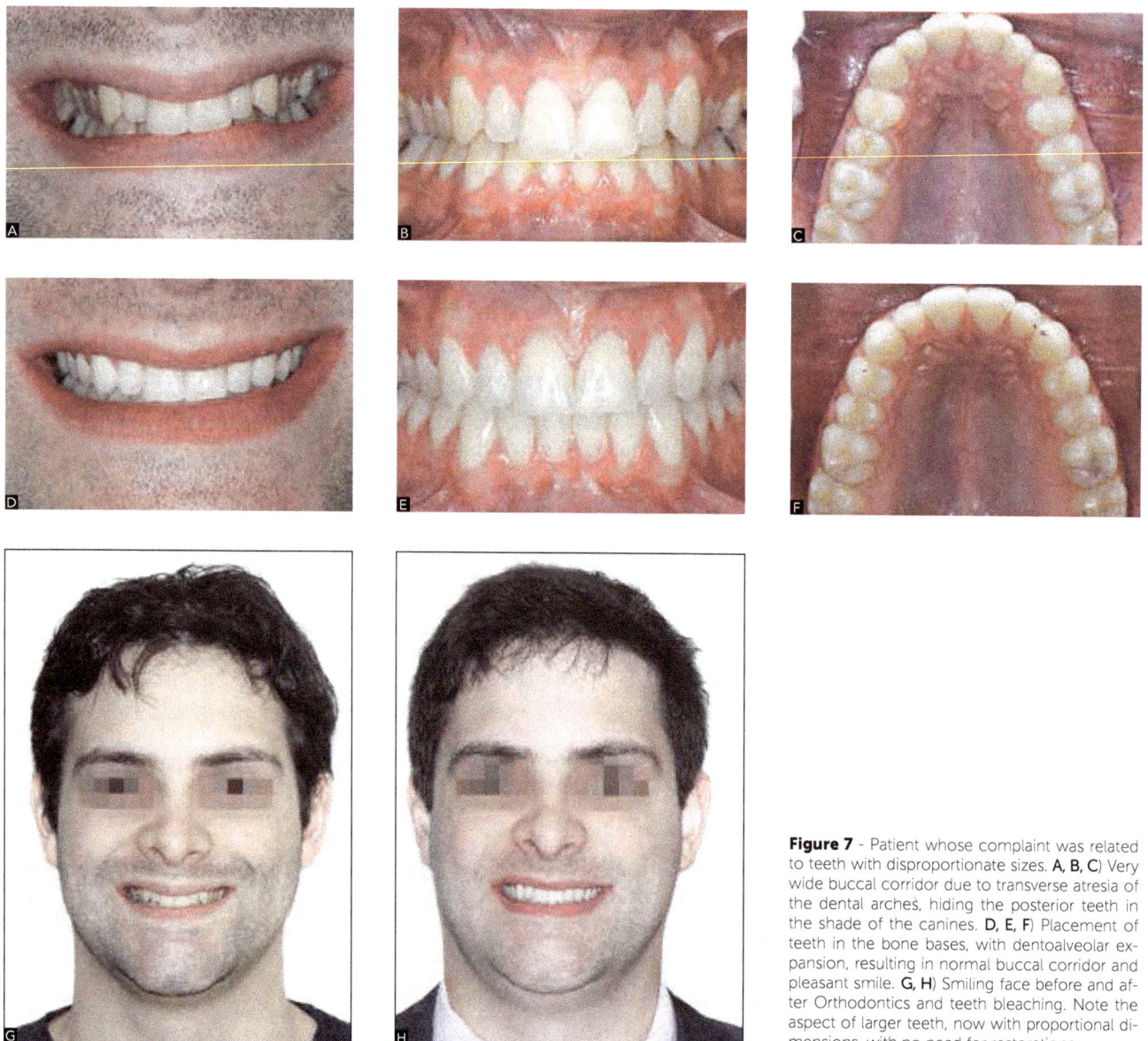

Figure 7 - Patient whose complaint was related to teeth with disproportionate sizes. **A, B, C)** Very wide buccal corridor due to transverse atresia of the dental arches, hiding the posterior teeth in the shade of the canines. **D, E, F)** Placement of teeth in the bone bases, with dentoalveolar expansion, resulting in normal buccal corridor and pleasant smile. **G, H)** Smiling face before and after Orthodontics and teeth bleaching. Note the aspect of larger teeth, now with proportional dimensions, with no need for restorations.

In this case, when the professional is concerned about placing the teeth well implanted into the bone base, there is anatomical integrity and the contact points are correctly established, which automatically generates the best optical response to light propagation. The orthodontist must achieve the expression of what naturally occurs when a normal occlusion is exposed in different situations of speech and smile.[1,10,50] Figure 8 shows the behavior of light, considering the normality in dental alignment and in the arch shape, with maximum reflection of light in the anterior areas and a progressive increase of light deflection in the distal direction, which does not return to the observer's retina.

However, there are situations in which the professional might have to intervene in a different manner, specially when there are limitations for teeth positioning in the bone base, which is common in cases of transverse skeletal asymmetry. We oftentimes face asymmetric mandibular growth, which generates mandibular laterognathism, displacing the entire lower bone base to one side, a situation defined as prevalent in the population, according to Duthie et al.[17] Many times, this happens due to late expression of growth, a nightmare in orthodontic clinic that can lead cases that were under clinical control to orthognathic surgery. In less dramatic cases, asymmetry may be disguised, which compromises the ideal position of the teeth in the bone base. In these cases, the teeth in the upper arch have their crowns buccally tipped, following the mandibular laterognathism. At the same time, the teeth on the same side of the mandible are lingually tipped.[42] Specially in the upper arch, this buccal tipping is biologically recommended because of its thinner gingival tissue, specially in the upper canines and first premolars regions.[43] In the case of misaligned bone bases, should the ideal torques be established, the canine root would be moved against the thin buccal bone plate, significantly reducing the thickness of the periodontium and increasing the risk of periodontal recession. Even if not immediate, periodontal recession may occur in the long-term due to canine positioning and volume, since it is the tooth that is most susceptible to trauma caused by toothbrushing.[61]

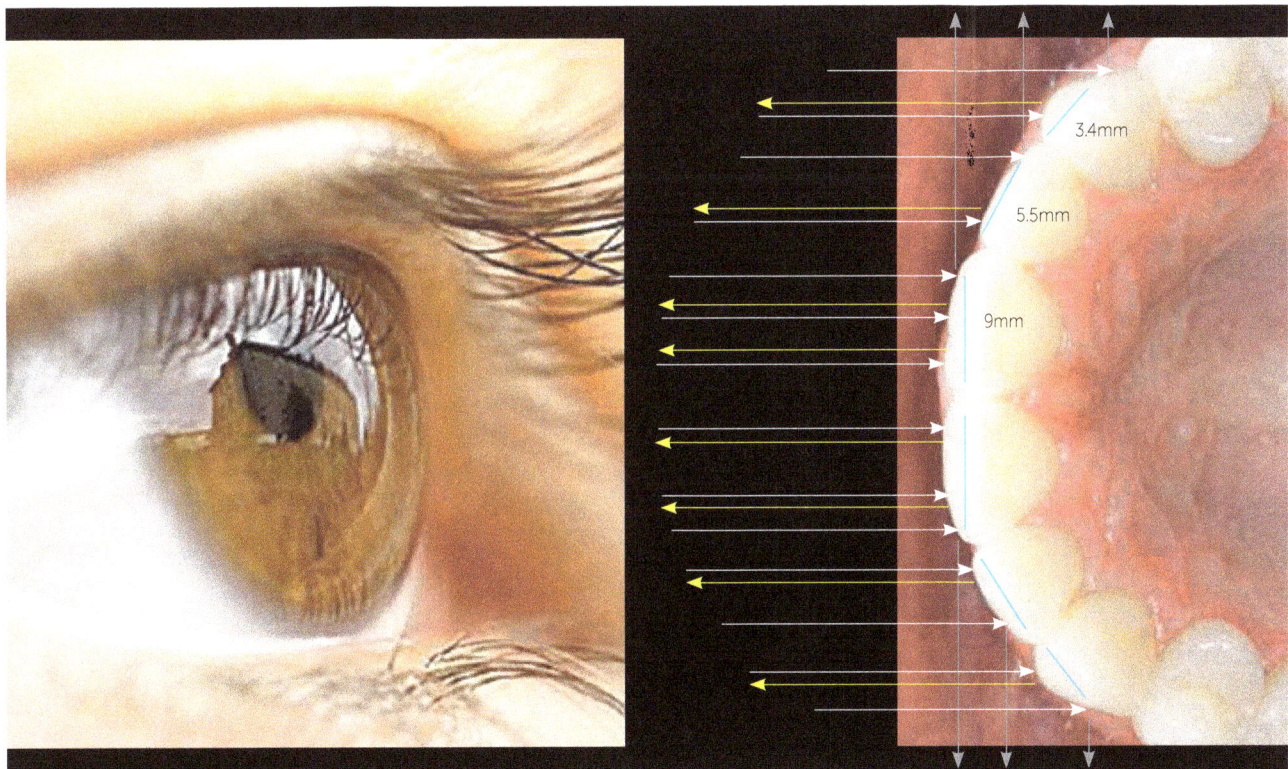

Figure 8 - Virtual width. Behavior of light focusing on anterior teeth (white arrows). Phenomenon that defines the virtual width, in which the central incisors, with larger flat area (blue line), reflect nearly all the light (yellow arrows); while on the canine, with a little more than ⅓ of the area that generates reflection of light, the deflection of light (gray arrows) predominates, which is explained by its position in the arch and convex anatomy.

According to Karring et al[24] even in teeth not orthodontically moved, a periodontuim with no alveolar bone is often found, by dehiscence or fenestration; therefore, a solid periodontal evaluation is recommended before inserting thick rectangular wires.[8,9]

In order to reverse the esthetical impairment of a canine buccal crown torque, procedures that lead to optical illusion can be used, an esthetical disguise that is essential in cases of orthodontically compensated skeletal asymmetry (Fig 9). The base of the procedure is an ameloplasty that hides the distal part of the buccal surface of the buccally tipped canine. It is necessary to divide the buccal surface into two and wear out the distal part of the crown with finishing burs, accentuating the curvature in the crown anatomy until there is no reflection of light and it is in the shade, due to light deflection. After one half of the buccal

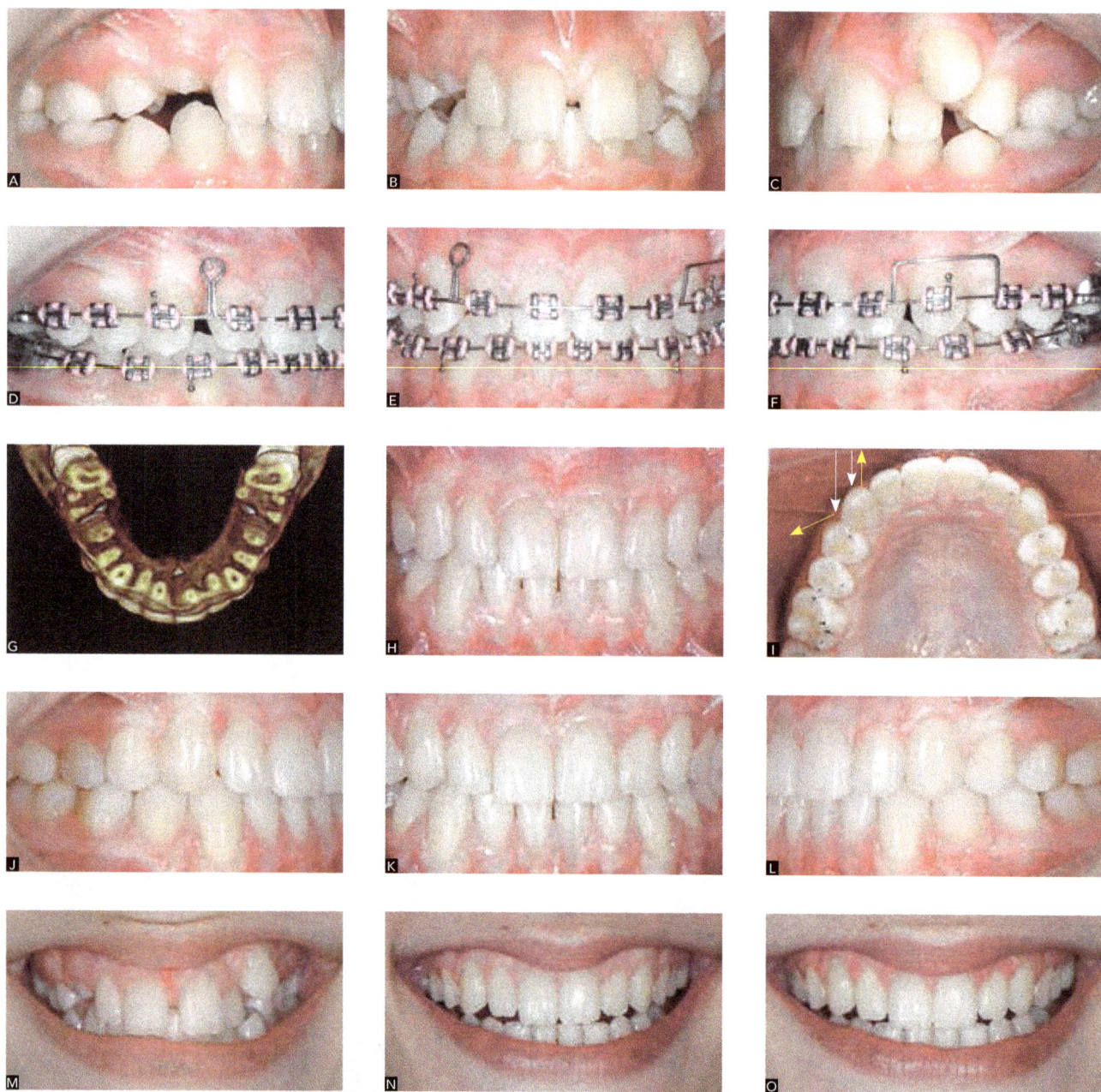

Figure 9 - Patient, whose mother had mandibular asymmetry, underwent orthodontic-surgical treatment. **A, B, C)** Transverse maxillary atresia, with crowding and deviation of the midlines. **D, E, F)** Orthodontic treatment with arch of midline correction. **G)** Tomographic slice, top view of the maxilla, showing minimum thickness of alveolar bone in the canine buccal surface. **H)** Final photograph of the treatment, with evident inappropriate torque of tooth #13, because buccal root movement was avoided due to periodontal risk. **I)** Ameloplasty on the distal half of the buccal surface of tooth #13, reducing reflection of light (arrows), with effect of optical illusion, reducing the virtual width of this tooth. **J, K, L)** Final result of the occlusion. Smile before (**M**) and after treatment (**N**), torque of tooth #13 was compensated. **O)** Smile after ameloplasty, virtually reducing tooth #13 due to the smaller flat area exposed to light.

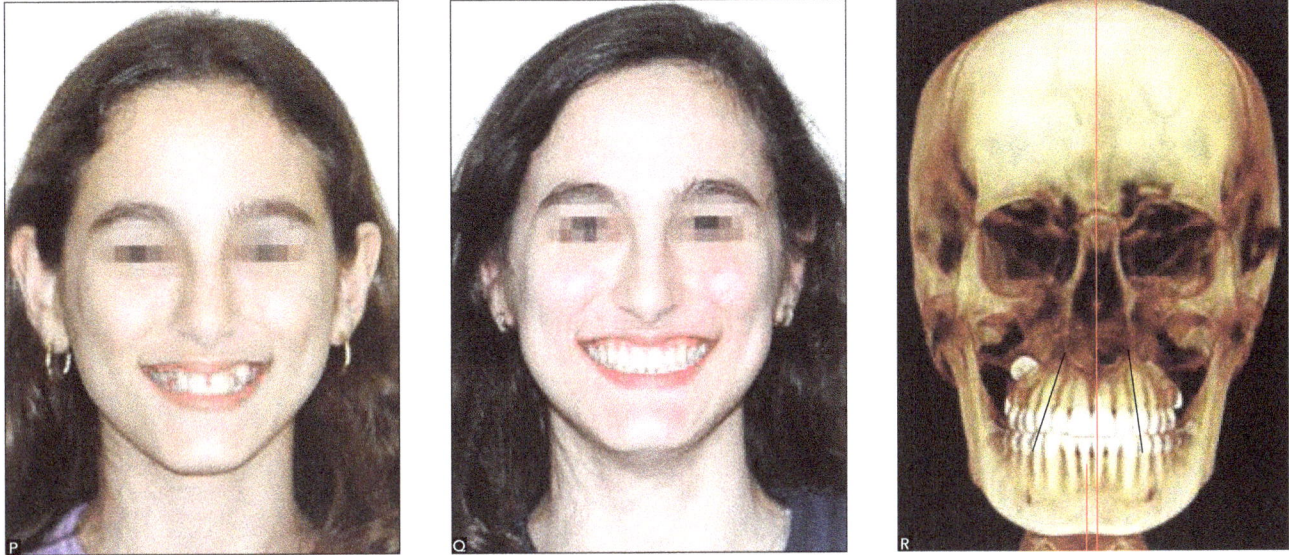

Figure 9 (continuation) - Smile before (**P**) and after treatment (**Q**). **R**) Tomography obtained after treatment, showing the different torques on the upper canines, adequate to mandibular asymmetry.

surface of the canine has been "hidden", polishing with abrasive rubbers is performed and the use of sodium fluoride at 0.05% is prescribed for daily mouthwash.

VIRTUAL HEIGHT OF CROWNS

A reasoning similar to the optical explanation that defines the virtual width must be applied to the virtual height. In other words, there is an alteration on the amount of light reflected over the patient's clinical crown, a difference between real and virtual height. (Fig 10) This difference is directly related to the torque of the upper anterior teeth that deflect most of the light emitted on the clinical crowns: upwards, when torque is excessive; or downwards, when the crowns are retroclined. A similar effect occurs when the occlusal plane is too posteriorly inclined or too flat.[53]

The correction or control of anterior teeth torques defines the success in obtaining the best expression of the dimensions of the dental crowns, when exposed to light.[47] Special attention must be given to torque control in cases in which there will be great retraction of anterior teeth, quite common in Class II division 1 patients, treated with upper first premolars extractions. Third order bend should be emphasized in the retraction arches or high torque brackets should be used at this stage.

Cephalometry is traditionally used for evaluation of torques in anterior teeth and, based on these data and on the treatment strategy, the orthodontic mechanics is

defined, with greater or minor concerns over root control. As long as it is correctly obtained, the procedure of reading the light generated by the flash of the camera used for intraoral photograph is also employed. According to Masioli,[38] the correct position for frontal intraoral photograph is with the center of the photograph coinciding with the intersection of the mid sagittal plane with the occlusal plane. In order to obtain natural head position, the camera lens must be directed perpendicularly to the coronal plane of the patient's head and parallel to the Camper's plane whereas the focus must be established between the upper central incisor and the canine (Fig 11).

When the incisors present ideal torques, in natural head position, the flash is reflected to the maximum in the middle of the clinical crowns of these teeth. The flash cervically displaced indicates that the incisors have insufficient lingual root torque (Fig 12B), while the light displaced to the incisal edge indicates upper incisors with excessive lingual root torque. This perception and the routine of photographing the evolution of treatment, not only enhances professional learning, but avoids excessive exposure of the patient to radiation.

Considering this information, patients with Class II division 2 or Angle Class I malocclusion, who have labial musculature with accentuated tonus and usually present excessive overbite and retroclination of upper incisors, are specially esthetically benefited when the anterior teeth

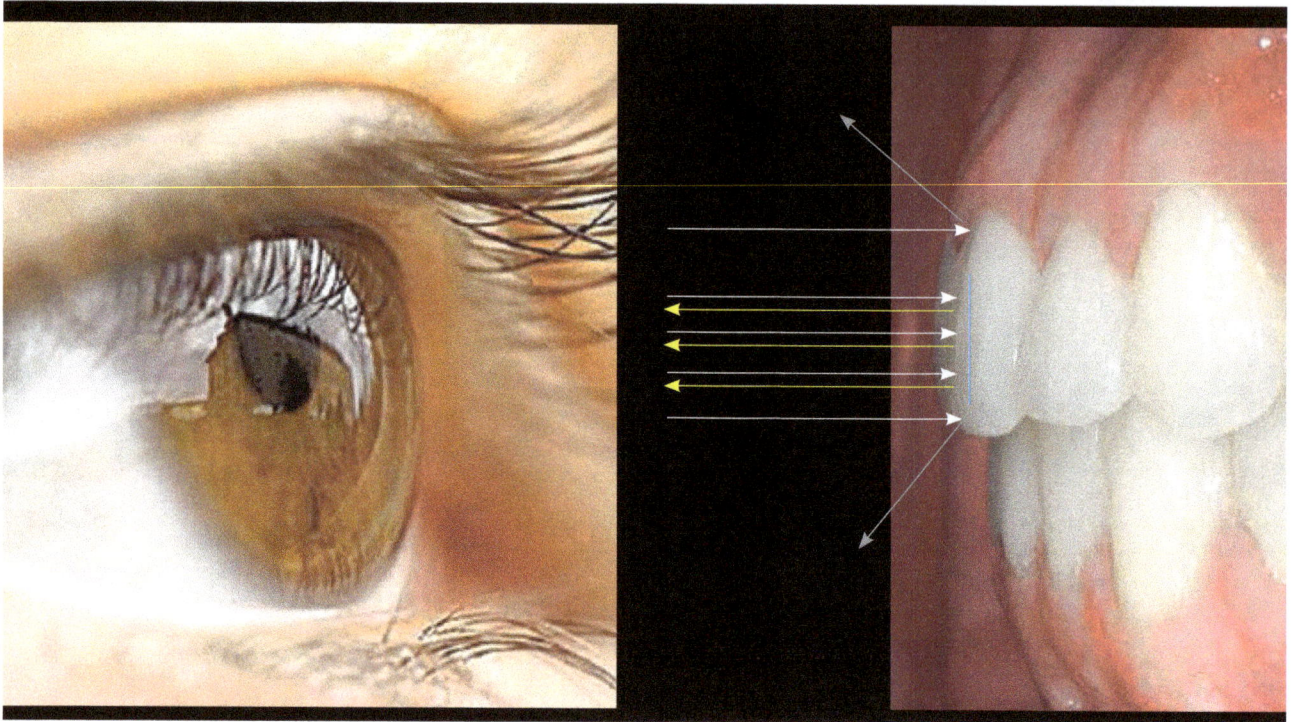

Figure 10 - Virtual height. Behavior of light focusing on anterior teeth (white arrows). Phenomenon that defines the virtual height: if the tooth is with adequate torque, the flat surface of the tooth is large and is at the center of the crown (blue line), reflecting most of the light that focuses (white and yellow arrows). The cervical and the incisal borders generate deflection of light (gray arrows).

are positioned at their correct tipping in the bone base. This finding can be seen in Figure 12 which reveals that during correction of malocclusion, significant improvements occurred in the torques of anterior teeth, which was easily perceived by the area in the crown where there was flash light reflected, migrating from the cervical to the middle of the upper incisor crowns.

Moreover, dental double protrusions are examples of how the appearance of the size of anterior teeth can be improved by orthodontic treatment. Figure 13 presents an adult female patient with excessive incisor proclination, but with a pleasant facial profile. In order to avoid extractions and, specially, the loss of lip support, it was decided to correct the excessive anterior teeth torques with the minimum retraction of these teeth. The patient was treated with controlled tipping, with movements lingually performed in the incisor crowns and maintenance of root apices in position. This way, all necessary spaces were obtained with generous interproximal wear on the posterior teeth, associated with temporary anchorage devices. Thus, an increase in the virtual height of these teeth was obtained with expanded reflection of light, since their buccal surfaces were buccally inclined, exposing a larger flat area of the clinical crowns to light, which is more pleasant and natural. [12,26,36]

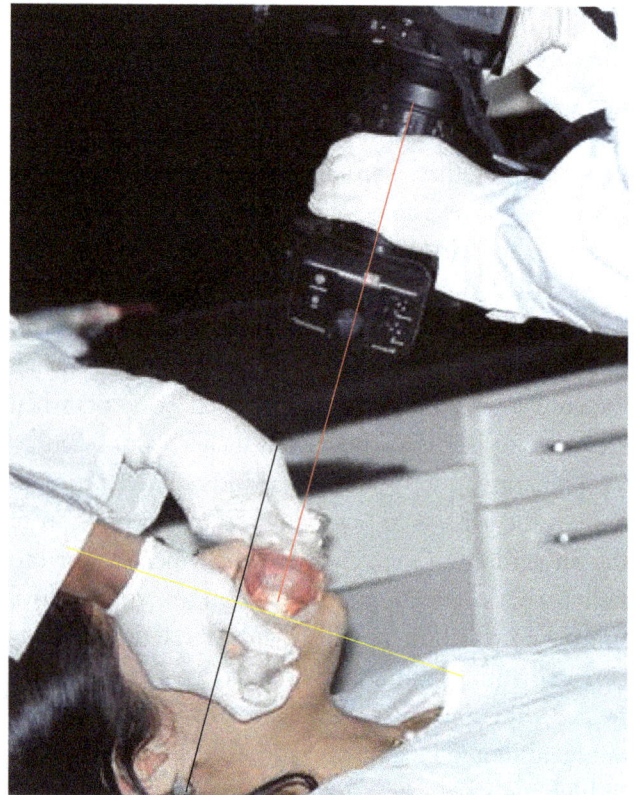

Figure 11 - Frontal intraoral photograph. Note that the lens are directed towards the central incisors, perpendicular to the coronal plane of the patient's head. The lens must also be parallel to Camper's plane (tragus – wing of the nose), defined as the natural postural plane, different from the occlusal plane, which may vary with treatment and may influence the expression of dental torques.

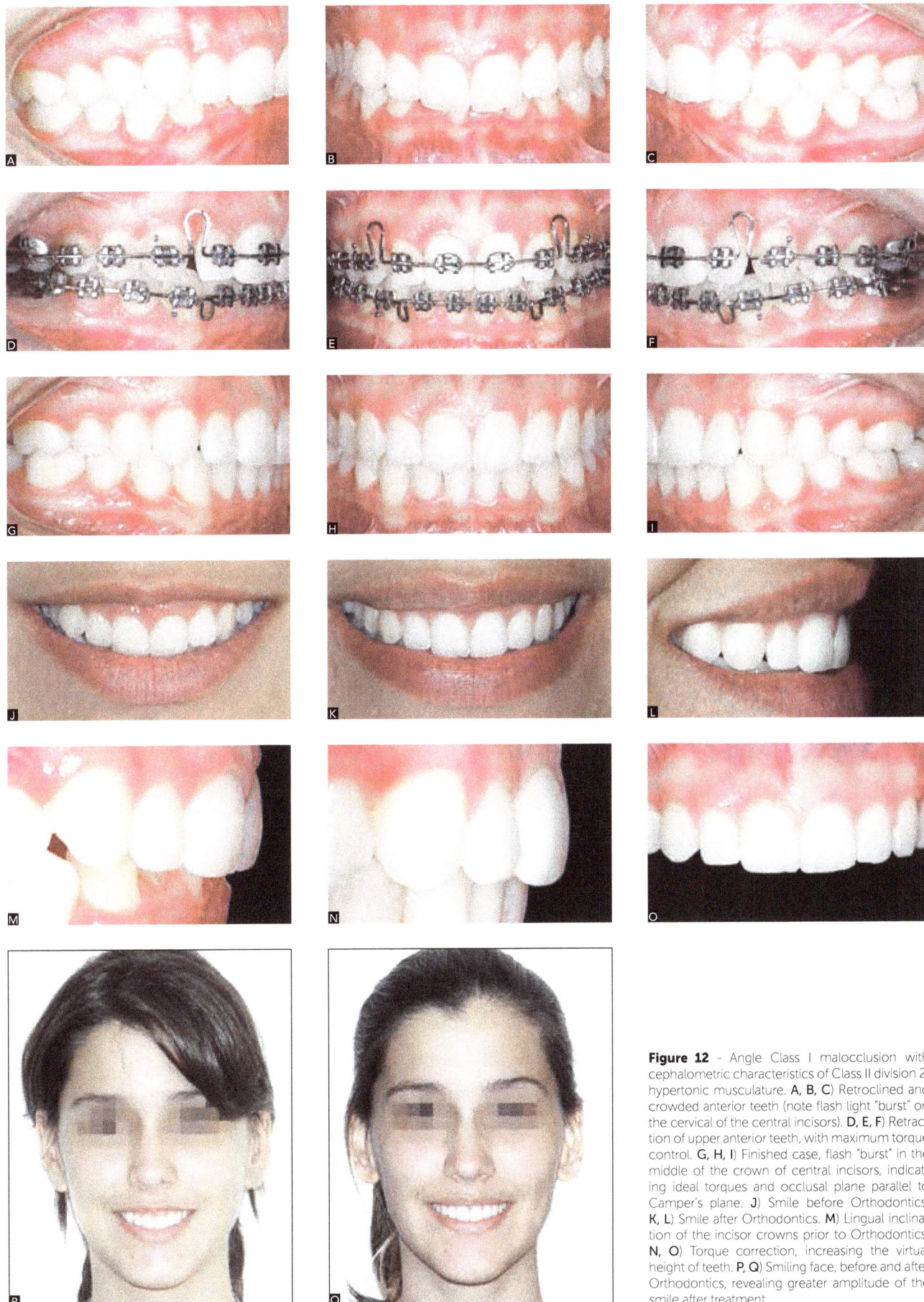

Figure 12 - Angle Class I malocclusion with cephalometric characteristics of Class II division 2, hypertonic musculature. **A, B, C)** Retroclined and crowded anterior teeth (note flash light "burst" on the cervical of the central incisors). **D, E, F)** Retraction of upper anterior teeth, with maximum torque control. **G, H, I)** Finished case, flash "burst" in the middle of the crown of central incisors, indicating ideal torques and occlusal plane parallel to Camper's plane. **J)** Smile before Orthodontics. **K, L)** Smile after Orthodontics. **M)** Lingual inclination of the incisor crowns prior to Orthodontics. **N, O)** Torque correction, increasing the virtual height of teeth. **P, Q)** Smiling face, before and after Orthodontics, revealing greater amplitude of the smile after treatment.

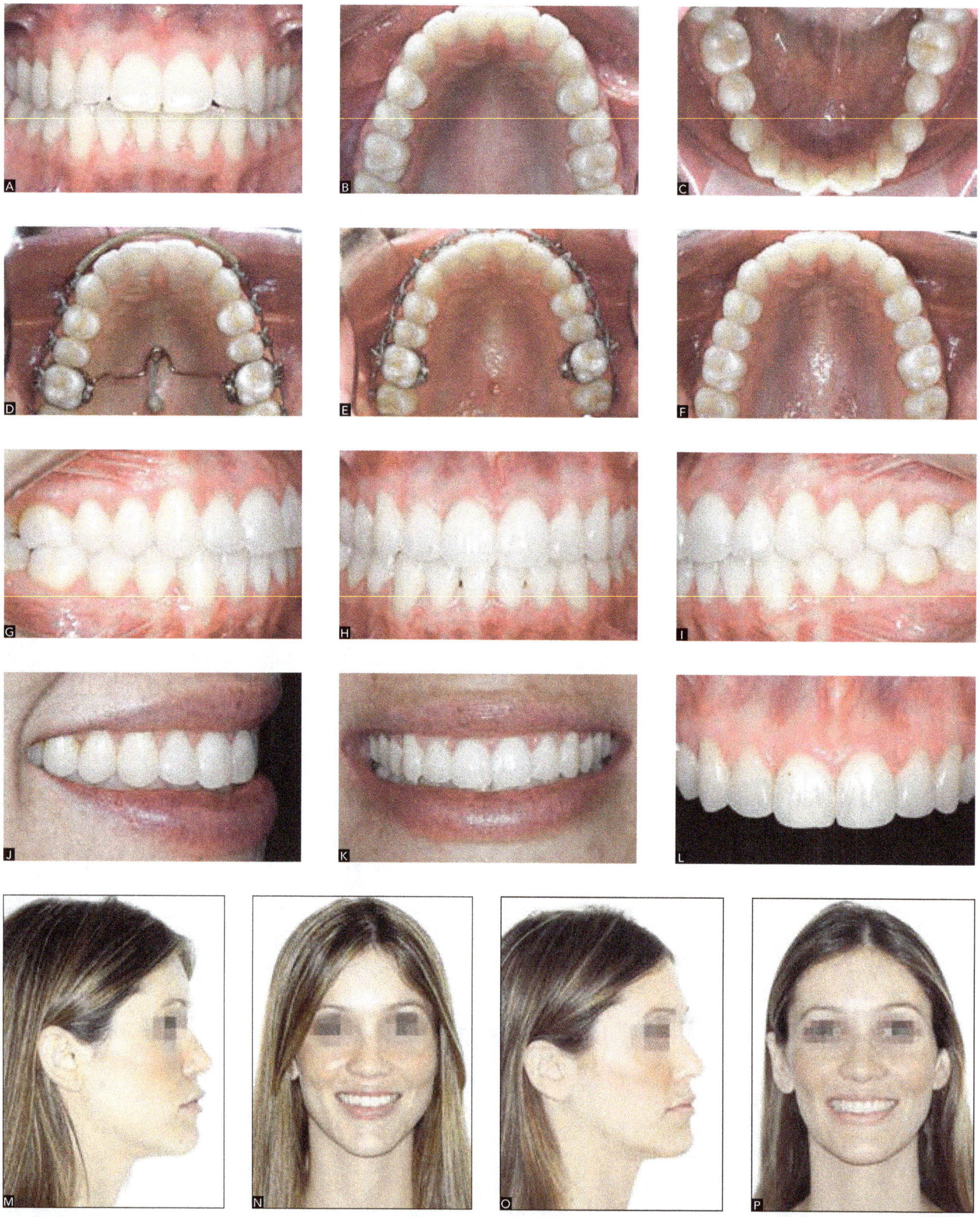

Figure 13 - Patient with Class I malocclusion, in good initial intercuspation. **A, B, C)** Dental double protrusion, with proclination of incisors revealed by the flash "burst" on the incisal surface of the upper central incisor. Large posterior teeth. **D)** Mini-implant on the palate, used as anchorage for retraction. **E, F)** After generous interdental wear on posterior teeth, the incisors were retracted, and the shape of the arches was maintained. **G, H, I)** Results after Orthodontics, with the "burst" of light in the middle of the crown of incisors. **J, K, L)** More pleasant smile as a result of torque correction and teeth positioned in the bone bases. **M, N)** Facial profile and smile before treatment, indicating minimum retraction of the lips. **O, P)** Face in profile and smile by the end of the treatment, enhancing the patient's beauty.

DOMINANCE OF CENTRAL INCISORS

A concept that has been strongly settled in oral prosthetic rehabilitation, specially advocated by Kina and Bruguera,[25] states that the central incisors must be dominant in the smile in order to provide unity, strength, joviality and sensuality. In a dental composition, the dominance of central incisors is considered natural. Previous studies show that human perception is deviated to the upper central incisors and, when their dominance on the face is increased or emphasized, people are considered as younger and more attractive.[25,54]

The studies carried out by King et al[27] showed the preference of dentists, orthodontists and laypeople for the incisal edge of the lateral incisors always being above the incisal plane, on average 0.5 mm, not exceeding 1 mm. This is the pattern used in Orthodontics, with the contour of the incisal edges of the upper anterior teeth following the curvature of the lower lip on the smile.[32,49,62]

Some authors[25,26] of the Dental Prosthesis field work with greater distances and, therefore, the smile curvature becomes more accentuated. The search for joviality based on dental dimensions has generated some excess, but the orthodontist cannot ignore the trends and convictions of other specialties in Dentistry. With some judgment, and after discussing the theme with the patient and the oral rehabilitation colleague, good results can be obtained with the use of porcelain veneers (Fig 14).

Another procedure employed by Dental Prosthesis, and discussed in the previous special article, is the recommendation of increasing the flat surface area on the morphology of the prosthetic anatomy of the central incisors, expanding the reflection of light and contributing to the dominance of central incisors on the facial dynamic.[1,19,36,55]

HEIGHT OF CONTACT POINTS

There are some procedures that can really make a difference on the results of treated cases. Smile symmetry and amplitude were already discussed in this article and must be associated with the sensation of depth and naturality when placing the contact points.

The golden ratio is applied to the height of the contact points of the anterior teeth.[41,50,52] The contact point between central incisors must correspond to 50% of the height of the crown of these teeth, and must gradually distally reduce, turning into 40% of this height at the contact point between central and lateral incisors, and 30% of this height at the contact point between lateral

incisor and canine. According to Kina and Bruguera,[25] a hypothetical line connecting the ends of the anterior contact points must be parallel to the horizontal lines of the face and to the edge of the lower lip in order to establish a cohesive and harmonious unity of the smile (Fig 15). These lines and proportions were also used in the determination of the "six horizontal smile lines", emphasized by Câmara[11] and widely used for smile analysis.

There are three ways to achieve this proportion:

1) Prosthetic increase — selective for the height of the crowns of anterior teeth: as it has been previously mentioned, the procedures of Restorative Dentistry and, specially, the porcelain veneers are some of the options that have been increasingly used and resistant to time.[2,26]

2) Gingivectomy including the papilla (Fig 16) — the correction of the gingival contour and the ideal height/width proportion of the teeth must be conciliated so as to intervene in the height of the interdental papilla. In this case, the intervention emphasizes the existence of more than 5 mm of distance between the alveolar bone crest and the contact point, a condition that is established to avoid the opening of black spaces in the interdental spaces.[59]

3) Ameloplasty, performed in two ways — increasing the contact area by interdental wear, or reducing the contact area of the incisal edges, altering the incisal spaces.[52] The interdental embrasures form interdental angles which, according to Magne and Belser,[37] are shaped as an inverted "V", narrower between the central incisors, asymmetric between central and lateral and large between lateral incisor and canine (Fig 17).

When the shape of the interincisal angles are changed by ameloplasty, the professional must also consider if it is desirable to change the shape of the teeth, making them rounder, with wider interincisal angle spaces (Fig 18). Women can be specially benefited with this procedure, while marked angles are masculine characteristics that are desired by the evaluators.[4] The patient must be consulted before this procedure is performed, and the simulation of the future shape of the teeth, drawn with a black dermographic pen, is recommended.

TEETH / PERIODONTIUM RELATION

The discovery of the importance that "pink esthetics" has on the results of dental treatments is not recent, and the definition of normality has nearly established

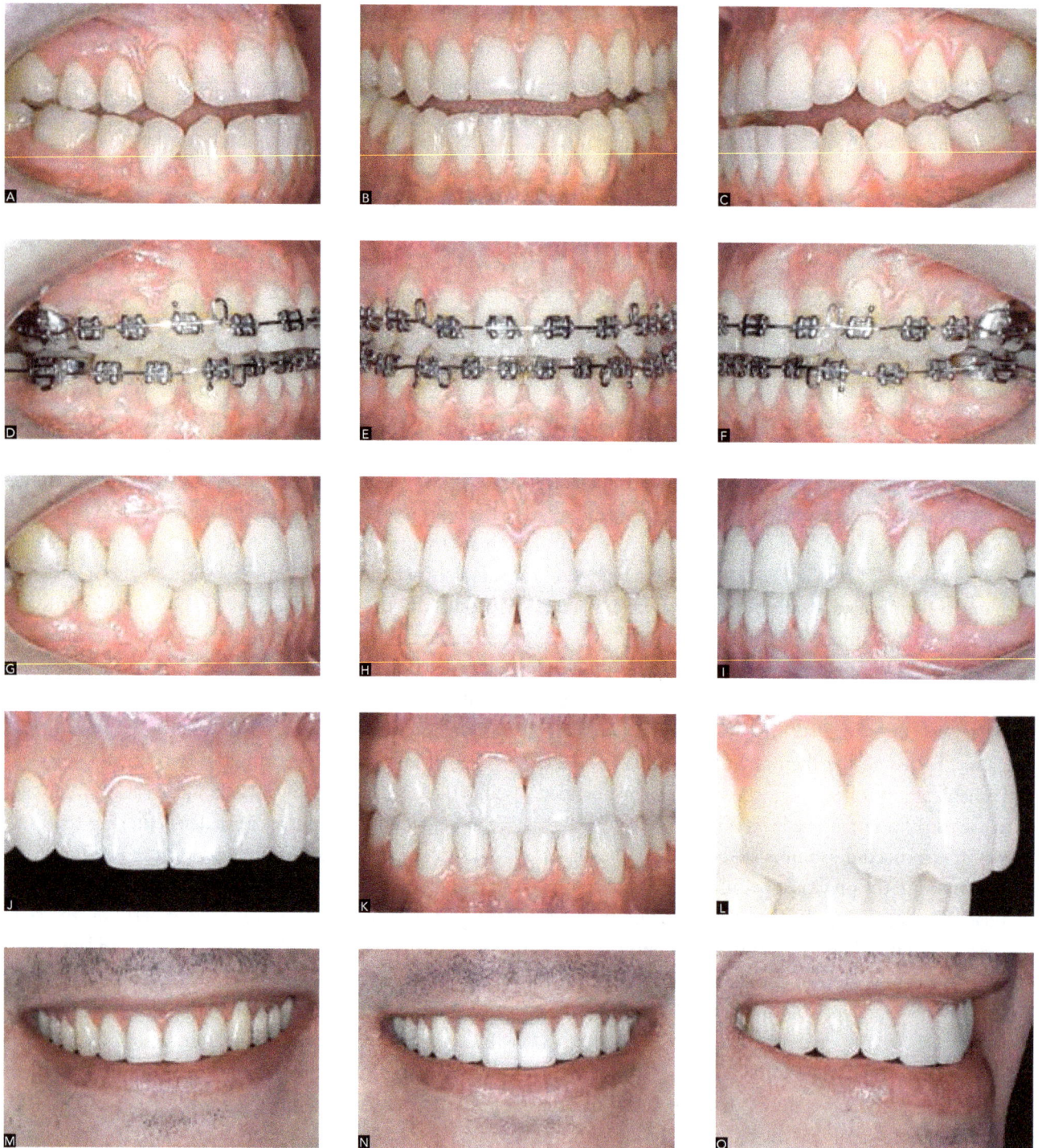

Figure 14 - Class III patient with anterior open bite, referred to orthodontic-surgical treatment. **A, B, C**) Initial intraoral photographs, revealing loss of height of central incisors, probably caused by chemical erosion. **D, E, F**) Occlusion established after surgical procedure with maxillary advancement. **G, H, I**) Result after Orthodontics, in which satisfactory occlusion can be noted, but with incisal curve almost flat. **J, K, L**) Final result of the patient's microesthetics, with dominance of the central established by means of porcelain veneers. **M**) Smile after Orthodontics, and before the veneers. **N, O**) Repercussion on miniesthetics (smile), after veneers on teeth #11 and #21: a younger smile.

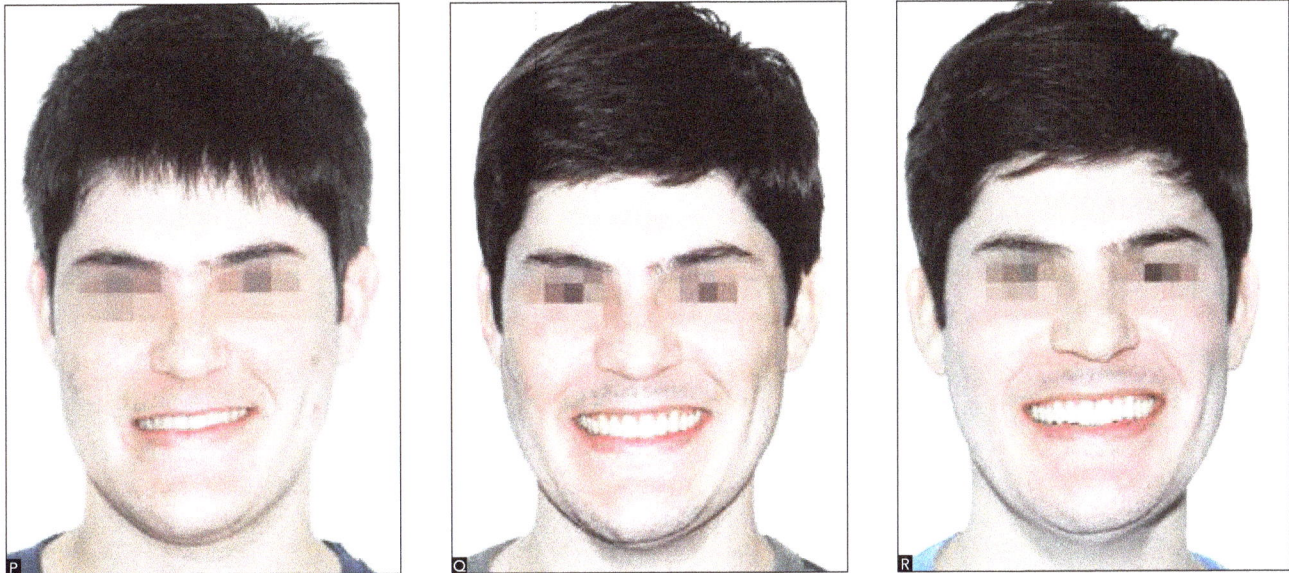

Figure 14 (continuation) - P, Q, R) Macroesthetics (smiling face), sequence of events (left to right): before treatment, after Orthodontics, after veneers.

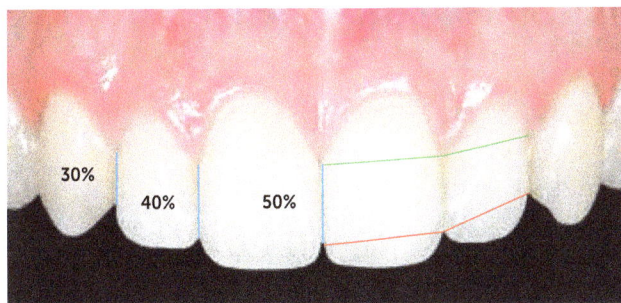

Figure 15 - Ideal heights of contact points. Between the central incisors, it must be half of the height of the crown of these teeth, decreasing distally, at each contact, always in relation to the central incisor. Guiding lines connecting the apices of the papillae (red) and the lower ends of the contact points (green), emphasized by Câmara.[11]

a consensus among professionals that deal with esthetics.[1,11,12,13,26,28,34,48,51,61,63] There is an integration between the factors that determine microesthetics, so that when ideal dental proportions and dimensions are established, the relations between the heights of the crowns of upper anterior teeth also define the adequate gingival contour. Furthermore, the problems tend to be correlated, and the solution becomes the intervention on the position of teeth and dental anatomy, alteration of the anatomy of the periodontium or both procedures.

Gingival contour

Kokich, Nappen and Shapiro[28] established the parameters that must be sought to obtain gingival contour, with the gingival margin of canines and upper central incisors at the same level, and the margin of upper lateral

incisors 1 mm below those. (Fig 17) The margin of the lateral at the same height of the central is considered acceptable, provided that, in prosthetic procedures, color and shade effects are established to reduce the virtual height of lateral incisors.[13,40]

Evidently, the gingival contour must be considered as esthetically important if there is gingival exposure at smiling, specially when the smile line is high.[57]

When the gingival contour is asymmetric, with difference in the height/width proportion, three situations, with distinct possibilities of performance, must be considered, as described below.

1) If the teeth are higid and the incisal edges are correctly leveled: there is a difference in height between the clinical and anatomical crowns of the tooth, usually related to the excess of gingival tissue. In this case, by means of a periodontal probe, it is noticeable that the gingival sulcus is deep or that he periodontal biological space is excessive. This happens when the keratinized gingiva is thick and did not migrate apically, which defines a partial eruption of the tooth; or when there was gingival hyperplasia, which is very common for orthodontic treatment, specially for patients with poor oral hygiene.[33,61]

In these cases, the patient must be referred to a periodontist for augmentation of the clinical crown of anterior teeth, performed by means of gingivectomy. Depending on the width of the keratinized gingiva area, a gingival flap associated with bone recontouring might be necessary.[28] The amount of periodontal

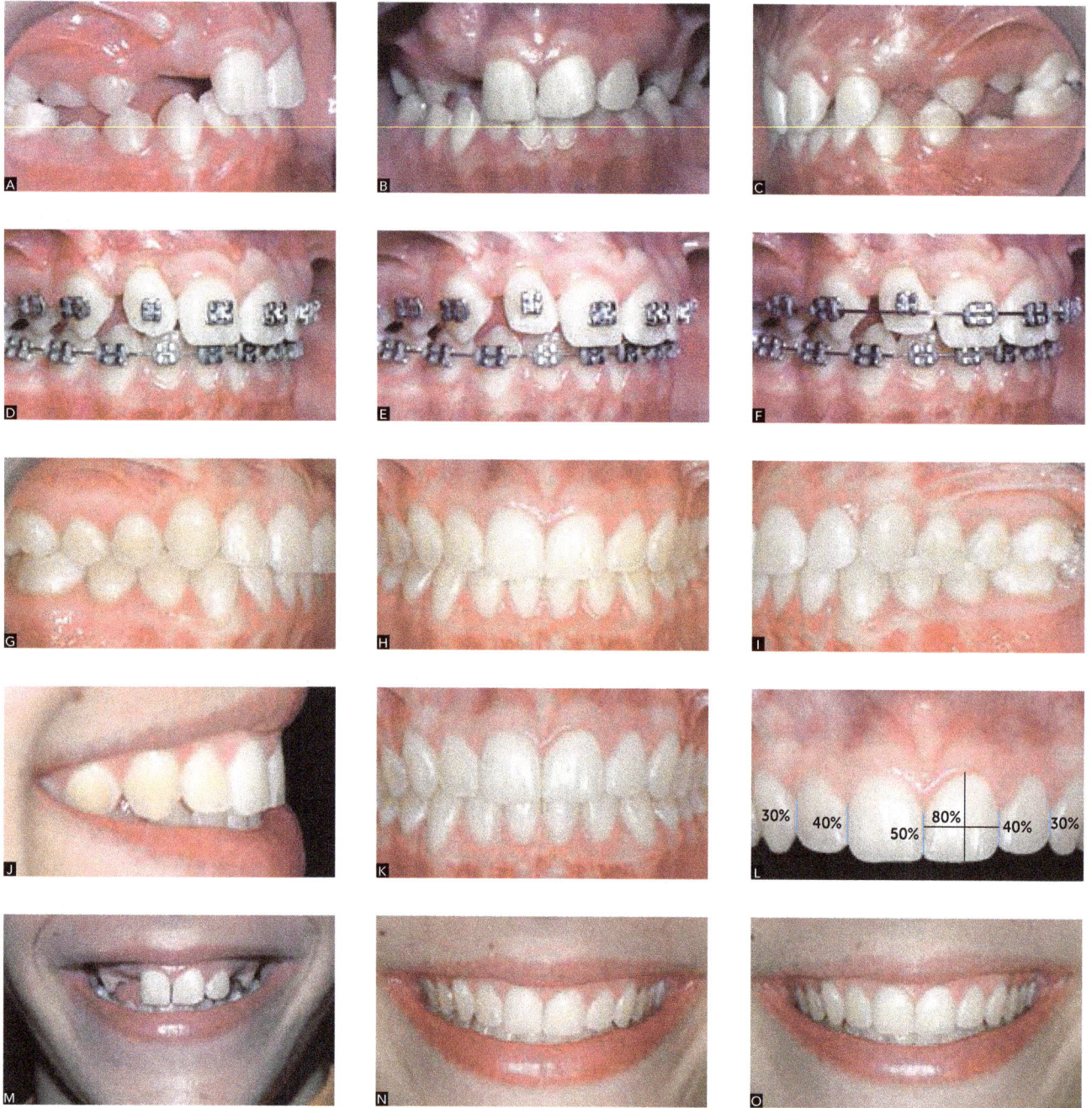

Figure 16 - Adolescent patient, with impacted canine and lateral incisors, without space. **A, B, C**) Maxilla with atresia, leading to right posterior crossbite, upper midline deviated to the right. **D, E, F**) After the lateral incisor had been forcefully extruded, ameloplasty was performed on the incisal surface in addition to cervically rebonding the bracket, allowing greater extrusion and correction of the gingival contour. **G, H, I**) Result obtained after Orthodontics, with satisfactory occlusion, but with difference in the height of the contact points and gingival contour of the left upper central incisors. **J, K, L**) Results after gingivectomy, including the papilla between teeth #21 and #22, to redimension the crown of tooth #21 and the contact point. **M**) Smile before Orthodontics. **N**) Smile after Orthodontics. **O**) Smile harmony after gingivectomy.

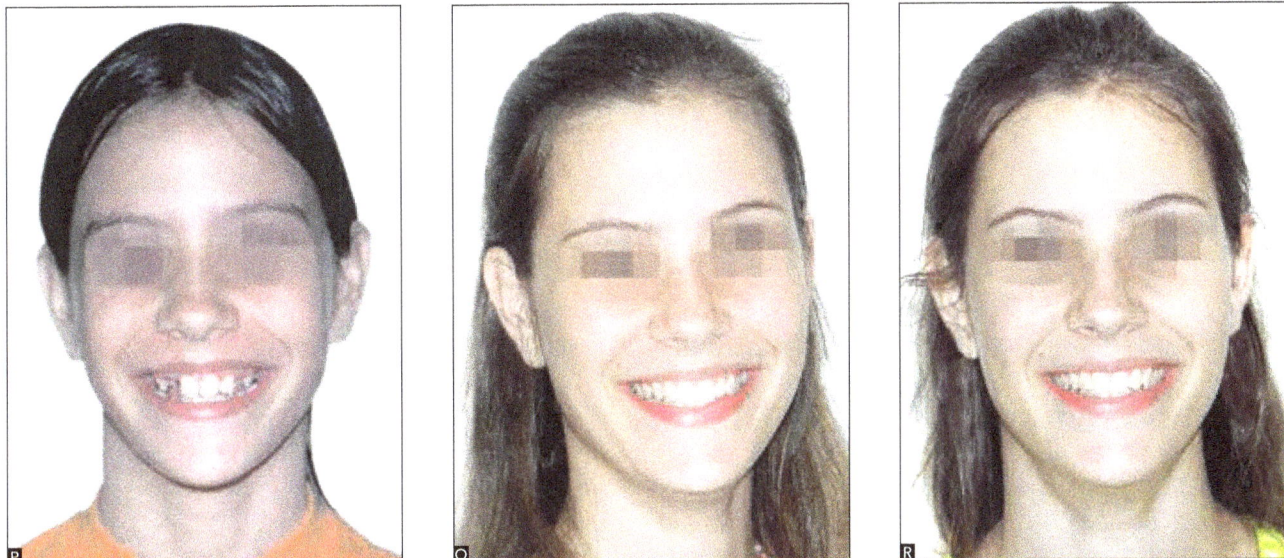

Figure 16 (continuation) - Smile before (**P**) and after orthodontic treatment (**Q**). R) Smile harmony after gingivectomy.

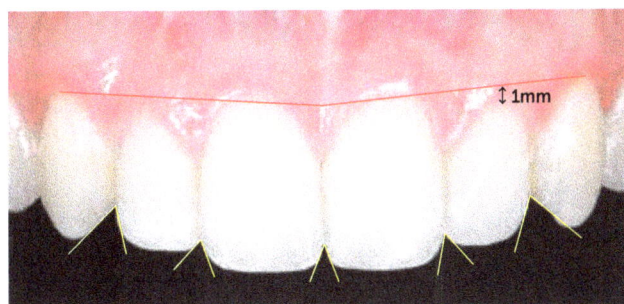

Figure 17 - Gingival contour and spaces. The red line shows the gingival contour, with lateral incisor 1 mm below the apical limit of the contour of the central incisor and the canine. In yellow, the conformation in inverted "V" in the interdental spaces, defined as: narrow between central incisors, asymmetric between central and lateral, and large between the lateral incisor and canine.

tissue that will be removed corresponds to what is enough to establish the best height/width proportion, along with the best gingival contour relation. In higid teeth, the exposure of the entire anatomical crown is recommended.

It is worth noting that, after surgery, the tooth seems to be greater in height in comparison to what it will actually be after three months, which is the period necessary for the operated gingiva to recover and for the gingival sulcus to be restored, reducing the crown height in nearly 2 mm. Patients with gingival smile are specially benefited by this procedure.

2) If the teeth are not higid: there usually is asymmetric wear of the incisal edges, associated with compensatory extrusion of these teeth, together with the entire periodontium of the compromised tooth. In these cases, the leveling of cementoenamel junctions must be carried out with individualized intrusion movements.[30,34] The appliance must be placed in compliance with the need for gingival contour correction, and not the leveling of incisal edges.[62] It is very important to emphasize that the intruded tooth needs to be retained for, at least, six months in its position, waiting for the turnover of the periodontal ligament, when the stretched collagen and elastic fibers are rearranged, reducing the risk of relapse. The importance of Orthodontics for the solution of periodontal and prosthetic problems was clearly exposed in the systematic review published by Gkantidis, Christou and Topouzelis.[21]

Esthetic restorative procedures will be necessary to establish the relation of incisal edges and dental proportions by means of composite or provisional resin during orthodontic finishing. It is also important to consider that there might be accumulation of gingival tissue with the intrusion of the tooth, which will indicate that a gingivectomy procedure should be performed at least three months before the definitive prosthetic work is performed.[63]

3) If there is a bone defect: usually associated with a history of periodontal disease or localized gum recession, making the gingival edge of a tooth to move apically. In this case, slow dental extrusion is indicated,

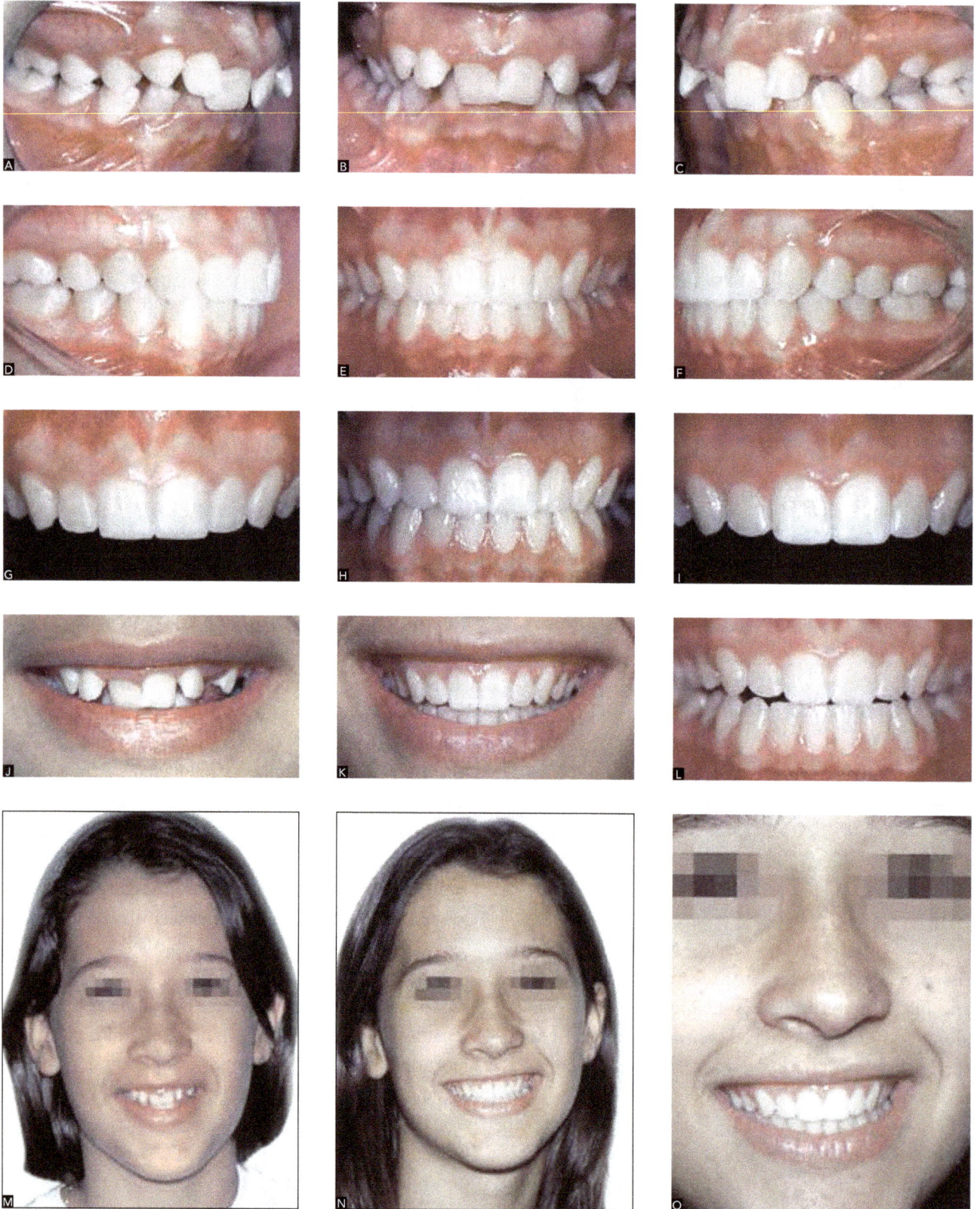

Figure 18 - Angle Class II division 2 malocclusion. **A, B, C**) Retroclined upper central incisors and overbite, characteristics of malocclusion. **D, E, F, G**) Treated case, with good arch relationship, the aspect of fused teeth on the upper central incisors calls our attention because of the very large contact point. **H, I**) After ameloplasty, which increased the incisal spaces, resulting in reduction in the height of the contact points between the central incisors, and their progressive distal decrease. **J, M**) Smile before treatment. **K, L, N, O**) Smile after Orthodontics and ameloplasty, resulting in rounder incisal edges and larger spaces.

followed by wear of the incisal edge.[21] In order to use the root of the extruded tooth, the limit of extrusion is the minimum crown/root relation (1:1). The tooth can be slowly extruded above this limit, with its extraction previously planned and with the aim of achieving alveolar bone and/or gingival soft tissue gain for posterior placement of implant.[30,57] Current scientific evidence reveals that additional studies are warranted so as to obtain predictability of periodontal response for correction of bone defects through orthodontic movement.[46]

One of the greatest concerns about gingival contour is with regard to implants and facial growth. It is known that the end of growth, which was believed to be at 16 years of age for girls and 18 years for boys, in fact does not happen. There is a late growth, with sudden changes, which is especially important for young adults between 17 and 23 years of age, that must be considered.[5] The consequences of vertical growth for gingival contour are known. Unlike the teeth, the implants do not follow the displacement of maxillary bones, producing important asymmetry on gingival and incisal contours (Fig 19). In these cases, the esthetic concern is even greater because implant substitution, of which gingiva migrates apically as time goes by, is not a simple procedure, and may generate a bone defect that is difficult to solve. The decision on placing implants in the anterior region must consider the height of the patient's smile line and, in particular, estimate the vertical facial growth.[60]

Mishandling orthodontic treatment may cause potential gingival defects when there is buccal root movement, especially in critical areas or in patients with thin periodontal biotype.[43] On average orthodontic treatments, periodontal recession and alveolar bone loss are minimum (0.03 mm and 0.13 mm, respectively), as showed in the systematic review published by Bollen et al.[6]

Zenith

The gingival zenith is the highest point of the gingival contour curvature, and may vary significantly in anterior teeth.[62] Sarver[50] presents as norm that the ideal position of the apex of the gingival contour of the lateral incisor would be in the center of the crowns, along the long axis of the tooth; while it is distally displaced on the central incisor and canine.

In recent research, Chu et al.[13] quantified the position of the gingival zenith of upper anterior teeth in a periodontally healthy population: 1 mm distal to the line that divides the middle of the crown, following the long axis of the tooth, on the upper central incisor; 0.4 mm distal to the line that divides the middle of the crown, following the long axis of the lateral incisor; and at the center of the line that represents the long axis of the upper canine (Fig 20).

The zenith can be orthodontically defined by the position of the bracket bonded to the upper anterior teeth or second-order bends on orthodontic wires, also known as artistic bends that define the mesiodistal tippings of these teeth. On the other hand, if we consider the mesiodistal angulation patterns which are used for the anterior teeth, the greatest tipping is established for the lateral incisors and canines which have the zenith less distally displaced if compared to the central incisor. The limit of what is esthetically pleasant for zenith deviations, in relation to the center of the upper central incisor, seems to be 2 mm, coinciding with a mesial tipping of 10 degrees from the long axis of these teeth.[22]

Prosthetically, the volume of the crown may contribute to the apical displacement of the gingival margin, and the coloration or shade in the cervical region of the tooth may generate the optical illusion of the most apical part of the gingival contour of each tooth — which is not simple, specially due to the need for a refined interaction between the technician in prosthesis and the prosthodontist.[37]

Definitely, the zenith represents an intrinsic characteristic of the periodontium and, therefore, can be more easily modified by periodontal surgery, with clinical crown augmentation; or recovering, in cases of periodontal recession. The stability of the position defined by the periodontist depends on respecting the periodontal biological space and the architecture of the alveolar bone crest which can be defined by bone recontouring.[18] Chu[15] emphasizes the use of the proportionality gauge developed by him for this purpose, using the vertical point, which defines 3 mm of interval between the colors of the two segments that compose the end of the instrument to guide the professional on establishing the alveolar bone limit in the cervical area of periodontally modified teeth (Fig 5).

Maximum symmetry on the placement of the zenith is recommended, specially on the upper central incisors due to the proximity established between them as well as to the facial midline.[25]

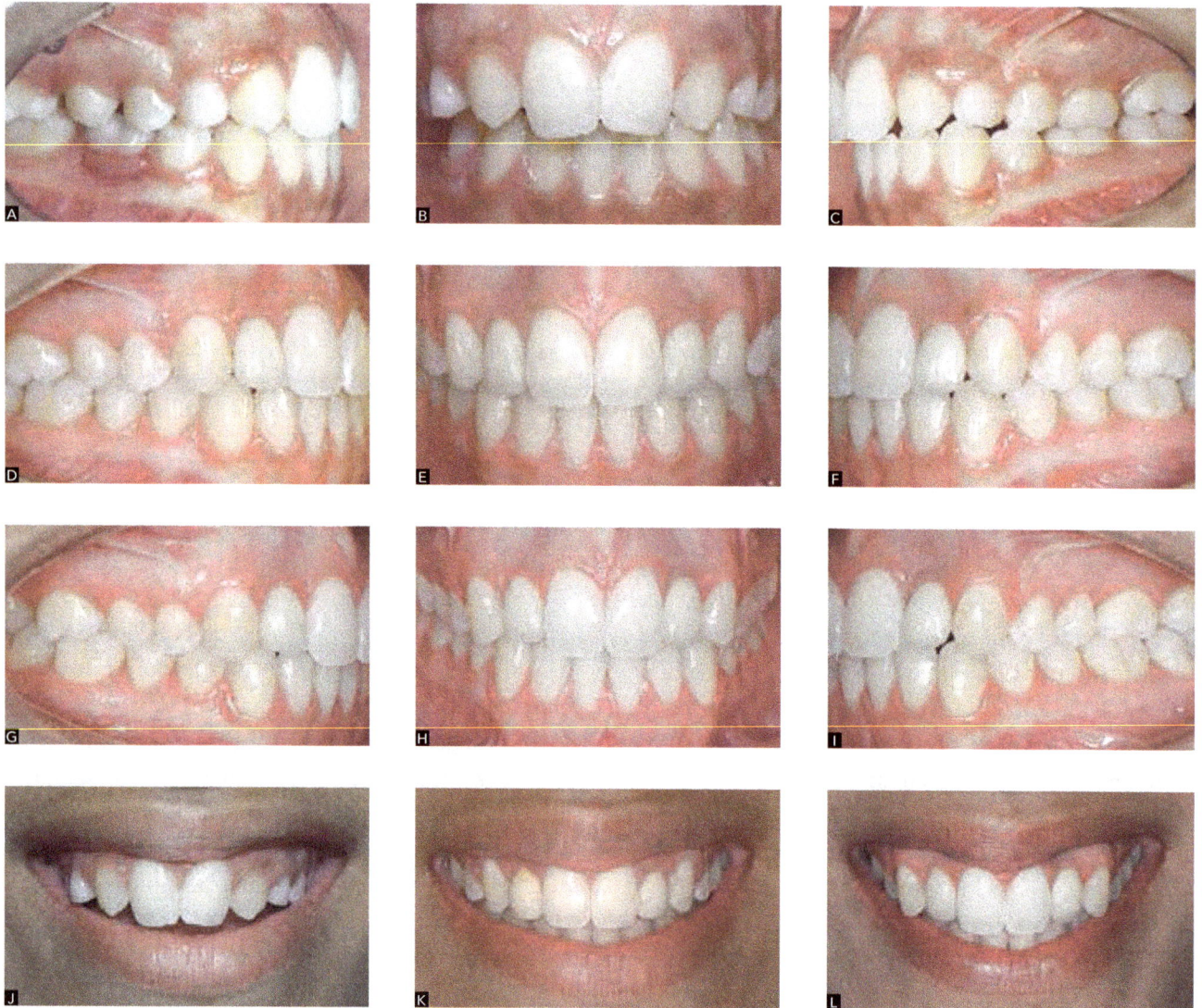

Figure 19 - Patient with agenesis of upper lateral incisor, who decided for dental implant. **A, B, C)** Initial photographs, showing the mesialization of permanent upper canines and the prolonged retention of deciduous canines. **D, E, F)** Orthodontic correction opening spaces by distalization of canines for placement of osseointe-grated implants and crowns, at 20 years of age. **G, H, I)** 26-year-old patient: note that the levels of gingival and incisal contour of the implants rose at least 1 mm. **J, K, L)** Sequence of photographs of the smile in different moments: before treatment, soon after Orthodontics with implants, and 6 years after implant placement, with canines quite marked by the infraocclusion of lateral incisors.

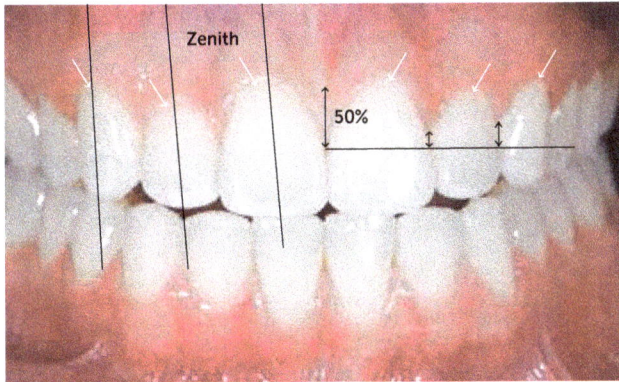

Figure 20 - Zenith and gingival papillae. Arrangement of the zenith defined by the inclinations of the long axis of the upper anterior teeth: in the middle of the canine, 0.5 mm distal to the lateral incisor, and 1 'mm distal to the central incisors (white arrows). Papilla between the central incisors filling the space until half of the height of the crowns of these teeth and gradually reducing, in height, to distal.

Height of the papilla / black spaces

The gingival papilla must apically fill from the interdental space to the contact point, being extended to half of the height of the upper central incisor, and following a position that is gradually more apical from the midline on, conferring a natural and beautiful aspect to the smile (Fig 20).

When the distance between the roots is shorter than 0.3 mm, it affects the presence of the proximal bone and, therefore, is usually accompanied by the absence of the interdental papillae On the other hand, greater interradicular spaces, as in the diastema, are usually associated with short and flattened papillae.

Tarnow, Magner and Fletcher[59] showed that the interdental papilla is present in 98% of the cases in which the cervical limit of the interdental contact is located up to 5 mm from the alveolar bone crest. When the distance from the contact point to the bone crest is of 6 mm, there is nearly 50% of chance of black space; and with 7 mm of distance, the presence of interdental papilla filling the space is found in only 27% of the cases. Therefore, it is possible to predict the appearance of black interdental spaces, which are especially common in patients with triangular teeth, when severe crowding is corrected or when there is bone loss by periodontitis.

Orthodontics has used the procedure of interdental wear for the closure of these spaces, changing the dental shape and, thus, approximating the contact point of teeth and the alveolar bone crest.[33,53,61] This procedure, extremely common among orthodontists, may lead to other undesirable esthetic consequences. Interdental wear changes two determinants of esthetics: 1) height/width proportion of the crowns, possibly generating excessively narrow teeth, and 2) increase in the height of the contact point, breaking the golden ratio of the smooth reduction in the distal direction.

A good guide to define the correct attitude towards interdental black spaces is, in ascending order of procedure:

1) Interproximal wear until the width of the incisor is not smaller than 80% of its width, in which case 75% is acceptable for naturally elongated teeth and faces.

2) Restorations or porcelain veneers changing the dental anatomy up to the limit of proportions in height of the contact points.

3) Periodontal surgery with graft to increase the height of the papilla, which is left as a last resource due to the fact that the prognosis is not always favorable.

The case presented in Figure 21 shows the closure of the pathological diastema in a periodontally compromised patient, followed by wear up the limit of the dental proportions, and finishing with veneers that closed the interdental black spaces.

PROPORTIONS BETWEEN DENTAL ARCHES (BOLTON DISCREPANCY)

A special part of this article was reserved to discuss a fundamental and specific procedure of Orthodontics, which is the analysis of Bolton discrepancy.[7] Additionally, it aimed at discussing the clinical development of this problem of high prevalence in the population, equally distributed in both genders and in different ethnicity and types of malocclusion.[23]

Although it is seen as a mathematical calculation for orthodontic planning that aims at establishing a better relation of the mesiodistal dimensions between the upper and lower arches, the discrepancy of dental volume must be carefully considered. Attenuating this difference is fundamental to establish satisfactory dental intercuspation, but, on the other hand, the problem can also be aggravated by wrong professional decisions. The fact that the measurements taken in models to define dental volume discrepancy show poor reliability deserves attention, with regard to measurement errors in cases of crowding over 3mm.[56]

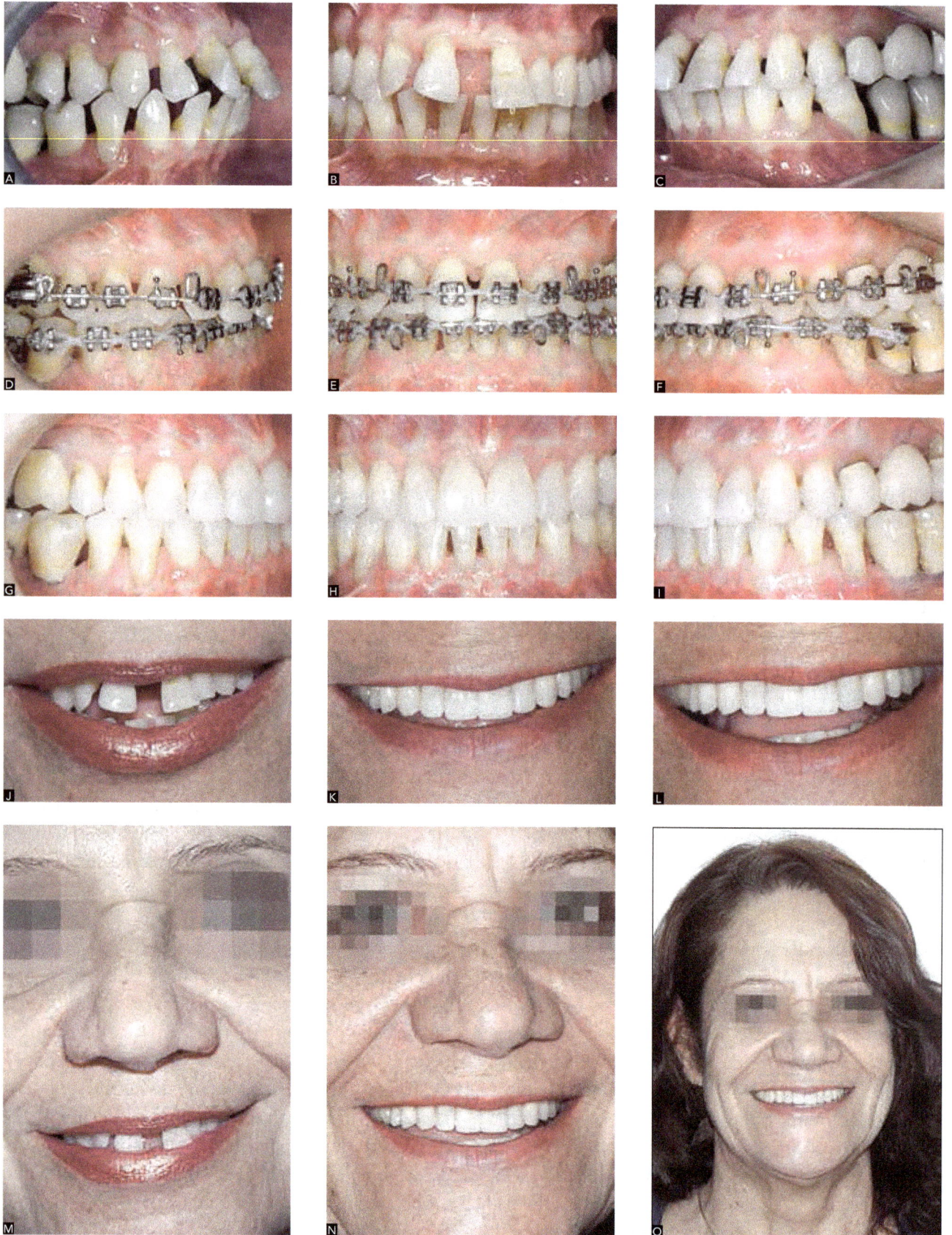

Figure 21 - Patient with history of aggressive periodontitis which was periodontally treated and controlled. **A, B, C)** Initial malocclusion, with dental loss, pathological tooth migration and multiple diastema. **D, E, F)** Ongoing orthodontic treatment, with interdental wear at the limit of the height x width proportion, for closure of black spaces, within the best dental proportion. Posterior teeth still in provisional, with precarious anatomy. **J, M)** Smile before orthodontic treatment. **K, L, N, O)** Smile after perio-ortho-prosthetic integrated treatment, in several amplitudes and approaches.

Dental volume addition was described in the first part of this article, with space opening performed to restore dental width (Fig 3). Most of the times, the professional decides to reduce dental volume in one of the arches by means of interdental wear or atypical extractions.

Decisions on incisors extractions should be previously tested by physical or virtual set-up, because the calculations do not contemplate the buccolingual thickness of the incisal edges. Moreover, small differences may be disguised by differentiated torques and variations of overbite.[29] The orthodontist may cause a large Bolton discrepancy when extraction of a lower incisor is planned (usually recommended to treat lower anterior crowding) and not previously tested. In extreme cases, a new malocclusion would be created by the orthodontist, which would result in a contracted lower arch, canines without contact and accentuated overjet and overbite.

The attenuation of the Bolton discrepancy by means of wear also needs to be considered, because, in cases in which the dimensions of upper incisors are at the limit of the height/width dental proportion or present square-shaped crowns, the wear is quite limited, for it causes dangerous root proximity and quite extensive contact points in the cervico-incisal height.[29] The Bolton discrepancy is an important and decisive finding for orthodontic treatment and, beyond numbers, it presents clinical unfolding. Because it is a mathematical estimate, its clinical implications must be considered. Some logical rules can be used to guide the orthodontist's conduct, showing the problem and solving it as the treatment evolves.

Clinically, the best treatment option should privilege molar intercuspation as the first step of treatment. After the distobuccal cusp of the upper first molar is occluded between the lower first and the second molars, the spaces are closed backwards, and some situations may appear:

1) If the relation is canine Class II after premolars have been distalized and occluded: it shows upper posterior excess, and it can be solved with interproximal wear on the mesial surface of the first molar; mesial and distal of premolars; and on the distal surface of upper canines.

2) If the relation is canine Class III after premolars have been distalized and occluded: it shows lower posterior excess, and it can be solved with interpoximal wear

on the mesial surface of the first molar; mesial and distal of premolars; and on the distal of lower canines.

3) If overjet or anterior crossbite persists after premolars have been distalized and occluded, and after canine occlusion has been defined: it shows lower anterior excess, and it can be solved with interproximal wear on the mesial surface of the canines and on the mesial and distal surface of lower incisors.

4) If overjet persists after premolars have been distalized and occluded, and after canine occlusion has been defined: it shows upper anterior excess, and it can be solved with interproximal wear on the mesial surface of canines and on the mesial and distal surfaces of upper incisors — respecting the ideal symmetry and proportions. In this case, the lack of lower anterior dental volume must be verified and the need for incisor clinical crown augmentation must be considered.

Clinical conditions may present a blend of these possibilities of solution, and the excess may also be by quadrants, with asymmetry between the right and left sides. A careful analysis of the relation of the inclined planes of the teeth in the clinical evaluation, as well as in the analysis of models, can determine if there is significant Bolton discrepancy, without the necessity of applying any formulas, as shown in Figure 22.

CONCLUSIONS

Microesthetics comprises treatment approaches that are more directly related to Orthodontics and other dental specialties that deal with esthetics. Mastering it must be part of the foundations on which a dentist's fine practice is based. The challenge is to use all the parameters available, those emphasized by the different specialties of Dentistry, and apply these concepts in each treated case. It is not a single detail that defines excellence, but the sum of many of them. This article aimed at describing the ideal dental proportions and dimensions, and their interaction with the periodontium, which shall be considered by the orthodontist for treatment finishing. Many of these aspects are out of the spectrum of changes that the orthodontic appliance could provide and totally dependent on the intervention of periodontists and prosthetists. Therefore, it is necessary to gather concepts and define patterns that must be followed by the team of professionals in order to avoid wasting time with unnecessary or contradictory procedures.

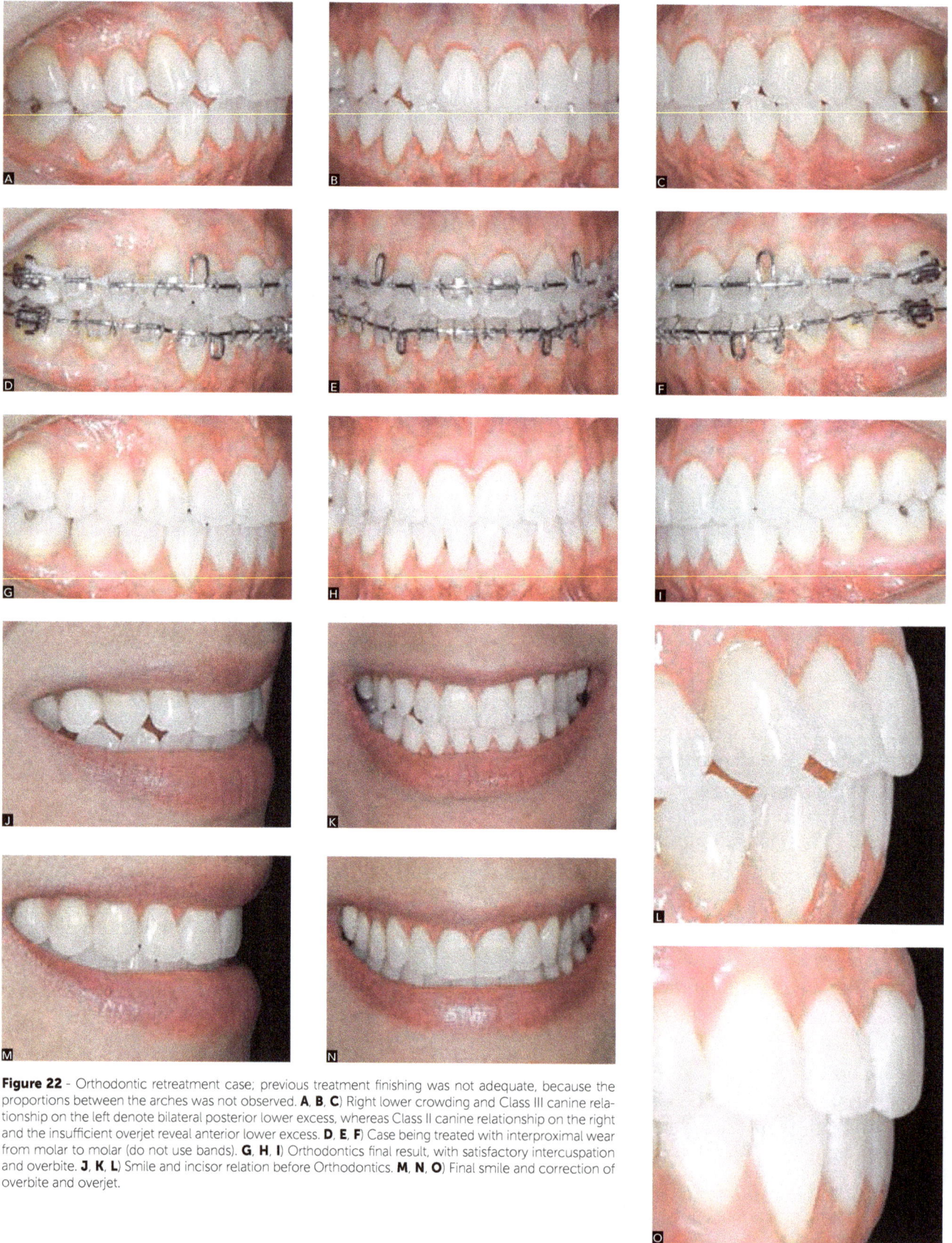

Figure 22 - Orthodontic retreatment case; previous treatment finishing was not adequate, because the proportions between the arches was not observed. **A, B, C)** Right lower crowding and Class III canine relationship on the left denote bilateral posterior lower excess, whereas Class II canine relationship on the right and the insufficient overjet reveal anterior lower excess. **D, E, F)** Case being treated with interproximal wear from molar to molar (do not use bands). **G, H, I)** Orthodontics final result, with satisfactory intercuspation and overbite. **J, K, L)** Smile and incisor relation before Orthodontics. **M, N, O)** Final smile and correction of overbite and overjet.

On the clinical tables of cases approved by the American Board of Orthodontics (ABO) and by the Brazilian Board of Orthodontics (BBO), which are presented in meetings, is the phrase: "All cases orthodontically treated have some defects, and the cases herein exposed represent the effort of the professionals to achieve the certification of excellence." This means that the complete excellence in all treated cases should always be sought, even if it is utopian. If all cases are prepared as if they were presented to the BBO exam, many of them would certainly not achieve the excellence degree for many reasons, but there would be an orthodontist who is much better in his clinical performance, ready to achieve the certification of excellence.

Microesthetics must not be seen in isolation, but as the key to achieve a pleasant smile (miniesthetics) and a harmonious face (macroesthetics). The greatest concern must always be the patient, with his desires not only granted, but overcome by the professional. Our concerns and actions are measured in millimeters, but can make all the difference to people's quality of life. To raise one's self-esteem by means of integrated dental treatment could be considered an objective, that may be referred to as "hyper-esthetics".

ACKNOWLEDGEMENTS

The authors would like to thank and honor Vincent G. Kokich who represented not only the search for excellence in Orthodontics, with his brilliant articles and lectures, but mainly the critical thinking and the search for the best scientific evidence that must guide the decisions that we need to make every day in our clinics. Special acknowledgements to Telma Martins de Araújo, Lícia Pacheco Teixeira and Gabriela Cassaro de Castro for the precious help on the elaboration of this work.

REFERENCES

1.　Adolfi D. Natural esthetics. Chicago: Quintessence; 2003.

2.　Adolfi D. Functional, esthetic, and morphologic adjustment procedures for anterior teeth. Quintessence Dent Technol. 2009;32:153-68.

3.　Al-Johany SS, Alqahtani AS, Alqahtani FY, Alzahrani AH. Evaluation of different esthetic smile criteria. Int J Prosthodont. 2011;24(1):64-70.

4.　Anderson KM, Behrents RG, McKinney T, Buschang PH. Tooth shape preferences in an esthetic smile. Am J Orthod Dentofacial Orthop. 2005;128(4):458-65.

5.　Behrents RG. Growth in aging craniofacial skeleton. Monograph 17 - Craniofacial Growth Series, Center for Human Growth and Development. Ann Arbor, Michigan: The University of Michigan; 1985.

6.　Bollen AM, Cunha-Cruz J, Bakko DW, Huang GJ, Hujoel PP. The effects of orthodontic therapy on periodontal health: a systematic review of controlled evidence. J Am Dent Assoc. 2008;139(4):413-22.

7.　Bolton WA. Disharmony in tooth size and its relation to the analysis and treatment of malocclusion. Angle Orthod. 1958;28(3):113-30.

8.　Brandão RCB, Brandão LBC. Ajuste oclusal na Ortodontia: por que, quando e como? Rev Dental Press Ortod Ortop Facial. 2008;13(3):124-56.

9.　Brandão RCB. Entrevista com Roberto Carlos Bodart Brandão. Rev Dental Press Ortod Ortop Facial. 2009;14(6):19-41.

10.　Câmara CALP. Estética em Ortodontia: diagramas de referências estéticas dentárias (DRED) e Faciais (DREF). Rev Dental Press Ortod Ortop Facial. 2006;11(6):130-56.

11.　Câmara CALP. Estética em Ortodontia: seis linhas horizontais do sorriso. Dental Press J Orthod. 2010;15(1):118-31.

12.　Chiche GJ, Pinault A. Estética em próteses fixas anteriores. 1a ed. São Paulo: Ed Santos; 1996.

13.　Chu SJ, Tan JH-P, Stappert, CFJ, Tarnow, DP. Gingival zenith positions and levels of the maxillary anterior dentition. J Esthet Restor Dent. 2009;21(2):113-20.

14.　Chu SJ. Range and mean distribution frequency of individual tooth width of the maxillary anterior dentition. Pract Proced Aesthet Dent. 2007;19(4):209-15.

15.　Chu SJ. A biometric approach to predictable treatment of clinical crown discrepancies. Pract Proced Aesthet Dent. 2007;19(7):401-9.

16.　Dürer A. The art of measurement. San Francisco: Alan Wofsy Fine Arts; 1981.

17.　Duthie J, Bharwani D, Tallents RH, Bellohusen R, Fishman L. A longitudinal study of normal asymmetric mandibular growth and its relationship to skeletal maturation. Am J Orthod Dentofacial Orthop. 2007;132(2):179-84.

18.　Fletcher P. Biologic rationale of esthetic crown lengthening using innovative proportion gauges. Int J Periodontics Restorative Dent. 2011;31:523-32.

19.　Fradeani M. Esthetic analysis: a systematic approach to prosthetic treatment. Chicago: Quintessence Books; 2004.

20.　Gillen RJ, Schwartz RS, Hilton TJ, Evans DB. An analysis of selected normative tooth proportions. Int J Prosthodont. 1994;7(5):410-7.

21.　Gkantidis N, Christou P, Topouzelis N. The orthodontic-periodontic interrelationship in integrated treatment challenges: a systematic review. J Oral Rehabil. 2010;37(5):377-90.

22.　Janson G, Branco NC, Fernandes TM, Sathler R, Garib D, Lauris JR. Influence of orthodontic treatment, midline position, buccal corridor and smile arc on smile attractiveness. Angle Orthod. 2011;81(1):153-61.

23.　Johe RS, Steinhart T, Sado N, Greenberg B, Jinge S. Intermaxillary tooth-size discrepancies indifferent sexes, malocclusion groups, and ethnicities. Am J Orthod Dentofacial Orthop. 2010;138(5):599-607.

24.　Karring T, Nyman S, Thilander B, Magnusson I. Bone regeneration in orthodontically produced alveolar bone dehiscences. J Periodontal Res. 1982;17(3):309-15.

25.　Kina S, Bruguera A. Invisível: restaurações estéticas cerâmicas. 1a ed. Maringá: Dental Press; 2007.

26.　Kina S, Romanini JC. Harmonia. Rev Dental Press Estét. 2007;4(2):67-88.

27.　King KL, Evans CA, Viana G, BeGole E, Obrez A. Preferences for vertical position of the maxillary lateral incisors. World J Orthod. 2008;9(2):147-54.

28.　Kokich VG, Nappen DL, Shapiro PA. Gingival contour and clinical crown length: their effect on the esthetic appearance of maxillary anterior teeth. Am J Orthod. 1984;86(2):89-94.

29.　Kokich VG, Shapiro PA. Lower incisor extraction in orthodontic treatment. Angle Orthod. 1984;54(2):139-53.

30.　Kokich VG, Spear FM. Guidelines for managing the orthodontic-restorative patient. Semin Orthod. 1997;3(1):3-20.

31. Kokich VG, Spear FM. Interdisciplinary management of anterior guidance: a case report. Adv Esthet Inter Dent. 2007;3(3):2-6.

32. Kokich VG. Esthetics and anterior tooth position: an orthodontic perspective. Part I: crown length. J Esthet Dent. 1993;5(1):19-23.

33. Kokich VG. Esthetics: the Orthodontic-Periodontic restorative conection. Semin Orthod. 1996;2(1):21-30.

34. Kokich VG. Excellence in finishing: modifications for the perio-restorative patient. Semin Orthod 2003;9(3):184-203.

35. Kokich VO Jr, Kiyak HA, Shapiro PA. Comparing the perception of dentists and lay people to altered dental esthetics. J Esthet Dent. 1999;11:311-24.

36. Lombardi RE. The principles of visual perception and their clinical application to denture esthetics. J Prosthet Dent. 1973;29(4):358-82.

37. Magne P, Belser U. Bonded porcelain restorations in the anterior dentition: a biomimetic approach. Chicago: Quintessence; 2001.

38. Masioli M. Fotografia odontológica. 2a ed. Porto Alegre: Artmed; 2010.

39. Mattos C, Santana RA. Quantitative evaluation of the spacial displacement of the gingival zenith in the maxillary anterior dentition. J Periodont. 2008;79(10):1880-5.

40. Mayekar SM. Shades of color: illusion or reality? Dent Clin North Am. 2001;45(1):155-72.

41. Morley J, Eubank J. Macro esthetic elements of smile design. J Am Dent Assoc. 2001;132(1):39-45.

42. Mucha JN. As limitações do tratamento ortodôntico não-cirúrgico. In: Medeiros PJ, Medeiros PP. Cirurgia ortognática para ortodontista. São Paulo: Ed. Santos; 2004. p. 29-56.

43. Müller HP, Eger T. Masticatory mucosa and periodontal phenotype: a review. Int J Periodontics Restorative Dent. 2002;22(2):172-83.

44. Naini FB, Moss JP, Gill DS. The enigma of facial beauty: esthetics, proportions, deformity, and controversy. Am J Orthod Dentofacial Orthop. 2006;130(3):277-82.

45. Orce-Romero A, Iglesias-Linares A, Cantillo-Galindo M, Yañez-Vico RM, Mendoza-Mendoza A, Solano-Reina E. Do the smiles of the world's most influential individuals have common parameters? J Oral Rehabil. 2013;40(3):159-70.

46. Rotundo R, Nieri M, Iachetti G, Mervelt J, Cairo F, Baccetti T, Franchi L, Prato GP. Orthodontic treatment of periodontal defects. A systematic review. Prog Orthod. 2010;11(1):41-4.

47. Sarver DM, Ackerman MB. Dynamic smile visualization and quantification: Part 2. Smile analysis and treatment strategies. Am J Orthod Dentofacial Orthop. 2003;124(2):116-27.

48. Sarver DM, Ackerman MB. Dynamic smile visualization and quantification and its impact on orthodontic diagnosis and treatment planning. In:

The art of smile: integrating Prosthodontics, Orthodontics, Periodontics, Dental Technology and Plastic Surgery. Chicago: Quintessence; 2005. p. 99-139.

49. Sarver DM. The importance of incisor positioning in the esthetic smile: the smile arc. Am J Orthod Dentofacial Orthop. 2001;120(2):98-111.

50. Sarver DM. Principles of cosmetic dentistry in orthodontics: Part 1. Shape and proportionality of anterior teeth. Am J Orthod Dentofacial Orthop. 2004;126(6):749-53.

51. Sarver DM. Soft-tissue-based diagnosis and treatment planning. Clin Impress. 2005;14(1):21-6.

52. Sarver DM. Enameloplasty and esthetic finishing in orthodontics: identification and treatment of microesthetic features in Orthodontics. Part 1. J Esthet Restor Dent. 2011;23(5):296-302.

53. Sarver DM. Enameloplasty and esthetic finishing in orthodontics: differential diagnosis of incisor proclination - the importance of appropriate visualization and records Part 2. J Esthet Restor Dent. 2011;23(5):303-13.

54. Schillinburg HT, Kaplan MJ, Grace CS. Tooth dimensions. A comparative study. J South Calif Dent Assoc. 1972;40(9):830-9.

55. Schillinburg HT. Fundamentals of fixed prosthodontics. 3a ed. Chicago: Quintessence; 1997.

56. Shellhart WC, Lange DW, Kluemper GT, Hicks, EP, Kaplan AL. Reliability of the Bolton tooth-size analysis when applied to crowded dentitions. Angle Orthod. 1995;65(5):327-34.

57. Spear FM, Kokich, VG. A multidisciplinary approach to esthetic dentistry. Dent Clin North Am. 2007;51(2):487-505.

58. Sterrett JD, Oliver T, Robinson F, Fortson W, Knaak B, Russell CM. Width/length ratios of normal clinical crowns of the maxillary anterior dentition in man. J Clin Periodontol. 1999;26(3):153-57.

59. Tarnow DP, Magner AW, Fletcher P. The effect of distance from the contact point to the crest bone of the presence or absence of the interproximal dental papilla. J Periodontol. 1992;68:995-6.

60. Thilander B. Orthodontic space closure versus implant placement in subjects with missing teeth. J Oral Rehabil. 2008;35 Suppl 1:64-71.

61. Zachrisson BU. Orthodontics and periodontics. In: Lindhe J, Karring T, Lang NP. Clinical Periodontology and Implant Dentistry. 3rd ed. Copenhagen: Blackwell Munksgaard; 1997. p. 741-93.

62. Zachrisson BU. Esthetic factors involved in anterior tooth display and the smile: vertical dimension. J Clin Orthod. 1998;32(7):432-45.

63. Zanetti GR, Brandão RCB, Zanetti LSS, Castro GC, Borges Filho FF. Integração orto-perio-prótese para correção de assimetria gengival: relato de caso. Rev Dental Press Estét. 2008;5(4):104-15.

23

Deformation of elastomeric chains related to the amount and time of stretching

Denise Yagura[1], Paulo Eduardo Baggio[2], Luiz Sérgio Carreiro[3], Ricardo Takahashi[3]

Objective: To investigate a potential relationship between degree of stretching and resulting permanent deformation of elastomeric chains (ECs) as well as whether or not stretching time has any bearing on the degree of permanent deformation. **Methods:** Five-module segments of closed elastomeric chains manufactured by 3M Unitek were stretched to 10-100% of their original length in devices especially designed for this purpose, remaining submerged in artificial saliva at 37 ± 1° C and were removed sequentially after 1, 2, 3 and 4 weeks. Upon removal, each segment was measured and, once recorded the values, were statistically analyzed with the purpose of assessing the degree of permanent deformation. **Conclusions:** It was concluded that permanent deformation is directly proportional to the degree of stretching of the ECs assessed. The mean percentages found were 8.4% to 10% of stretching, and exceeding 20% (21.3%) when stretched by 40%, and reaching 56.6% permanent deformation when stretched 100% of their original length. Finally, the highest percentage of permanent deformation occurred during the first week and was not statistically significant after this period.

Keywords: Elastomers. Tensile strength. Permanent deformation.

» The authors report no commercial, proprietary or financial interest in the products or companies described in this article.

[1] Graduated in Dentistry, School of Dentistry of Barretos. Specialist in Orthodontics. Londrina State University (UEL).
[2] Associate Professor, Graduate Program Director in Orthodontics, UEL.
[3] Associate Professor, UEL.

Denise Yagura
Rua Visconde de Nassau, 650 – Apto 802 – Zona 07
CEP: 87.020-0230 – Maringá/PR – Brazil
E-mail: denise_yagura@hotmail.com

INTRODUCTION AND LITERATURE REVIEW

Among the various force-producing mechanisms used in orthodontics to move teeth as physiologically as possible through the alveolar bone, elastomeric chains (ECs) are undoubtedly the most widely employed in daily practice.[14,15]

EC insertion and removal requires little chair time and is not dependent on patient compliance. Furthermore, ECs are inexpensive and compatible with soft tissues.[8] When stretched, ECs generate elastic potential energy that can be transformed into mechanical energy, which in turn produces tooth movement. Given that they are made from amorphous polyurethane-based polymers, ECs exhibit characteristics of both rubber and plastic, which accounts for their elasticity.[5] The polymers are composed of primary and secondary links with weak molecular attraction that initially display a spiral pattern. When this pattern is subjected to the application of forces it undergoes deformation, causing ECs to be arranged linearly through crosslinking. The weak secondary links allow the spiral pattern to be transformed into a linear pattern while recovery of the initial structure becomes possible by means of crosslinking.[16] Permanent deformation occurs when the polymer is stretched beyond its elastic limit, causing disruption of crosslinks. However, certain factors influence EC performance, such as rapid force decay after stretching, i.e., inability to develop constant forces for an extended period of time, thereby impairing their effectiveness.[1,3,7,13,14,16] Additionally, ECs are influenced by temperature variations, salivary pH and the degree of stretching to which they are subjected.[14] In the oral environment, ECs absorb water, saliva and pigments, eventually undergoing chemical degradation, which results in the weakening of intermolecular forces, thereby decomposing their internal links. This leads to the onset of force decay processes, lack of dimensional stability and permanent deformation, making it difficult to determine the actual force magnitude being delivered to a given tooth.[3] Therefore, this *in vitro* study aimed to investigate the potential relationship between degree of stretching and resulting permanent deformation of elastomeric chains (ECs), as well as determine whether or not stretching time has any bearing on the degree of permanent deformation of ECs.

MATERIAL AND METHODS

For this research, closed gray ECs (CK Chain Spool - 3M Unitek), were carefully sectioned into segments of five modules each, with an initial length of 10 mm, ignoring the two ends of the segments, whose function was only to facilitate EC stretching. Four acrylic plates were fabricated and perforated for the insertion of 20 stainless steel pins with 0.2 cm diameter and 1.5 cm length arranged in parallel in 10 pairs with increasing distance between them in 1.0 mm increments, starting from 1.1 cm and ending with 2.0 cm. Ten EC segments were fitted to each pair of pins with the aid of a Mathieu needle holder, and were thus stretched to 10-100% of their original length. To prevent the pins from approaching each other due to the tension produced in stretching the ECs, a pin of equal length was fitted between all pairs of pins as shown in Figure 1. The plates were immersed in a stainless steel case containing artificial saliva with the following composition: Calcium 1.5 mmol L-1, Phosphate 0.9 mmol L-1, KCL 150 mmol L-1 in cacodylate buffer, 0.1 mol L-1 pH 7.0, Fluorine 0.05 mg/mL (1.1 mL solution/mm²). This case was kept closed and in water bath at 37 ± 1° C in a soaking tub (Fig 2). These plates were first identified with a black OHP marker pen, according to the duration of the experiment. It is noteworthy that the water level was kept below the stainless steel lid, thus preventing contamination of the artificial saliva. Subsequently, the plates were removed sequentially after 1, 2, 3 and 4 weeks. Once retrieved from the saliva and blotted dry, each elastomeric segment was fitted to a measuring device especially made for this purpose consisting of a pin fixed to a wooden base, covered with graph paper (Fig 2). One end of the EC was seated in the pin and its final length recorded on graph paper. Thereafter, the length of each EC was measured and recorded with a caliper. Each week, the artificial saliva was replaced. It was first pre-heated in a container up to a temperature of 37 ± 1 °C, thereby averting changes in temperature.

Data were statistically analyzed by analysis of covariance (ANCOVA) with the purpose of checking whether there was a statistically significant difference between time and degree of stretching. Level of significance was set at 5% (p = 0.0556), to identify possible differences between groups.

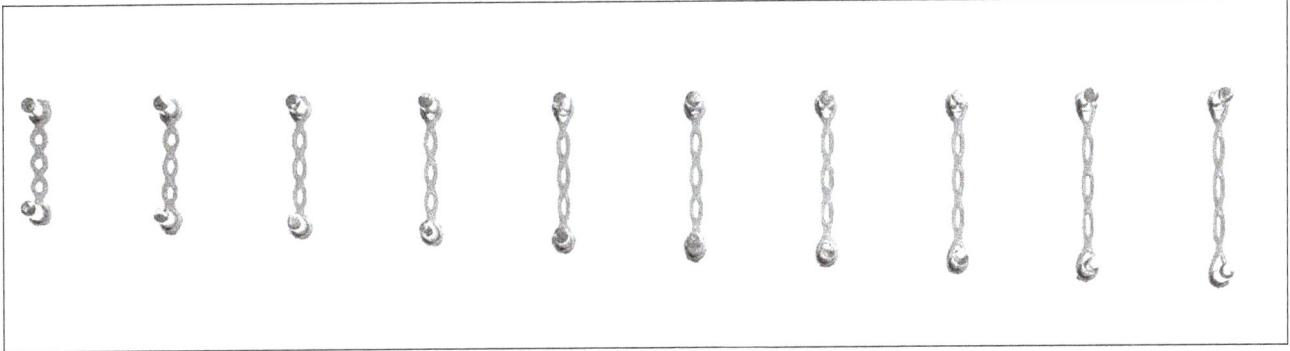

Figure 1 - Acrylic plate with stretched elastomeric chains.

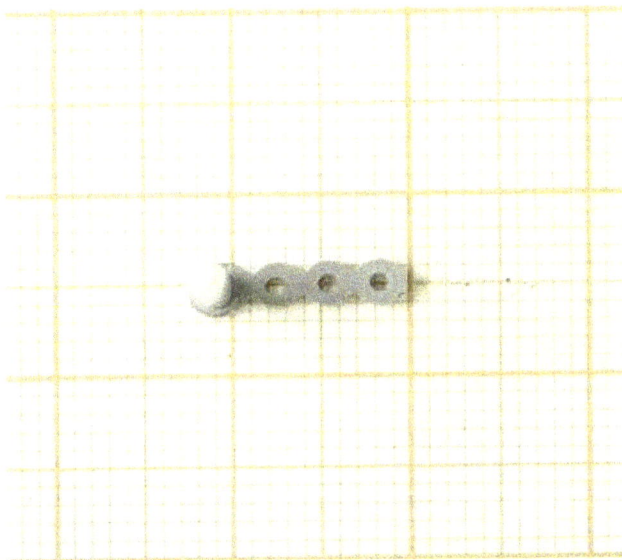

Figure 2 - Soaking tub used in the experiment.

RESULTS

Overall, it was found that permanent deformation of ECs was proportional to increases in stretching (Table 5). However, it was found that the mean deformation observed in the second, third and fourth weeks differed significantly from the mean stretching observed in the first week. No statistically significant differences were found in comparing the second to the third, the second to the fourth as well as the third to the fourth weeks (Table 7).

The results found in each week, according to time and degree of stretching, are presented in Tables 1, 2, 3 and 4; mean and standard deviation values reflecting the behavior of the variable *deformation* according to week and degree of stretching are shown in Table 5.

In order to assess to what extent the mean deformation was similar in all weeks, the test of equality of inclination coefficient was applied with a 5% level of significance (p = 0.0556). This was necessary because the hypothesis which assumed that the mean deformation in at least one week was influenced by the percentage separation between the pins was rejected. The magnitude of these differences can be seen in Table 6, in the inclination coefficient column. Table 6 also shows the mean stretching throughout the levels of separation for each week. The term *intercept* refers to the estimated mean deformation in millimeters in each week, irrespective of distance. The expression *inclination coefficient* refers to the mean change in one distance unit (10%). In the first week, regardless of distance, a mean deformation of 0.0479 mm per 10% stretching was found, i.e., in order to reach a mean deformation of 10% to 50% stretching, or 20% to 60%, one can simply multiply 0.0479 mm by 5, and a deformation of 0.23 mm is obtained. In the second week, the deformation was 0.0564 mm, in the third was 0.0530, and in the fourth, 0.0544 mm.

Based on the analysis of covariance (ANCOVA), it was found initially that, for all weeks, the mean deformation depends linearly (Fig 3) on the percentage of pin stretching (p < 0.001), i.e., in at least one of the weeks the mean deformation was influenced by the percentage of pin stretching (independent variable).

Since the hypothesis of lack of parallelism is not rejected yet, the mean elongations were compared between weeks (distances between the adjusted straight lines). These results can be seen in Figure 4.

Table 1 - Results, in mm, obtained after stretching for one week.

1st week					STRETCHING (mm) Initial length = 10 mm					
Trial	10%	20%	30%	40%	50%	60%	70%	80%	90%	100%
1	10.7	11.2	11.5	11.9	12.5	13.0	13.2	13.8	14.5	15.0
2	10.7	11.1	11.3	12.0	12.1	13.0	13.3	13.7	14.6	15.1
3	10.8	11.0	11.5	12.0	12.5	13.0	13.2	13.9	14.5	15.0
4	10.7	11.1	11.5	12.0	12.3	13.0	13.2	13.9	14.6	15.0
5	10.7	11.1	11.5	12.0	12.4	13.0	13.2	13.8	14.6	15.0
6	10.7	11.0	11.5	12.0	12.5	13.0	13.3	13.7	14.6	15.1
7	10.7	11.1	11.5	12.0	12.5	13.0	13.3	13.7	14.5	15.1
8	10.7	11.2	11.5	12.0	12.5	13.0	13.2	13.8	14.5	15.0
9	10.7	11.1	11.4	12.0	12.5	13.0	13.2	13.8	14.6	15.0
10	10.7	11.1	11.5	12.0	12.5	13.0	13.2	13.9	14.5	15.1

Table 2 - Results, in mm, after stretching for two weeks.

2nd week					STRETCHING (mm) Initial length = 10 mm					
Trial	10%	20%	30%	40%	50%	60%	70%	80%	90%	100%
1	10.9	11.0	11.9	12.0	12.9	13.0	13.7	14.4	15.4	16.4
2	10.8	11.0	11.9	12.0	12.8	13.0	13.9	14.4	15.0	15.9
3	10.9	11.3	11.6	12.5	12.8	13.0	13.9	14.4	15.0	15.9
4	10.8	11.0	11.6	12.0	12.8	13.0	13.9	14.4	15.2	15.9
5	10.9	11.1	11.7	12.0	12.8	13.0	13.9	14.4	15.2	15.9
6	10.9	11.2	11.9	12.0	12.9	13.0	13.8	14.4	15.4	16.1
7	10.8	11.3	11.9	12.0	12.9	13.0	13.9	14.4	15.0	16.3
8	10.9	11.1	11.9	12.0	12.8	13.0	13.8	14.4	15.0	15.9
9	10.8	11.0	11.9	12.0	12.8	13.0	13.8	14.4	15.0	16.0
10	10.9	11.0	11.9	12.0	12.8	13.0	13.9	14.4	15.0	15.9

Table 3 - Results, in mm, after stretching for three weeks.

3rd week					STRETCHING (mm) Initial length = 10 mm					
Trial	10%	20%	30%	40%	50%	60%	70%	80%	90%	100%
1	10.9	11.1	11.9	12.0	12.8	13.0	13.9	14.1	15.0	15.7
2	10.9	11.1	11.9	12.0	12.5	12.9	13.9	14.1	15.0	15.7
3	10.9	11.1	11.9	12.0	12.8	13.0	13.8	14.1	15.0	15.7
4	10.9	11.1	11.9	12.0	12.6	13.0	13.9	14.1	15.0	15.7
5	10.9	11.1	11.9	12.0	12.8	13.0	13.8	14.1	15.0	15.7
6	10.9	11.1	11.9	12.0	12.7	12.9	13.9	14.1	15.0	15.7
7	10.9	11.1	11.9	12.0	12.8	13.0	13.9	14.1	15.0	15.7
8	10.9	11.1	11.9	12.0	12.8	13.0	13.8	14.1	15.0	15.7
9	10.9	11.1	11.9	12.0	12.5	13.0	13.9	14.1	15.0	15.7
10	10.9	11.1	11.9	12.0	12.8	13.0	13.9	14.1	15.0	15.7

Table 4 - Results, in mm, after stretching for four weeks.

4th week					STRETCHING (mm) Initial length = 10 mm					
Trial	10%	20%	30%	40%	50%	60%	70%	80%	90%	100%
1	10.9	11.5	12.0	12.1	12.9	13.3	14.0	14.5	15.1	15.8
2	10.9	11.4	12.0	12.2	12.9	13.3	14.0	14.8	15.0	16.0
3	10.9	11.4	11.9	12.2	12.9	13.0	14.0	14.7	15.5	15.9
4	10.9	11.4	11.9	12.2	12.9	13.1	14.0	14.7	15.3	15.9
5	10.9	11.4	12.0	12.2	12.9	13.2	14.0	14.8	15.0	15.9
6	10.9	11.5	12.0	12.2	12.9	13.2	14.0	14.6	15.5	16.0
7	10.9	11.4	12.0	12.9	12.9	13.0	14.0	14.5	15.1	15.9
8	10.9	11.4	12.0	12.9	12.9	13.3	14.0	14.7	15.3	15.8
9	10.9	11.4	12.0	12.9	12.9	13.3	14.0	14.8	15.0	15.9
10	10.9	11.5	12.0	12.9	12.9	13.0	14.0	14.8	15.2	15.9

Table 5 - Mean and standard deviation values, in mm, for each degree of stretching vs. week combination.

Stretching	1st week Mean ± SD	2nd week Mean ± SD	3rd week Mean ± SD	4th week Mean ± SD	Mean ± SD
10%	10.71 ± 0.03	10.86 ± 0.05	10.90 ± 0.00	10.90 ± 0.00	10.84 ± 0.08
20%	11.10 ± 0.07	11.10 ± 0.12	11.10 ± 0.00	11.43 ± 0.05	11.18 ± 0.16
30%	11.47 ± 0.07	11.82 ± 0.13	11.90 ± 0.00	11.98 ± 0.04	11.79 ± 0.21
40%	11.99 ± 0.03	12.05 ± 0.16	12.00 ± 0.00	12.47 ± 0.37	12.13 ± 0.28
50%	12.43 ± 0.13	12.83 ± 0.05	12.71 ± 0.13	12.90 ± 0.00	12.72 ± 0.20
60%	13.00 ± 0.00	13.00 ± 0.00	12.98 ± 0.04	13.17 ± 0.13	13.04 ± 0.10
70%	13.23 ± 0.05	13.85 ± 0.07	13.87 ± 0.05	14.00 ± 0.00	13.74 ± 0.31
80%	13.80 ± 0.08	14.40 ± 0.00	14.10 ± 0.00	14.69 ± 0.12	14.25 ± 0.34
90%	14.55 ± 0.05	15.12 ± 0.17	15.00 ± 0.00	15.20 ± 0.19	14.97 ± 0.28
100%	15.04 ± 0.05	16.02 ± 0.19	15.70 ± 0.00	15.90 ± 0.07	15.66 ± 0.40
Mean	12.732	13.105	13.026	13.264	13.03
SD	1.39	1.65	1.54	1.58	1.55

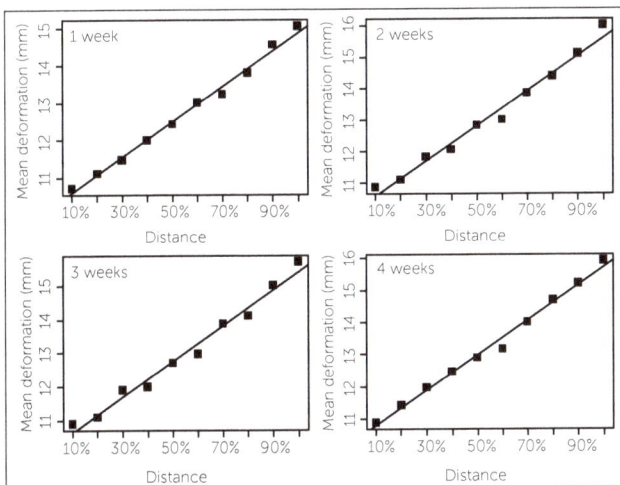

Figure 3 - Dispersion of mean deformation vs. distance. The straight line shows adjustment by least squares.

Table 6 - Estimates of parameters for adjusted models.

Week	Intercept	Inclination coefficient	R²
1st Week	12.732 (0.004)*	0.0479 (0.0014) *	0.9919
2nd Week	13.105 (0.076) *	0.0564 (0.0027) *	0.9805
3rd Week	13.026 (0.073) *	0.0530 (0.0025) *	0.9796
4th Week	13.264 (0.051) *	0.0544 (0.0018) *	0.9905

R^2 = Adjusted determination coefficient; * standard deviation.

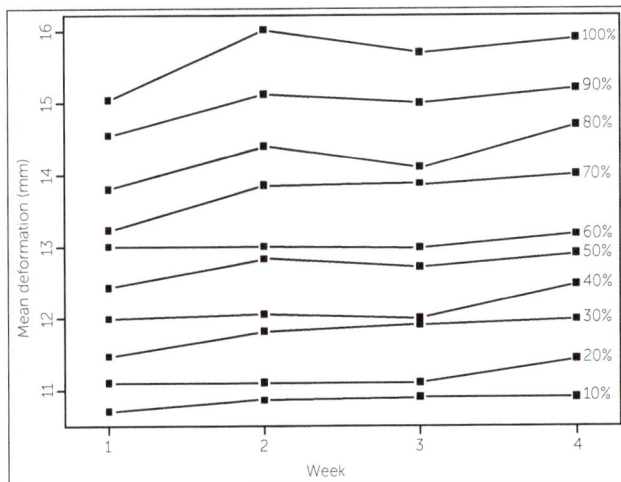

Figure 4 - Mean deformation, over the weeks, for each of the distances.

Table 7 - Comparison between mean deformations.

	1st week	2nd week	3rd week	4th week
1st Week		0.0004*	0.0037*	< 0.0001*
2nd Week	0.0004*		0.4086	0.1012
3rd Week	0.0037*	0.4086		0.0165*
4th Week	< 0.0001*	0.1012	0.0165*	

* = Statistically significant difference.

In comparing the mean deformations, statistically significant differences were detected only in the first week, compared to the others. Table 7 demonstrates a comparison between mean deformations in all weeks.

In this study it was found that the percentage of force decay rises as immersion time increases. However, a reversal – though not statistically significant – was observed between the means of the second and third weeks (Table 5 and Fig 4).

DISCUSSION

To be effective in their function, ECs should produce an appropriate magnitude of force for a certain period of time.[10] However, it is known that ECs cannot generate constant forces for a long period of time since their elastic properties are altered over time, causing permanent deformation and, consequently, loss of tension. The inability of elastic materials to return to their original size after undergoing substantial deformation and releasing the tensile forces applied to them, is defined as plastic, or permanent, deformation.[4] The effects of this plastic deformation are manifested by the decrease of these materials' ability to deliver forces.[15]

In the present study, EC behavior was evaluated weekly over a period of 4 weeks — the interval between patient visits,[4,8,9,12,17] as this time period coincides with the average period when orthodontists usually replace the patient's elastics.[2] The time factor is of paramount importance for ECs, since it is known that one of their main properties, i.e., the dissipation of forces with constant magnitude during their clinical application, is directly influenced by the time period during which they are employed, given a loss of tension and consequent force decay.[18] In the present study, a statistically significant difference was noted between the mean deformation of the first week and the others (Table 7), which suggests - without considering the biology of tooth movement – that it is convenient to change ECs weekly, since comparisons between the second and third weeks, between the third and fourth weeks, and between the second and fourth weeks, showed no significant differences. However, it is recommended that ECs be replaced every 3 weeks.[6,13] Furthermore, ECs should not be used for longer than 4 weeks, not only due to force decay but also due to difficulties in oral cleaning, with the resulting accumulation of food debris.[13]

Additionally, EC use should not exceed a period of 6 weeks as ECs eventually lose, on average, 30% of their initial force. Besides, there is an increase in the accumulation of plaque and chemical interaction with food and oral fluids.[11]

Regarding immersion time in artificial saliva, the rate of force decay increases with time,[1,9,24] as concluded in this study. Although not significant statistically, a reversal was also observed between the means of the second and third weeks (Table 5 and Fig 5).

As regards the degree of elongation undergone by ECs, force decay is proportional to the degree of stretching to which the ECs are subjected,[1] in agreement with the findings of this study (Table 5 and Fig 4). For example, it became evident that, as shown in Table 1, 10% stretching yielded a mean deformation of approximately 8.4%, whereas 100% stretching caused the deformation to increase to 56.6%. Thus, from a clinical standpoint, an issue could be raised: How much stretching is recommended to (a) achieve a low rate of permanent deformation, and (b) apply forces that are as constant as possible? Based on the results of this study, it would be reasonable to suggest 30% stretching, which would provide a mean deformation of about 17.9%. However, it should be emphasized that this argument is only applicable to 3M Unitek ECs which were analyzed here, since ECs can vary in thickness, elastic property, manufacturing process, adding pigments or fluorine and distance between modules. These factors, acting alone or in conjunction, will certainly influence both the forces delivered and the degree of permanent deformation undergone by these materials. Therefore, professionals who use ECs should be aware of the various issues and types of materials addressed in this study, and act accordingly.

The use of a tension gauge is advised to measure the initial force since certain closed chains — when stretched to 100% of their original length — can produce excessive forces, approaching 450 grams. It is therefore recommended to stretch these ECs between 50% and 75% of their original length. However, there are ECs which, when stretched to 100% of their original length, produce acceptable magnitudes of force (approximately 300 grams).[3] Based on this, professionals are advised to stock in their offices

ECs with at least three different distances between modules, provided they have the same thickness and are manufactured by the same company. This would allow the application of the desired force magnitude, taking into consideration the degree of stretching recommended by this study (30%).

Furthermore, a permanent deformation of 50% to 60% was observed when the ECs were stretched to 100% of their original length. These percentages resemble those found for American Orthodontics (54%) ECs.[15] However, the percentages found for 3M Unitek (76%) ECs[15] differ from those found in this study.

While a simulation was made of the oral environment, it should be stressed that in an *in vivo* study, a wide range of factors such as the patient's diet, the composition of their saliva, presence of bacterial enzymes, masticatory forces, tooth movement, distance of force application, presence of fluoride and temperature changes could affect the mechanical performance of ECs, thereby altering the results obtained in this study.

CONCLUSION

Based on the results it can be conclude that:

1) A direct relationship was found between degree of stretching and permanent deformation of the ECs evaluated.

2) The mean stretching percentages found were 8.4% to 10%, exceeding 20% (21.3%) when stretched by 40%, and reaching 56.6% permanent deformation when stretched to 100% of their original length.

3) The highest percentage of permanent deformation occurred during the first week, and was not statistically significant after this period.

REFERENCES

1. Andreasen GF, Bishara SE. Comparison of alastik chains with elastics involved intra-arch molar to molar forces. Angle Orthod. 1970;40(3):151-8.

2. Araújo FBC, Ursi WJS. Estudo da degradação da força gerada por elásticos ortodônticos sintéticos. Rev Dental Press Ortod Ortop Facial. 2006;11(6):52-61.

3. Baty DL, Storie DJ, Fraunhofer JA. Synthetic elastomeric chains: a literature review. Am J Orthod Dentofacial Orthop. 1994;105(6):536-42.

4. Bishara SE, Andreasen GF. Comparison of time related forces between plastic alastiks and latex elastics. Angle Orthod. 1970;40(4):319-28.

5. Cardoso MA, Mendes AM. Avaliação das forças liberadas por elásticos ortodônticos em cadeia esterilizados com soluções de glutaraldeído. Rev Ortod Gaúch. 2001;5(2):100-11.

6. Eliades T, Eliades G, Watts DC. Structural conformation of in vitro and in vivo aged orthodontic elastomeric modules. Eur J Orthod. 1999;21(6):649-58.

7. Ferreira JJ, Caetano MTO. A degradação de força de segmentos de elásticos em cadeia de diferentes tamanhos: estudo comparativo in vitro. J Bras Orthodon Ortop Facial. 2004;9(51):225-33.

8. Ferriter JP, Meyer CE, Lorton L. The effect of hydrogen ion concentration on the force-degradation rate of orthodontic polyurethane chains elastics. Am J Orthod Dentofacial Orthop. 1990;98(5):404-10.

9. Fraunhofer JA, Coffelt MTP, Orbell GM. The effects of artificial saliva and topical fluoride treatments on the degradation of the elastic properties of orthodontic chains. Angle Orthod. 1992;62(4):265-74.

10. De Genova DC, McInnes-Ledoux P, Weinberg R, Shaye R. Force degradation of orthodontic elastomeric chains — A product comparison study. Am J Orthod. 1985;87(5):377-84.

11. Howard RS, Nikolai RJ. On the relaxation of orthodontic elastic threads. Angle Orthod. 1979;49(3):167-72.

12. Kuster R, Ingervall B, Burgin W. Laboratory and intra-oral tests of the degradation of elastic chains. Eur J Orthod. 1986;8(3):202-8.

13. Lu TC, Wang WN, Tarng TH, Chen JW. Force decay of elastomeric chain — A serial study Part II. Am J Orthod Dentofacial Orthop. 1993;104(4):373-7.

14. Matta ENR, Chevitarese O. Avaliação laboratorial da força liberada por elásticos plásticos. Rev Soc Bras Ortod. 1997;3(4):131-6.

15. Matta ENR, Chevitarese O. Deformação plástica de elásticos ortodônticos em cadeia: estudo in vitro. Rev Soc Bras Ortod. 1998;3(5):188-92.

16. Martins MM, Mendes IM, Côrte Real MLNP; Goldner MTA. Elásticos ortodônticos em cadeia: revisão da literatura e aplicações clínicas. Rev Clin Ortod Dental Press. 2006;5(5):71-8.

17. Mundstock KS, Beltrame KP, Mundstock CA. Avaliação da força dos alastiques em cadeia num período de 0 a 28 dias. Rev Assoc Paul Espec Ortod Ortop Facial. 2003;1(3):29-33.

18. Rock WP, Wilson HJ. Force reduction of orthodontic elastomeric chains after one month in the mouth. Br J Othod. 1986;13(3):147-50.

24

Short-term efficacy of mandibular advancement splint in treatment of obstructive sleep apnea-hypopnea syndrome

Calliandra Moura Pereira de Lima[1], Laurindo Zanco Furquim[2], Adilson Luiz Ramos[3]

Objective: The aim of the present study was to determine the short-term efficacy of treatment for snoring and obstructive sleep apnea-hypopnea syndrome (OSAHS) using a mandibular advancement splint. **Methods:** The sample comprised 20 patients (13 men and 7 women; mean age = 48 years; mean body mass index = 27.07) with OSAHS. Polysomnograms were performed before and 60 days after mandibular advancement splint therapy. **Results:** There was a significant reduction in the apnea-hypopnea index (AHI) following treatment (mean pretreatment AHI = 20.89 ± 17.9 *versus* mean posttreatment AHI = 4.43 ± 3.09) ($p < 0.05$). The snoring reduced and the sleep efficiency improved, as registered by polysomnograms ($p < 0.05$). **Conclusions:** The sleep quality improved in patients using mandibular advancement splint. Further studies evaluating long-term effects are needed.

Keywords: Sleep apnea syndrome. Snoring. Polysomnography.

» The authors report no commercial, proprietary or financial interest in the products or companies described in this article.

[1] Specialist in Orthodontics, State University of Maringá (UEM/Brazil).
 MSc student in Health, Federal University of Santa Maria (UFSM/Brazil).
[2] PhD in Oral Patology, Bauru Dental School. Head Professor of Orthodontics, UEM/Brazil.
[3] PhD in Orthodontics, São Paulo State University (UNESP/Brazil).
 Head Professor of Orthodontics, UEM/Brazil.

Calliandra Moura Pereira de Lima
Rua 7 de Setembro, 2500 – Centro – Campo Grande/MS - Brazil
CEP: 79.020-310 – E-mail: calli.pereira@bol.com.br

INTRODUCTION

Snoring and sleep apnea stand out among the 84-catalogued diseases related to sleep disorders, affecting 10% of the population worldwide. More than 15 million Brazilians snore. With regard to sex, the proportion of men to women is 10:1, as men are more prone to the buildup of fat in neck and abdominal region[16].

Sleep is essential to the homeostasis and restoration of the organism, including the central nervous system. Sleep is a dynamic physiological process involving the loss of consciousness and inactivation of the voluntary musculature, and is reversible through the effect of stimuli (tactile, auditory, somatosensory).[9]

Obstructive sleep apnea is a chronic, progressive respiration disorder involving the periodic interruption of breathing during sleep.[28] This condition is characterized by the apposition of the tongue and soft palate on the lateral and posterior walls of the oropharynx, causing the collapse of these structures. The reduction in or complete absence of airflow varies with the severity of the obstruction, normally occurring from 5 to 10 seconds as well as 5 to 10 times during sleep. Once the individual becomes hypoxemic, he/she awakens and the airways become unblocked. The individual then falls asleep again and the event is repeated. The repetitive effort to maintain air passing through the airways causes a 30% increase in volume and flaccidity of these structures.[27]

Snoring is defined as an inspiratory noise caused by friction of the soft tissues of the oropharynx due to partial obstruction of the upper airways. It is estimated that 35% of habitual snorers can develop obstructive sleep apnea-hypopnea syndrome (OSAHS).[10] The main etiological factors of OSAHS are muscle hypotonicity (due to alcohol, drugs, muscle relaxants, sedentary lifestyle, ageing and mouth breathing), obesity (increase in adipose tissue in the upper torso and cervical region), increased volume of respiratory secretion, hypertension, hypertrophy of the tonsils and uvula, dorsal decubitus position during sleep, retrognathia and macroglossia.[7,9,10,11,27]

OSAHS is considered a public health problem due to the related cardiovascular problems and the risk of work-related and traffic accidents stemming from daytime sleepiness and consequent mistakes when making decisions. OSAHS is also related to a poor quality of life, with the deterioration of neurocognitive aspects and subsequent negative repercussions on family/social relations and intellectual/professional production.[9]

Depending on the severity of the condition, treatment can range from behavior modification to surgical procedures.[7,23] Behavior modification includes sleep posture, weight loss, the suspension of alcohol and sedatives, and sleep hygiene.[7,9,22] Patients who sleep in a dorsal decubitus position snore more loudly and experience a worsening in apnea events. This is due to the posterior movement of the dorsum of the tongue, soft palate and palatine uvula, thereby causing obstruction. It is therefore recommended that patients sleep in the lateral decubitus position.[9,16,22] Sleep hygiene consists of healthy attitudes and practices aimed at promoting continuous, efficient sleep, leading to a reduction in daytime sleepiness. Such practices include regular times for going to sleep and waking up, regular physical exercise (but not close to bedtime), light eating with a minimal interval of two hours prior to sleep, avoiding substances with caffeine and/or nicotine at least four hours prior to sleep, limiting the use of alcohol to the minimum and adapting the environment to favor restful sleep by avoiding incompatible activities, such as watching television, snacking and using the telephone.[9,27]

Intraoral mandibular advancement appliances to treat primary snoring problems and mild OSAHS are derived from functional orthopedic appliances, which are used in the treatment of retrognathia in patients in growth phase.[7-11,23,24,25] These appliances have been employed as a treatment alternative for patients with moderate to severe sleep apnea who are intolerant to the use of continuous positive airway pressure (CPAP).[1,2,7-13,21,23,24,25]

This study focused in short-term efficacy and acceptance of a mandibular advancement splint (intraoral appliance) as an aid in the treatment of snoring and obstructive sleep apnea-hypopnea syndrome.

METHODS

The present study received approval from the Ethics Committee of the State University of Maringá (UEM/Brazil) and all subjects signed terms of informed consent agreeing to participate in the study. The sample was selected from 30 patients who sought treatment of snoring and sleep apnea between June 2006 and June 2007 at Dental Press Educational Center (Maringá/PR, Brazil). Seven were excluded due to excessive tooth loss leading to difficulty in adapting the splint, active periodontal disease, craniofacial disorders, upper airways obstruction or systemic disease. Three patients abandoned treatment one day after the installation of the appliance, reporting considerable discomfort. Thus, the sample consisted of 20 patients between 32 and 60 years of age (mean = 48 years), 13 of whom were male (65%) and 7 were female (35%). Either the participants themselves or their spouses (which was more frequently the case) reported snoring or interrupted breathing during sleep.

All patients underwent polysomnography prior and 60 days after installation of the mandibular advancement splint (nighttime use). All exams were obtained from Neuromap 40i equipment (Neurotec, Itajubá-MG, Brazil) over an average of seven hours. Polysomnograms recorded AHI, snoring events, sleep efficiency, minimal oxygen saturation and heart arrhythmia.

Body mass index (BMI) was also recorded before and after polysomnograms.

The mandibular advancement splint used included an advancement tube-pin system (modified removable MPA, Coelho Filho, 1995).[6,23] The tube-pin connects the upper and lower plates to promote the forward movement of the mandible. Intermaxillary elastic bands (1/8-in) were placed on the hooks of the acrylic plates for better fixation of the mandible in a more forward position (Figs 1, 2 and 3).

The acrylic plates were limited to an average of 3 mm of functional free space to avoid neuromuscular discomfort.[9,11] The appliances were constructed with the greatest possible mandibular advancement of each patient without discomfort.

The Wilcoxon test was used to compare pre and posttreatment findings, at 5% significance level.

RESULTS

Table 1 shows comparison between AHI results at pre and post-advancement splint therapy exams. Table 2 demonstrates snoring recorded at pre and post-therapy evaluations. Table 3 presents BMI, minimum O_2 saturation and sleep efficiency at the two experimental times. Table 4 shows arrhythmia records before and after splint therapy.

DISCUSSION

As reported in the literature,[5,8,12,13,17,18,19,21,25,26,28,29] the mean apnea-hypopnea index (AHI) reduced significantly among the patients in the present study, that underwent intraoral splint therapy (mandibular advancement device). Mean AHI reduced from 20.89 ± 17.9/hour to 4.43 ± 3.09/hour.

Efficacy of mandibular advancement splint therapy has been related to AHI reduction. In mild to moderate OSAHS the treatment success using intraoral devices could range from 80 to 90%. However, in severe cases this kind of therapy successfully treats 50 to 60%, with partial efficacy.[7] The present study corroborates those data. After treatment, 15 patients had no apnea or less than 5/hour, four had mild apnea (5 to 15/hour) and one had moderate apnea (15 > AHI < 30/ hour) (p < 0.05). Among those patients who presented severe OSAHS in pretreatment phase (n = 5), two went to mild after treatment, one went to moderate, and two were considered successfully treated (AHI < 5).

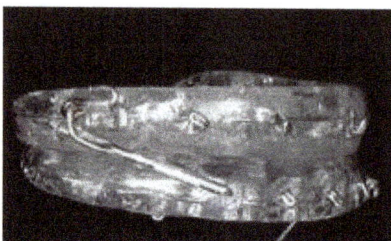

Figure 1 - Mandibular advancement splint used.

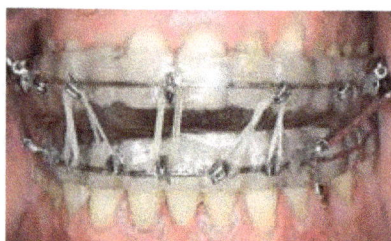

Figure 2 - Frontal intraoral view of mandibular advancement splint.

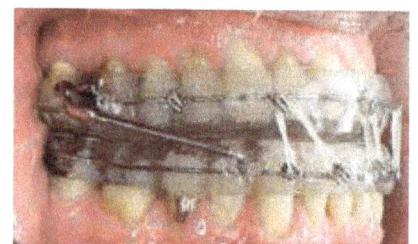

Figure 3 - Lateral intraoral view of mandibular advancement splint.

Table 1 - Pretreatment and posttreatment mean apnea-hypopnea index (AHI), and level of severity distribution.

AHI	pretreatment	posttreatment	significance
$\overline{X} \pm SD$	20.89 ± 17.46	4.43 ± 3.09	*
Absent (AHI < 5) (n)	0	15	*
Mild (5 > AHI < 15) (n)	9	4	*
Moderate (15 > AHI < 30) (n)	6	1	*
Severe (AHI > 30) (n)	5	0	*

* $p < 0.05$.

Table 2 - Pretreatment and posttreatment snoring severity.

Snoring	pretreatment	posttreatment	significance
Absent (n)	0	6	*
Mild (n)	4	13	*
Moderate (n)	9	1	*
Severe (n)	7	0	*
Total (n)	20	20	

* $p < 0.05$.

Table 3 - Mean and standard deviation of pretreatment and posttreatment BMI, minimum SO_2 and sleep efficiency.

	pretreatment	posttreatment	
	$\overline{X} \pm SD$	$\overline{X} \pm SD$	p
BMI	27.07 ± 4.49	27.65 ± 4.33	0.109 (ns)
SO_2	84.3 ± 9.33	92.75 ± 2.4	0.009 (ns)
Sleep efficiency (%)	83.58 ± 7.58	88.13 ± 4.45	0.033*

* $p < 0.05$.

Table 4 - Presence of pretreatment and posttreatment heart arrhythmia.

Arrhythmia	pretreatment	posttreatment	significance
Yes (n)	3	0	n.s.
No (n)	17	20	n.s.
Total (n)	20	20	

Among those patients who presented moderate OSAHS before treatment (n = 6), two presented mild and four presented AHI less than five after treatment. All patients presenting mild OSAHS before treatment (n = 9) were considered treated after the use of mandibular advancement splint.

In the present study the severity of the snoring reduced significantly, as documented by the polysomnograms, which revealed the absence of snoring in 6 patients (30%), while 13 exhibited mild snoring (65%) and only 1 patient exhibited moderate snoring (5%) ($p < 0.05$). Snoring could remain at some level although AHI reduces.[7,13]

Saturated O_2 went from 84.3±9.33 to 92.75±2.4, however with no statistical significance ($p > 0.05$). The quantitative sleep efficiency improved from 83.58 ± 7.58 to 88.03 ± 4.45 ($p < 0.05$). There were no significant changes in BMI. Three patients exhibited pretreatment heart arrhythmia, whereas no patients exhibited heart arrhythmia during the post-treatment polysomnogram, although this data were not statistically significant. In general, those data confirm the benefits of related AHI reduction by using intraoral appliance.

It was reported that mandibular advancement appliance prevent the collapse of the upper airways during sleep by maintaining the mandible in a protrusive position, exerting extrusive forces and lingual movement on the upper anterior teeth, and mesial and vestibular movement on the lower anterior teeth, with significant long-term occlusal changes.[14,15,20] It was also reported that the use of a mandibular advancement appliance alters the configuration of the upper airways, with a decrease in the length of the palate and an increase in the area of the pharynx, likely due to a loss of edema caused by snoring and repetitive apnea events.[3,4]

Although some dental alterations and other side effects may be undesirable in certain patients, the effective treatment of a life-threatening condition, such as OSAHS, is believed to supersede the maintenance of referential occlusion. Even in the presence of large dental movements, interruption of the treatment with an oral appliance should only occur when the patient accepts another treatment modality, such as continuous positive airway pressure equipment for the upper airways.[7,8,14,15]

Patients who require treatment for OSAHS are generally over 40 years of age, which is when periodontal disease begins to become aggravated. Thus, prospective studies involving a detailed periodontal evaluation are needed to determine a possible predicting factor of dental movement.[14]

As an oral appliance for the treatment of OSAHS is a life-long approach and the consequences of its use beyond six years are unknown, periodic clinical and radiographic exams are required to monitor the effects, which are at times beneficial and other times harmful, depending on facial pattern and pretreatment occlusion.

It is suggested that clinicians should be cautious in dental practice when treating patients with apnea using oral appliances if they have an ample anteroposterior airway and alteration in weight during treatment.[17]

Despite the positive results found in the present study, follow-up of these patients is necessary for determining

long-term results regarding the snore and sleep apnea and side effects stemming from treatment.

CONCLUSIONS

Sleep quality improved in patients using mandibular advancement splint, but further studies evaluating long-term effects are needed.

REFERENCES

1. Almeida FR, Bittencourt LR, de Almeida CI, Tsuiki S, Lowe AA, Tufik S. Effects of mandibular posture on obstructive sleep apnea severity and the temporomandibular joint in patients fitted with an oral appliance. Sleep. 2002 Aug 1;25(5):507-13.

2. Almeida FR, Lowe AA, Tsuiki S, Otsuka R, Wong M, Fastlicht S, Ryan F. Long-term compliance and side effects of oral appliances used for the treatment of snoring and obstructive sleep apnea syndrome. J Clin Sleep Med. 2005 Apr 15;1(2):143-52.

3. Almeida FR, Lowe AA, Sung JO, Tsuiki S, Otsuka R. Long-term sequellae of oral appliance therapy in obstructive sleep apnea patients: Part 1. Cephalometric analysis. Am J Orthod Dentofacial Orthop. 2006;129(2):195-204.

4. Almeida FR, Lowe AA, Otsuka R, Fastlicht S, Farbood M, Tsuiki S. Long-term sequellae of oral appliance therapy in obstructive sleep apnea patients: Part 2. Am J Orthod Dentofacial Orthop. 2006;129(2):205-13.

5. Blanco J, Zamarrón C, Abeleira Pazos MT, Lamela C, Suarez Quintanilla D. Prospective evaluation of an oral appliance in the treatment of obstructive sleep apnea syndrome. Sleep Breath. 2005;9(1):20-5.

6. Coelho Filho CM. Mandibular protraction appliance for Class II treatment. J Clin Orthod. 1995;29(5):319-39.

7. Dal-Fabbro C, Chaves Jr CM, Tufik S. A Odontologia na Medicina do Sono. 376p. Maringá: Dental Press Editora; 1 ed. 2010.

8. Gotsopoulos H, Kelly JJ, Cistulli PA. Oral appliance therapy reduces blood pressure in obstructive sleep apnea: randomized, controlled trial. Sleep. 2004;27(5):934-41.

9. Ito FA, Ito RT, Moraes MN, Sakima T, Bezerra MLS, Meirelles RC. Condutas terapêuticas para tratamento da Síndrome da Apnéia e Hipopnéia Obstrutiva do Sono (SAHOS) e da Síndrome da Resistência das Vias Aéreas Superiores (SRVAS) com enfoque no Aparelho Anti-Ronco. Rev Dental Press Ortod Ortop Facial. 2005;10(4):143-56.

10. Ito FA, Ito RT, Moraes MN, Sakima T, Bezerra MLS. Mecanismo de ação dinâmico do Aparelho Anti-Ronco (AAR): relato de um caso clínico. Rev Clin Ortod Dental Press. 2004;3(1):41-50.

11. Ito RT, Moreira ACM, Bronzi ES, Yoshida AH, Ito FA, Yoshida N, et al. Aparelho Anti-Ronco: um enfoque multidisciplinar. Rev Dental Press Ortod Ortop Facial. 2000;5(2):48-53.

12. Lamont J. O efeito de tipos de splints para avanço mandibular sobre o Ronco e a Apnéia Obstrutiva do Sono. Rev Dental Press Ortod Ortop Facial. 1999;1(2):74-5.

13. Lowe AA. Dental appliances for the treatment of snoring and obstructive sleep apnea. In: Kryger M, Roth T, Dement W. Principles and practice of sleep medicine. Philadelphia: W.B. Saunders; 2000. p. 929-39.

14. Marklund M, Franklin KA, Persson M. Orthodontic side-effects of mandibular advancement devices during treatment of snoring and sleep apnoea. Eur J Orthod. 2001 Apr;23(2):135-44.

15. Markland M. Predictors of long-term orthodontic side effects from mandibular advancement devices in patients with snoring and obstructive sleep apnea. Am J Orthod Dentofacial Orthop. 2006;129(2):214-21.

16. Orlando S. A parceria que promove um sono tranqüilo. Rev Bras Odontol. 2003;60(5):5-10.

17. Otsuka R, Almeida FR, Lowe AA, Ryan F. A comparison of responders and no responders to oral appliance therapy for the treatment of obstructive sleep apnea. Am J Orthod Dentofacial Orthop. 2006;129(2):222-9.

18. Otsuka R, Ribeiro de Almeida F, Lowe AA, Linden W, Ryan F. The effect of oral appliance therapy on blood pressure in patients with obstructive sleep apnea. Sleep Breath. 2006 Mar;10(1):29-36.

19. Otsuka R, Almeida FR, Lowe AA. The effects of oral appliance therapy on occlusal function in patients with obstructive sleep apnea: A short-term prospective study. Am J Orthod Dentofacial Orthop. 2007;131(2):176-83.

20. Pantin CC, Hillman DR, Tennant M. Dental side effects of an oral device to treat snoring and obstructive sleep apnea. Sleep. 1999;22(2):237-40.

21. Parker J. A prospective study evaluating the effectiveness of a mandibular repositioning appliance (PM Positioner) for the treatment of moderate obstructive sleep apnea. Sleep. 1999;22:230-1.

22. Paulin RF, Melo ACM, Ito RT, Sakima T, Reimão R. A apnéia obstrutiva do sono: considerações gerais e estratégias de tratamento. J Bras Ortodon Ortop Facial. 2001 dez.-2002 jan;6(36):488-92.

23. Ramos LVT, Furquim LZ. Aparelho para a apnéia obstrutiva do sono. Rev Clín Ortod Dental Press. 2004; 3(2):21-6.

24. Rider EA. Removable Herbst appliance for treatment of obstructive sleep apnea. J Clin Orthod. 1988;88(22):256-7.

25. Rose EC, Germann M, Sorichter S, Jonas IE. Case control study in the treatment of obstructive sleep — disordered breathing with a mandibular protrusive appliance. J Orofac Orthop. 2004;65(6):489-500.

26. Rose EC, Staats R, Virchow C Jr, Jonas IE. Occlusal and skeletal effects of an oral appliance in the treatment of obstructive sleep apnea. Chest. 2002;122(3):871-7.

27. Silveira M. A síndrome da apnéia obstrutiva do sono, o ronco e seu tratamento com o aparelho Apnout. J Bras Ortodon Ortop Facial. 2001;6(32):151-4.

28. Tan YK, L'Estrange PR, Luo YM, Smith C, Grant HR, Simonds AK, et al. Mandibular advancement splints and continuous positive airway pressure in patients with obstructive sleep apnea: a randomized cross-over trial. Eur J Orthod. 2002;24(3):239-49.

29. Tsuiki S, Almeida FR, Lowe AA, Su J, Fleetham JA. The interaction between changes in upright mandibular position and supine airway size in patients with obstructive sleep apnea. Am J Orthod Dentofacial Orthop. 2005;128(4):504-12.

25

Transverse effect of Haas and Hyrax appliances on the upper dental arch in patients with unilateral complete cleft lip and palate

Anna Júlia de Oliveira Façanha[1], Tulio Silva Lara[2], Daniela Gamba Garib[3], Omar Gabriel da Silva Filho[4]

Objective: The aim of the present study was to evaluate the transverse effect of rapid maxillary expansion in patients with unilateral complete cleft lip and palate while comparing the Haas and Hyrax appliances. **Methods:** The sample consisted of 48 patients divided into two groups: Group I – 25 patients treated with modified Haas appliance (mean age: 10 years 8 months); and Group II – 23 patients treated with Hyrax appliance (mean age: 10 years 6 months). Casts were taken during pre-expansion and after removal of the appliance at the end of the retention period. The models were scanned with the aid of the 3 Shape R700 3D scanner. Initial and final transverse distances were measured at cusp tips and cervical-palatal points of maxillary teeth by using the Ortho Analyzer™ 3D software. **Results:** The mean expansion obtained between cusp tips and cervical-palatal points for inter-canine width was 4.80 mm and 4.35 mm with the Haas appliance and 5.91 mm and 5.91 mm with the Hyrax appliance. As for first premolars or first deciduous molars, the values obtained were 6.46 mm and 5.90 mm in the Haas group and 7.11 mm and 6.65 mm in the Hyrax group. With regard to first molars, values were 6.11 mm and 5.24 mm in the Haas group and 7.55 mm and 6.31 mm in the Hyrax group. **Conclusion:** Rapid maxillary expansion significantly increased the transverse dimensions of the upper dental arch in patients with cleft palate, with no significant differences between the Hass and Hyrax expanders.
Keywords: Palatine expansion technique. Cleft palate. Dental arch.

[1] Specialist in Orthodontics, Hospital for Rehabilitation of Craniofacial Anomalies – São Paulo University (HRAC-USP).
[2] Professor of Interceptive Orthodontics (HRAC-USP).
[3] Full professor, School of Dentistry — University of São Paulo/Bauru. Professor of Orthodontics (HRAC-USP).
[4] MSc in Orthodontics, State University of São Paulo (UNESP).

» The authors report no commercial, proprietary or financial interest in the products or companies described in this article.

Tulio Silva Lara
Rua Sílvio Marchione, 3-20 – Vila Universitária – Bauru/SP — Brazil.
CEP: 17012-900 – E-mail: tuliolara@hotmail.com

INTRODUCTION

Unilateral complete cleft lip and palate simultaneously involves the primary and secondary palate and accounts for 30% of all clefts. This condition requires more extensive treatment, as the cleft divides the maxilla and the alveolar arch into two completely distinct segments.[1] Treatment initially involves primary functional and esthetic surgeries for the closing of the lip and palate, which have a long-term impact on mid face growth.[2,3] The patient is then followed up throughout the growth period until entering the orthodontic phase (end of the deciduous dentition phase).[4]

Primary surgeries of the lip and palate usually potentiate reductions in the transverse and sagittal dimensions of the upper arch as a consequence of the restricted growth of the mid face and the approximation of the initially separated maxillary segments.[3] These sagittal and transverse deficiencies of the upper alveolar arch is expressed already at the mixed dentition phase and tend to become aggravated in adolescence.[5] Thus, the task of orthodontists is to counteract the harmful effects of the altered facial growth also characterized by posterior and anterior cross bite — often found in patients with cleft lip and palate.[6]

Besides other occlusion issues,[7] posterior cross bite is the most common malocclusion in these patients, involving a single tooth or the entire dental arch, showing a tendency toward exacerbation from the mixed to the permanent dentition. Interceptive orthodontic interventions should be performed during the mixed dentition phase for correction of the compromised transverse dimension.[8] Moreover, the expansion of the upper arch also plays an important role in preparing the arch and cleft region for the secondary alveolar bone graft, which is performed at the end of the mixed dentition prior to the eruption of the permanent canine adjacent to the cleft region.[4]

Rapid maxillary expansion performed by means of a Haas or Hyrax appliance is the most common method employed at the Hospital for Rehabilitation of Craniofacial Anomalies (USP, Brazil) to increase the width of the maxilla. The main difference between the two appliances is the type of anchorage: tooth-supported with the Hyrax appliance and tooth-mucosa-supported with the Haas appliance.

The active expansion phase in patients with unilateral complete cleft lip and palate promotes distancing of the maxillary segments and widening of the cleft.[8] Expansion in these patients is not followed by bone formation at the median palatine suture, as it occurs in patients without cleft palate,[9] because the distancing of the maxillary halves occurs in the region of the cleft. Thus, retention should remain after the appliance is removed and until bone graft is performed. Expansion in such patients involves similar restrictions to those found in patients without cleft palate, as the other maxillary sutures offer considerable resistance to widening, requiring orthopedic appliances.

Motivated by the interest in evaluating the results of the expansion philosophy of the team at the Hospital for Rehabilitation of Craniofacial Anomalies/USP, the aim of the present prospective study was to assess alterations in the transverse dimension of the upper dental arch in patients with unilateral complete cleft lip and palate who have undergone rapid maxillary expansion, comparing the results achieved with the Haas and Hyrax appliances with the aid of digital models.

MATERIAL AND METHODS

This study was approved by the Hospital for Rehabilitation of Craniofacial Anomalies/USP Institutional Review Board (protocol 255/2010-SVAPEPE-CEP).

The sample consisted of 48 patients enrolled in the orthodontic sector of the hospital. All patients had unilateral complete cleft lip and palate, had undergone primary surgeries at an early age and were in the mixed dentition phase, exhibiting maxillary atresia with an indication for rapid maxillary expansion.

The patients were randomly divided into two groups. Group I comprised 25 patients treated with the modified Haas appliance (Fig 1A), with bands on the permanent molars and orthodontic clip bonded to the deciduous molars (16 males and 9 females; mean age: 10 years 8 months; age range: 8 years to 19 years and 2 months). Group II comprised 23 patients treated with the Hyrax appliance (Fig 1B) (13 males and 10 females; mean age: 10 years 6 months; age range: 8 years and 2 months to 18 years and 1 month). All patients underwent the same activation protocol. The expander was activated for seven days with 2/4 turns in the morning and 2/4 turns in the evening. Whenever necessary, further activation was performed until overcorrection was reached (palatine cusps of the upper molars occluding the vestibular cusps of the lower molars). Hooks for a facial mask were welded to the inverse traction of the maxilla for patients that also had sagittal discrepancy with good prognosis for orthopedic treatment.

After achieving overcorrection, the screw was stabilized with acrylic resin. The expander was maintained passive with a retention protocol for six months, after which the expander was removed and a fixed retainer was installed.

Dental cast of the maxillary arch were obtained at two different times: immediately before banding for the expander (T_1), and after the six-month period of retention immediately following the removal of the expander (T_2). The impressions were made with alginate and filled with Paris plaster. The dental casts were then scanned by a 3Shape R700 3D scanner (3Shape A/S, Copenhagen, Denmark), which reproduces a three-dimensional digital image based on laser beams scans projected over the plaster models in different directions. The Ortho Analyzer ™ 3D program was used to obtain the three-dimensional image of the scanned models, allowing frontal, lateral, posterior and occlusal visualization. The reference points were marked on the model in the occlusal view for the calculation of the distances between teeth. Figure 2 illustrates the measurements made on the digital models of the upper dental arches.

Analyses were performed by a single examiner. Sixty percent of the sample was analyzed a second time after a seven-day interval in order to determine the measurements reliability using the intraclass correlation coefficient (ICC) for which the following scores were used: 0.80 to 1.00 = excellent agreement; 0.60 to 0.80 = substantial; 0.40 to 0.60 = moderate; 0.20 to 0.40 = fair; 0 to 0.20 = discreet; and −1 to 0 = poor.

Mean, standard deviation (SD), maximum and minimum values were calculated. The paired Student's t-test was employed to determine statistically significant differences between the initial and final measurements of each group. The independent t-test was used for inter-group comparison. The level of significance was set at 5% ($p < 0.05$).

RESULTS
Tables 1 to 4 display the results of the measurement reliability and transverse distances measured on the models.

DISCUSSION
Cleft lip and palate occurs in the mid face and causes structural problems in the alveolar bone and maxilla. The urgent relationship with the malocclusion is demonstrated by the anatomic rupture that compromises the alveolar ridge as well as dental problems, such as

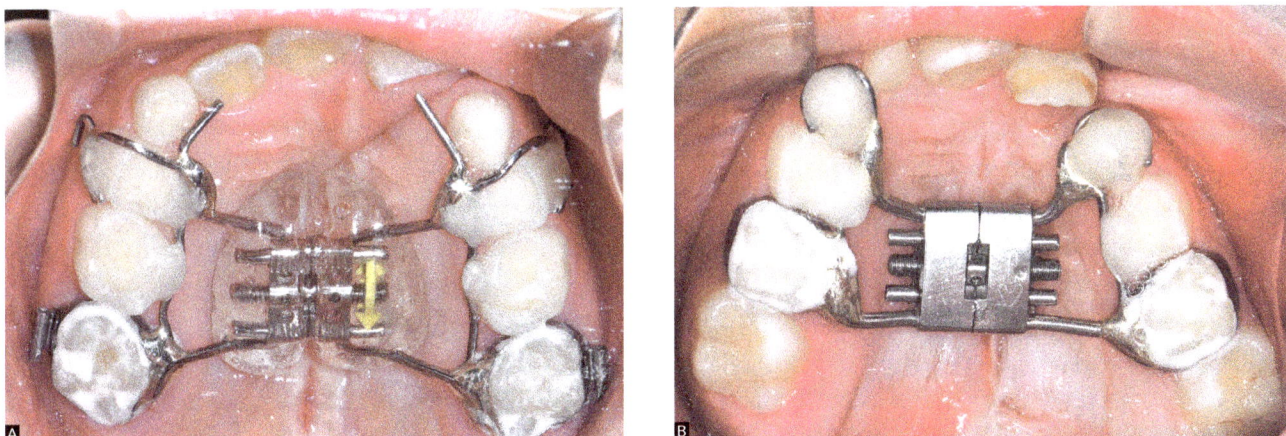

Figure 1 - Occlusal photographs of two patients from the sample illustrating both expanders: Modified Haas (A) and Hyrax (B)

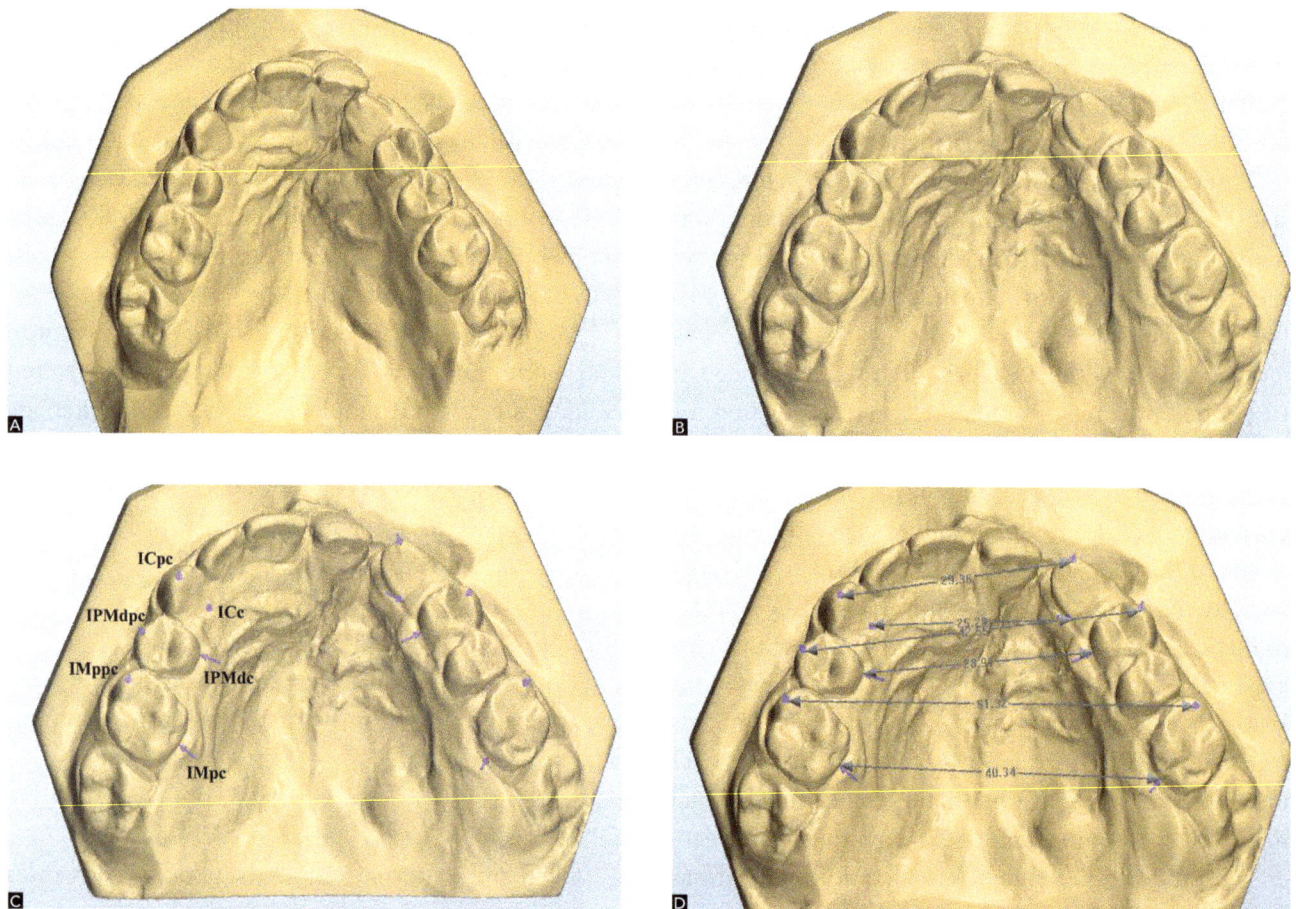

Figure 2 - Initial and final digital models showing the results of rapid maxillary expansion (**A** and **B**); reference points (**C**) and measurements made (**D**) on post-expansion models

agenesis and malpositioning, as well as sagittal and transverse maxillary difficiencies.[10] The treatment protocol adopted by the Hospital for Rehabilitation of Craniofacial Anomalies/USP for patients with unilateral complete cleft lip and palate emphasizes early surgical procedures (cheiloplasty and palatoplasty), with no orthopedic intervention in the preoperative or immediate postoperative periods. As a general rule, orthodontic treatment is initiated at the onset of the mixed dentition phase. Two reasons justify the lack of orthodontic intervention in the deciduous dentition phase: the instability of the early correction of cross bites, which leads to an excessively long treatment and retention time; and the fact that alterations in the shape of the dental arch and the occlusion are exacerbated in the mixed dentition phase.[11]

Expansion is the first step of orthodontic treatment (pre-alveolar bone graft). It aims at reestablishing the transverse dimensions of the atresic maxilla. The maxillary expander designed by Haas is the main appliance used for lateral repositioning of the collapsed maxillary processes[6] and follows the same activation protocol used for patients without cleft palate. In this phase, the inverse traction of the maxilla may be associated with the post-expansion period to revert cases of negative sagittal discrepancy, expressed by anterior crossbite.[12] The Hyrax appliance is also commonly used for maxillary expansion. The main difference between the two expanders is the acrylic support on the palate in the Haas appliance. However, both expanders are effective in increasing the transverse dimension of the maxilla. The choice of one over the other is based on the shape

Table 1 - Error of the method (Intraclass Correlation Coefficient).

Measure	ICC (Haas)		ICC (Hyrax)	
	Initial	Final	Initial	Final
ICpc	0.99	0.82	1.00	0.99
ICc	0.97	0.99	0.99	1.00
IPMdpc	0.91	1.00	0.99	1.00
IPMdc	0.99	0.99	1.00	1.00
IMppc	0.99	0.98	0.96	0.99
IMpc	1.00	0.99	1.00	0.99

Table 2 - Transverse distances measured on initial and final digital models and mean amount of expansion (Dif.) in millimeters for patients using the modified Haas expander.

Measure	Initial model Mean ± S.D.	Final model Mean ± S.D.	Dif.	p
ICpc	26.81 ± 3.13	31.60 ± 3.35	4.79	< 0.01*
ICc	21.15 ± 3.39	25.50 ± 3.76	4.35	< 0.01*
IPMdpc	35.39 ± 3.67	41.85 ± 4.22	6.46	< 0.01*
IPMdc	24.25 ± 3.03	30.15 ± 3.36	5.9	< 0.01*
IMppc	49.20 ± 3.91	55.31 ± 3.28	6.11	< 0.01*
IMpc	35.29 ± 2.84	40.54 ± 3.24	5.24	< 0.01*

* statistically significant difference (p < 0.05)

Table 3 - Transverse distances measured on initial and final digital models and mean amount of expansion (Dif.) in millimeters for patients using the Hyrax expander.

Measure	Initial model Mean ± S.D.	Final model Mean ± S.D.	Dif.	p
ICpc	24.63 ± 3.98	30.54 ± 2.95	5.91	< 0.01*
ICc	20.37 ± 2.96	26.28 ± 3.91	5.91	< 0.01*
IPMdc	33.10 ± 3.71	40.21 ± 3.96	7.12	< 0.01*
IPMdc	22.72 ± 3.59	29.37 ± 3.50	6.65	< 0.01*
IMppc	44.68 ± 4.26	52.23 ± 3.73	7.55	< 0.01*
IMpc	31.32 ± 3.90	37.63 ± 3.79	6.31	< 0.01*

* statistically significant difference (p < 0.05)

Table 4 - Comparison of modified Haas and Hyrax appliances groups regarding mean increase in transverse dimensions of the maxilla following rapid maxillary expansion.

Measure	Group Haas (n)	Group Hyrax (n)	Difference (mm)	P
ICpc	4.80 (18)	5.91 (18)	1.11	0.16 ns
ICc	4.35 (11)	5.91 (16)	1.56	0.06 ns
IPMdpc	6.46 (19)	7.11 (16)	0.65	0.48 ns
IPMdc	5.90 (19)	6.65 (16)	0.75	0.29 ns
IMppc	6.11 (24)	7.55 (22)	1.44	0.02*
IMpc	5.24 (24)	6.31 (21)	1.07	0.08 ns

ns = non-significant.
* statistically significant difference (p < 0.05).

of the patient's palate. Whenever the transverse width and depth allow, the Haas expander is the appliance of choice due to the anchorage provided by its acrylic portion. In the present study, the modified Haas expander was used, which differs from the original by the presence of two orthodontic bands instead of four, and by bonded orthodontic clips on the deciduous molars.

Following the tendency of using digital records in Orthodontics,[13] the evaluation of the transverse effect of the Haas and Hyrax expanders was performed with digital models, which offer advantages in terms of storage, retrieval, durability, diagnostic versatility and transmitting information.[14] Moreover, studies comparing digital and conventional models report considerable accuracy and reproducibility in the measurements of tooth width, overjet and overbite.[15] The ICC of the measurements obtained from the digital models by a single examiner on two different occasions demonstrate the reliability of the method (Table 1).

Both appliances were capable of restoring the adequate upper arch morphology and correcting the posterior cross bite (Figs 1 and 2). The results demonstrate significant increase (p < 0.0001) in all transverse dimensions measured (Tables 2 and 3), which is in agreement with findings reported in the literature.[16]

The increases in the inter-molar, inter-premolar or inter-deciduous molar and inter-canine widths were statistically significant in both groups. The group treated with the Haas expander had an increase in inter-molar distance of 6.11 mm on the tips of the mesiovestibular cusps, 5.24 mm on the palatine-cervical portion of the molars, and an increase in the inter-canine distance of 4.79 mm when measured on the cusps and 4.35 mm when measured on the palatine-cervical portion (Table 2). These values are similar to those reported by previous studies.[17,19] In a study involving digital models of 32 children without cleft palate and with unilateral or bilateral cross bite (16 children treated with the Haas expander and 16 treated with the Hyrax expander), the Haas group had an increase in inter-molar distance of 6.33 mm on the tips of the mesiovestibular cusps and 6.04 mm on the central sulcus of the first molars; an increase in the inter-canine distance of 2.27 mm when measured on the cusps and 4.74 mm when measured on the cervical portion.[20]

In the present study, the patients treated with the Hyrax expander had an increase in inter-molar distance of 7.55 mm on the tips of the mesiovestibular cusps and 6.31 mm in the palatine-cervical portion; an increase in the inter-canine distance of 5.91 mm when measured on the cusps or on the palatine-cervical portion (Table 3). These results are similar to findings reported in the literature for patients in the mixed dentition phase treated with the Hyrax expander.[19,21,23] However, another study reports larger increases (9.97 mm in inter-molar distance on the tips of the mesiopalatine cusps and 9.51 mm in the in the mesial portion of the central sulcus of the and 7.93 mm in the inter-canine distance when measured on the cusps and 6.29 mm when measured on the cervical portion).[20]

No statistically significant differences were found between groups in the comparison of the inter-molar and inter-canine distances obtained with the Haas or Hyrax appliances, except for the inter-molar distance measured on the tips of the cusps, which was greater in the Hyrax group (Table 4). This was likely due to the greater tooth tipping caused by this appliance.

Discrepant results are reported in the literature, with some studies reporting a greater increase in inter-molar and inter-canine distances using the Hyrax expander[20] and others reporting a greater tendency of vestibular tipping of molars using the Haas expander.[16] Both appliances generally demonstrate similar behavior regarding the expansion of the dentoalveolar region of the maxilla.[24] However, the Haas expander may cause greater vestibular tipping of the anchoring teeth (3.5° for the first molar) in comparison to the Hyrax expander (1.6°), although this is not a clinically relevant difference.[24]

CONCLUSIONS

- Rapid maxillary expansion using the modified Haas and Hyrax expanders proved efficient in increasing the transverse dimensions of the upper dental arch in patients with unilateral complete cleft lip and palate.

- No significant differences between appliances were found regarding the transverse effects produced by the modified Haas and Hyrax expanders in the present study.

REFERENCES

1. Silva Filho OG, Ferrari Júnior FM, Carvalho RM, Mazzottini R. A cirurgia ortognática na reabilitação do paciente portador de fissura unilateral completa de lábio e palato. Rev Dental Press Ortod Ortop Facial. 1998;3(4):51-70.

2. Silva Filho OG, Freitas JAS. Caracterização morfológica e origem embriológica. In: Trindade IEK, Silva Filho OG, organizadores. Fissuras labiopalatinas: uma abordagem interdisciplinar. São Paulo: Ed. Santos; 2007. cap. 2, p. 16-49.

3. Silva Filho OG, Ramos AL, Abdo RC. The influence of unilateral cleft lip and palate on maxillary dental arch morphology. Angle Orthod. 1992;62(4):283-90.

4. Cavassan AO, Silva Filho OG. Abordagem ortodôntica. In: Trindade IEK; Silva Filho OG. organizadores. Fissuras labiopalatinas: uma abordagem interdisciplinar. São Paulo: Ed. Santos; 2007. cap. 12, p. 213-38.

5. Athanasiou AE, Mazahery M, Zarrinnia K. Dental arch dimensions in patients with unilateral cleft lip and palate. Cleft Palate J. 1988;25(2):139-45.

6. Capelozza Filho L, Almeida AM, Ursi WJS. Rapid maxillary expansion in cleft lip and palate patients. J Clin Orthod. 1994;28(1):34-9.

7. Reis AC, Capelozza Filho L, Ozawa TO, Cavassan AO. Avaliação da angulação e inclinação dos elementos dentários em pacientes adultos jovens portadores de fissura transforame incisivo bilateral. Rev Dental Press Ortod Ortop Facial. 2008;13(1):113-23.

8. Long RE Jr, Semb GS, Shaw WC. Orthodontic treatment of the patient with complete lip and palate: lessons of the past 60 years. Cleft Palate Craniofac J. 2000 [Access in 2010 set 10];37(6). Available from: http://www.cpcjournal.org/doi/pdf/10.1597/1545569%282000%29037%3C0533%3AOTOTPW%3E2.0.CO%3B2.

9. Silva Filho OG, Lara TS, Silva HC, Bertoz FA. Comportamento da sutura palatina mediana em crianças submetidas à expansão rápida da maxila: avaliação mediante imagem de tomografia computadorizada. Rev Dental Press Ortod Ortop Facial. 2007;12(3):94-103.

10. Garib DG, Silva Filho OG, Janson G, Pinto JHN. Etiologia das más oclusões: perspectiva clínica (parte III) – fissuras labiopalatinas. Rev Clín Ortod Dental Press. 2010;9(4):30-6.

11. Abdo RCC, Silva Filho OG, Ramos AL. Comportamento do arco dentário superior de crianças fissuradas de lábio e palato, operadas – estudo longitudinal de 3 a 6 anos. Ortodontia. 1992;25(2):15-26.

12. Silva Filho OG, Capelozza Filho L, Wernech VA, Freitas JAS. Abordagem ortodôntica ao paciente com fissura unilateral completa de lábio e palato. Ortodontia. 1998;31(3):32-44.

13. Creed B, Kau CH, English JD, Xia JJ, Lee RP. A comparison of the accuracy of linear measurements obtained from cone beam computerized tomography images and digital models. Semin Orthod. 2011;17(1):49-56.

14. Joffe L. OrthoCAD: digital models for a digital era. J Orthod. 2004;31(4):344-7.

15. Santoro M, Galkin S, Teredesai M, Nicolay OF, Cangialosi TJ. Comparison of measurements made on digital and plaster models. Am J Orthod Dentofacial Orthop. 2003;124(1):101-5.

16. Weissheimer A. Efeitos imediatos da expansão rápida da maxila no sentido transversal, com os disjuntores tipo Haas e Hyrax, em tomografia computadorizada cone beam [dissertação]. Porto Alegre (RS): Pontifícia Universidade Católica do Rio Grande do Sul; 2008.

17. McNamara JA, Baccetti T, Franchi L, Herberger TA. Rapid maxillary expansion followed by fixed appliances: a long-term evaluation of changes in arch dimension. Angle Orthod. 2003;73(4):344-53.

18. Lima AL, Lima Filho RMA, Bolognese AM. Long-term clinical outcome of rapid maxillary expansion as the only treatment performed in class I malocclusion. Angle Orthod. 2005;75(3):416-20.

19. Oliveira NL, Da Silveira AC, Kusnoto B, Viana G. Three-dimensional assessment of morphologic changes of the maxilla: a comparison of 2 kinds of palatal expanders. Am J Orthod Dentofacial Orthop. 2004;126(3):354-62.

20. Mundstock KS. Estudo dos efeitos da expansão rápida de maxila em pacientes com mordida cruzada posterior tratados com aparelhos de Haas e de Hyrax [tese]. Araraquara (SP): Universidade Estadual Paulista; 2006.

21. Adkins MD, Nanda RS, Currier GF. Arch perimeter changes on rapid palatal expansion. Am J Orthod Dentofacial Orthop. 1990;97(3):194-9.

22. Chiavini PCR. Efeitos da expansão rápida da maxila com aparelho expansor tipo Hyrax: avaliação cefalométrica póstero-anterior em modelos de estudo [tese]. Araraquara (SP): Faculdade de Odontologia de Araraquara; 2004.

23. Ciambotti C, Ngan P, Durkee M, Kohli K, Kim H. A comparison of dental and dentoalveolar changes between rapid palatal expansion and nickel-titanium palatal expansion appliances. Am J Orthod Dentofacial Orthop. 2001;119(1):11-20.

24. Garib DG, Henriques JF, Janson G, Freitas MR, Coelho RA. Rapid maxillary expansion - Tooth tissue-borne versus tooth-borne expanders: a computed tomography evaluation of dentoskeletal effects. Angle Orthod. 2005;75(4):548-57.

26

Horizontal and vertical maxillary osteotomy stability, in cleft lip and palate patients, using allogeneic bone graft

Kelston Ulbricht Gomes[1], Wilson Denis Benato Martins[2], Marina de Oliveira Ribas[2]

Objective: This study was carried out to evaluate maxillary stability after orthodontic-surgical treatment of patients with cleft lip and palate. Cephalometric analysis was applied to two different groups, with and without allogeneic bone graft. **Methods:** The sample comprised 48 patients with cleft lip and palate. The test group comprised 25 patients who, after correction of maxillary position, received allogeneic bone graft at the gap created by Le Fort I osteotomy. The control group comprised 23 patients and its surgical procedures were similar to those applied to the test group, except for the use of bone graft. Manual cephalometric analysis and comparison between lateral teleradiographs, obtained at the preoperative phase, immediate postoperative phase and after a minimum period of six months, were carried out. **Results:** An higher horizontal relapse was observed in the control group ($p < 0.05$). There were no statistically significant differences in vertical relapses between test and control groups ($p > 0.05$). **Conclusion:** The use of allogeneic bone graft in cleft lip and palate patients submitted to Le Fort I osteotomy contributed to increase postoperative stability when compared to surgeries without bone graft.

Keywords: Orthognathic surgery. Oral surgery. Bone grafting.

» The authors report no commercial, proprietary or financial interest in the products or companies described in this article.

[1] PhD in Oral and Maxillofacial Surgery, Pontifical Catholic University of Paraná (PUC-PR).
[2] Professor of Dentistry at PUC-PR.

Kelston Ulbricht Gomes
Av. Silva Jardim, 2042 – Sala 1205 – Curitiba/PR, Brazil
CEP: 80250-200 – E-mail: kelstongomes@yahoo.com.br

INTRODUCTION

Cleft lip and palate deformities are amongst the most common congenital anomalies of the face.[1]

Cleft lip and palate surgery as well as orthodontic treatment are amongst the therapeutic possibilities for recovering patients' esthetics and function. In patients with cleft lip and palate, some occlusal deleterious situations such as teeth crowding and unilateral crossbite with segments collapse, open bite on the affected side and retrusion of the maxilla, are identified.[2-6]

After the growth spurt, orthognathic surgery is indicated to correct skeletal and dental discrepancies in patients who present dentofacial deformity.

Hirano and Suzuki[7] described potential aspects which are responsible for maxillary retrusion in adult cleft patients: Unfavorable muscular action due to scars caused by early surgeries in lip and palate, pharyngeal flaps and absence of teeth, which reduces occlusal stability.

The stability of orthognathic surgeries depends on the type and the extent of movements performed by the maxilla. Stability is considered difficult especially in patients with cleft lip and palate. Usually, these patients have undergone surgery in the soft and hard palate, which normally results in fibrosis, limiting the extent of both transverse and anteroposterior movements of the maxilla.[8-12]

In order to avoid relapses when treating dentofacial deformities in cleft patients, some authors suggest increasing the time of intermaxillary fixation during the postoperative phase, performing bimaxillary surgeries, using face masks with reverse traction of the maxilla and interpositioning bone grafts between the gaps created by maxillary advancement.[13,14,15]

A successful correction of dentofacial deformities depends on effective stabilization and prompt union of the repositioned bone segments. When there is a large area of contact between the segments, safe and satisfactory bone union is expected. When the contact area is small, there may be instability, relapse or fibrous union (pseudoarthrosis) between segments. In such cases, grafts are recommended. Some authors[16,17] suggest allogeneic bone graft in orthognathic surgery. However, in the aforementioned studies, allogeneic bone graft was performed in patients without cleft lip and palate.

The study of Precious,[18] in 2007, concluded that scars on the upper lip and on the palate interfere with nose, lips, soft adjacent tissues and skeletal development.

When intervention is performed with bone graft and correction of nasolabial musculature at the age of five or six years old, a symmetric function is established, which improves facial development. The primary muscle surgery improves growth and decreases the chances of undergoing orthognathic surgery.[19]

Nique et al[2] have studied the use of allograft bone for alveolar reconstruction in unilateral cleft patients. The receptor area was radiographically observed for a period of 3 to 6 months. The allograft bone is an excellent alternative to repair alveolar cleft, its use brings significant benefits for the patient, eliminating the morbidity of a second surgical site.

Garrison et al[19] evaluated twenty patients who were simultaneously submitted to both alveolar bone graft and Le Fort I osteotomy. The researchers evaluated the extent of maxilla relapse at the anteroposterior and vertical direction through lateral teleradiographs. They concluded that there was no significant change in the horizontal plan, however, in the vertical direction there was a great tendency to relapse. The intermaxillary fixation time lasted for eight weeks and mandibular fixation was used at the orbital rim and zygomatic crest. For the evaluation, cephalometry was adopted, the SN plan was traced and a perpendicular line was drawn from the Nasion. The researchers measured the distance from this line to point A in order to evaluate potential changes in the horizontal direction (anteroposterior). To determine the vertical movement, a line was drawn perpendicular to the SN up to the point A.

Another research, carried out by Heliovaara et al,[20] examined the causes of relapse through a retrospective analysis of 71 patients, 58 of which had unilateral and bilateral clefts. The mean advancement of the maxilla was 6.9 mm. Grafts were harvested from calvaria or mandible and there were used four miniplates for containing the maxilla as well as intermaxillary fixation which was kept during 6 weeks and maintained after releasing fixation with class III elastics. The researchers concluded that the type of cleft (unilateral or bilateral), the scars in the soft palate, muscle tension, adaptation and stability of bone segments are amongst the main causes of relapse in maxillary osteotomies. The occlusal stability is important to prevent relapses.

Hirano and Suzuki[7] evaluated one group comprised of 14 patients with cleft palate only and other group comprised of 11 patients with bilateral cleft lip and palate. The gaps created by Le Fort I osteotomy were filled with autogenous bone without applying intermaxillary fixation or surgical guide. Patients were evaluated through lateral teleradiographs and point A was used as the reference point. Patients were evaluated at pre- and immediate postoperative phases as well as one year after the surgery. The average relapse in the group with cleft palate only was 8.5% in the horizontal direction and 16.7% in the vertical direction. In the group with bilateral cleft, relapse was 9.4% horizontal, and 17.8% vertical. The authors suggest that the main factors for relapses are: the method used for fixating the osteotomized segments, neuromuscular adaptation, the extent of movement of the maxilla and previous orthodontic preparation.

Ianetti et al[21] evaluated the use of bimaxillary surgeries for minimizing potential relapses in patients with cleft lip and palate. They highlight intense scarring and soft tissue tension as being responsible for relapse. To reduce the relapse, authors suggest overcorrection of the maxilla; however, they warn that major advances of the maxilla can result in velopharynx incompetence. These conclusions were based on the evaluation of 15 patients who underwent combined bimaxillary surgery. In order to improve the stability of the maxilla, the authors suggest performing bone graft in the space created by Le Fort I osteotomy, with the indicated use of intermaxillary elastics for three weeks and the surgical guide being removed after six weeks. The stability evaluation was carried out by means of lateral teleradiographs, taken at the preoperative phase, six weeks, a year and two years after the surgery. The references were point A, the posterior nasal spine and point B. For cases in which only the maxilla was operated, relapse was of 25%, and in cases of maxillary and mandibular osteotomy, relapse was of 8%.[21]

In another study, conducted by Erbe et al,[22] cephalometric analysis was performed during immediate and late postoperative phases (39-110 months) for patients simultaneously undergoing both Le Fort I osteotomies for advancement and autogenous alveolar bone graft. Operative changes in the position of the maxilla were evaluated in vertical and horizontal directions. All parameters used in the cephalometric measurements were manually measured by one single examiner as an attempt to eliminate observer bias. Some reference points were difficult to identify; however, the careful observation of a series of lateral films of the head increased accuracy and the identification of reference points was made possible.

Even with surgical correction of the maxilla, some degree of relapse is expected due to the aforementioned shortcomings and peculiarities (previous surgery on the palate and lack of occlusal stability by the absence of teeth). Bone grafting performed in the space created by both osteotomy and correction of the position of the maxilla can reduce the occurrence of relapse.

Thus, the objective of this study was to evaluate horizontal and vertical stability of maxillary osteotomy using allogeneic bone graft in patients with cleft lip and palate.

MATERIAL AND METHODS

The stability of orthodontic-surgical treatment of patients with cleft lip and palate was evaluated through cephalometric analysis in two different groups, one with and another without the use of allogeneic bone graft.

The study was approved by the local Institutional Review Board under the number 0003716/10.

Material

The sample consisted of 48 patients with cleft lip and palate, submitted to surgery at the Assistance Center for Cleft Lip and Palate (CAIF) in Curitiba, Paraná, Brazil, from January 2006 to March 2009.

All patients underwent orthognathic maxillary surgery, performed with the Le Fort I technique, with rigid internal fixation and intermaxillary fixation lasting for an average of 4 (four) weeks. The test group (TG) consisted of 25 patients of both genders with unilateral and bilateral clefts, with an average age of 23.16 years. The surgeries were isolated in the maxilla or combined with mandibular surgeries. After the maxilla had been repositioned, allogeneic bone graft, from the Bank of Muscle and Bone Tissue of the Clinical Hospital from Federal University of Paraná, was inserted to fill the gaps created by the osteotomies.

The control group (CG) consisted of 23 patients of both genders with cleft lip and palate, unilateral and bilateral types, with an average age of 25.78 years. Surgical procedures were similar to those applied to the TG, except for the use of bone graft. In the selection of patients, those with cleft lip and palate who underwent orthognathic surgery from January 2006 to March 2009, of both sexes and aged above 18 years were included. Patients submitted to orthognathic surgery only in the mandible, as well as those who had undergone more than one orthognathic surgery were excluded. Patients who did not performed alveolar bone graft in childhood were also excluded.

Methods

a) A blind study in which manual cephalometric analysis of the lateral teleradiographs was carried out by one single examiner. Radiographs were obtained at the preoperative phase, immediate postoperative phase and after a minimum period of six months.

b) The records as well as the cephalometric analysis were carried out using advocated parameters and measures.[19,23] The anteroposterior position of the maxilla was determined by drawing the SN plan and a perpendicular line in relation to it, from the Nasion (Na) point. The distance from this line to point A was measured, determining the anteroposterior preoperative maxilla position which was compared to the postoperative position, over time (h) (Fig 1).

c) A perpendicular line was drawn from the SN plane towards point A in order to determine the preoperative vertical position of the maxilla which was compared to the postoperative position, over time (v) (Fig 1).

d) Having such reference points as guides, the maxillary tracing in the preoperative radiograph was superimposed over the first postoperative (immediate) radiograph. Tracings were repeated, resulting in horizontal and vertical linear values which correspond to the amount of movement obtained with surgery.

e) With a new radiograph obtained afterwards, at least 6 months after the first one, the process of comparison was repeated by means of superimposing the tracings. At this time, the immediate postoperative radiograph was used and the values for assessing the occurrence of relapse were obtained.

f) The purpose of these measurements was to linearly measure possible vertical and horizontal postoperative changes, over time, and relate them to the use of bone grafts.

RESULTS

Both groups (CG and TG) presented normal distribution with regard to the following variables: horizontal advancement, horizontal relapse, vertical movement and vertical relapse. The average horizontal advancement was similar in both groups. The average vertical movement was higher in TG than in CG (Table 1).

Horizontal relapse was higher in CG (p <0.05). There were no statistically significant differences in vertical relapses between TG and CG (p> 0.05) (Tables 2 and 3).

Variables such as gender, type of procedure and type of cleft did not influence the stability of the surgery in any group (p>0.05) (Figs 2, 3 and 4).

The CG had a follow-up period longer than the TG. However, despite this difference, there is no correlation between this variable and horizontal or vertical relapses (Pearson Correlation Coefficient p>0.05). (Table 4; Figs 5 and 6).

By using Pearson Correlation Coefficient it was obtained a p-value> 0.05, indicating that there is no correlation between the two variables. Therefore, despite the follow-up time of the group with graft was smaller than in the group with no graft, there was no correlation between this variable and relapse, both horizontal and vertical.

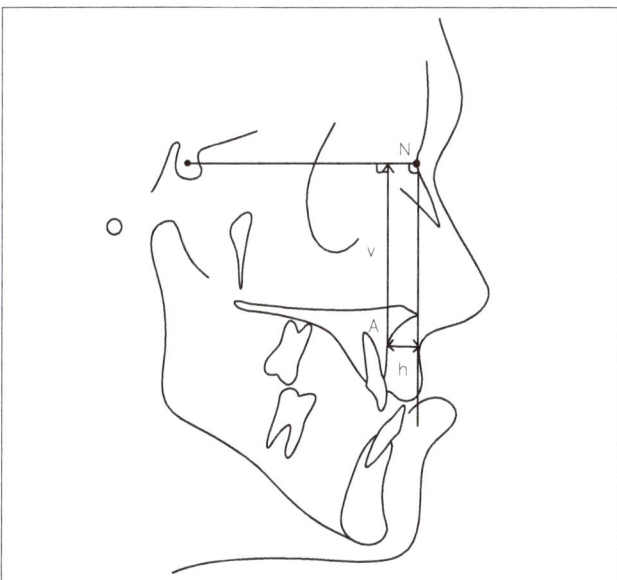

Figure 1 - Cephalometric tracings: reference lines and points used for evaluating postoperative results. S= Sella; N= Nasion; A= Point A; h= horizontal measurement; v= vertical measurement (Adapted from: Garrison et al[19]).

Table 1 - Descriptive statistics of variables according to each group.

Variable	Group	n	Mean ± SD	Median
Horizontal advancement (mm)	Without bone graft	23	5.52 ± 2.25	6.00
	With bone graft	25	5.44 ± 2.36	6.00
Horizontal relapse (mm)	Without bone graft	23	-1.09 ± 1.12	-1.00
	With bone graft	25	-0.36 ± 0.95	0.00
Vertical movement (mm)	Without bone graft	23	1.61 ± 2.76	2.00
	With bone graft	25	4.00 ± 3.54	3.00
Vertical relapse (mm)	Without bone graft	23	-0.30 ± 1.29	0.00
	With bone graft	25	-0.88 ± 1.48	0.00

Table 2 - Student's t-test carried out in order to assess whether the mean horizontal and vertical relapses are different from zero in the group without bone graft.

Group without bone graft		
Variable	n	Mean ± SD
Horizontal relapse (mm)	23	-1.087 ± 1.124
Vertical relapse (mm)	23	-0.304 ± 1.294

One-sample test Test value = 0			
Variable	T	D.F.	p-value
Horizontal relapse (mm)	-4.635	22	0.0001
Vertical relapse (mm)	-1.127	22	0.271

P-value< 0.05 indicates that the variable mean is different from zero.

Table 3 - Student's t-test carried out in order to assess whether the mean horizontal and vertical relapses are different from zero in the group with bone graft.

Group with bone graft		
Variable	n	Mean ± SD
Horizontal relapse (mm)	25	-0.360 ± 0.952
Vertical relapse (mm)	25	-0.880 ± 1.481

One-sample test Test value = 0			
Variable	T	D.F.	p-value
Horizontal relapse (mm)	-1.890	24	0.070
Vertical relapse (mm)	-2.970	24	0.006

P-value< 0.05 indicates that the variable mean is different from zero.

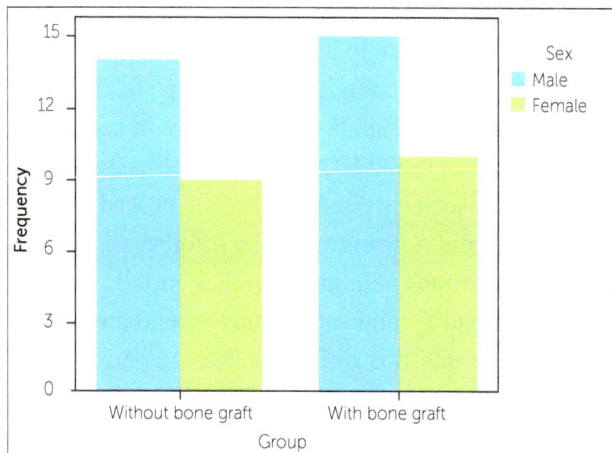

Figure 2 - Distribution frequency according to the variable sex.

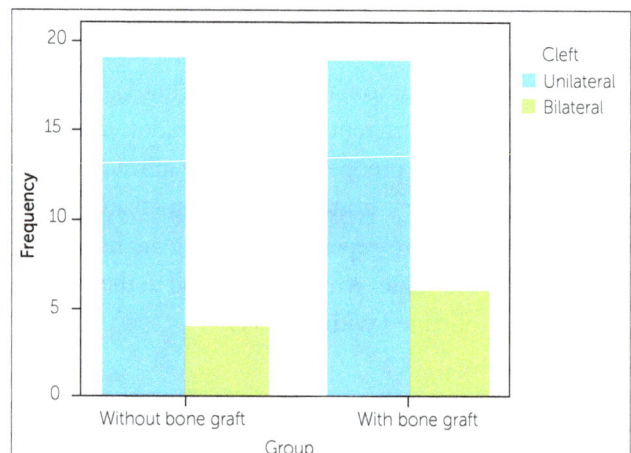

Figure 3 - Distribution frequency according to the variable type of cleft.

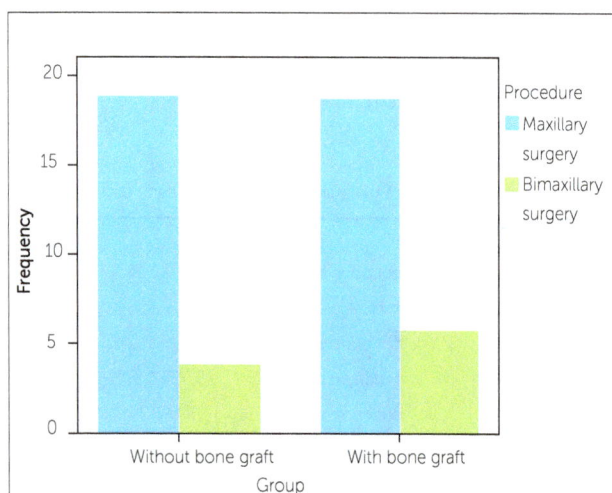

Figure 4 - Distribution frequency according to the variable type of procedure.

DISCUSSION

The authors agree with the literature regarding the instability of orthognathic surgery in patients with cleft lip and palate. The cause of instability is attributed to some variables such as several previous surgeries, fibrous tissue resulted from previous procedures, changes in dentition and muscle balance. At the same time, for non-cleft patients, stability and predictability in orthognathic surgery usually vary depending on the direction and magnitude of the surgical procedures, generally in that order of importance.[9,10]

The literature indicates a significant trend towards a higher number of postoperative relapses in cleft patients than in patients with non-cleft maxillary hypoplasia who underwent orthognathic surgery.[9,14]

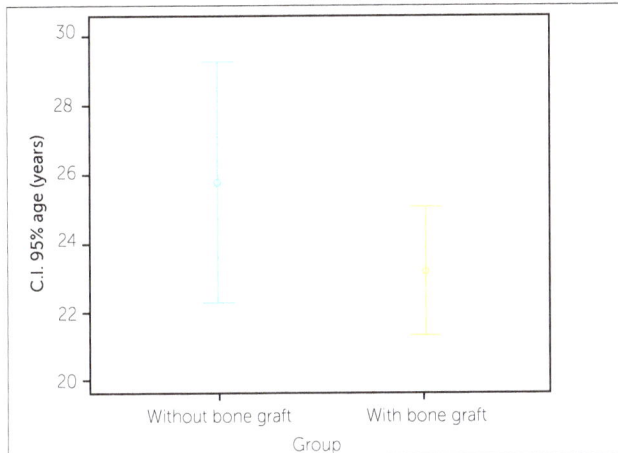

Figure 5 - Confidence interval with regard to age in each group.

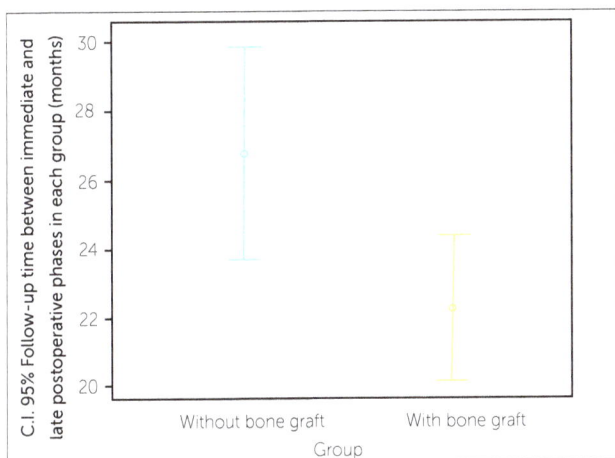

Figure 6 - Confidence interval with regard to postoperative follow-up period in each group.

Table 4 - Descriptive statistics of variables.

Variable	Group	n	Mean ± SD	Median
Age (years)	Without bone graft	23	25.78 ± 8.11	23.00
	With bone graft	25	23.16 ± 4.66	23.00
Follow-up time between immediate and late postoperative phases	Without bone graft	23	24.87 ± 11.37	23.00
	With bone graft	25	17.68 ± 8.38	17.00

Some authors suggested that to improve stability, a better, more effective and rapid healing should be provided by means of performing bone grafts adapted in the gaps created by the correction of the maxilla.[16,17] To evaluate the effectiveness of the grafting procedure, the authors proposed a study carried out by means of cephalometric analysis of patients undergoing orthognathic surgery.

Additionally, taking into account the benefits observed with the use of allogenic bone graft, the authors included in the study patients who had allogeneic graft-type only, since it is known that allogenic bone grafting offers several advantages such as easy handling, great amount of available material, cost reduction and, especially, decrease in patient's postoperative morbidity. Nique et al[2] studied the use of allograft in patients with alveolar defects and cleft lip and palate, obtaining good results for bone integration. Other authors have also had good results concerning allograft bone grafting in orthognathic surgery for non-cleft patients.[16,17]

As for the methods, the authors used those already described in the literature, for instance, radiographic evaluation by means of cephalometric analysis performed at three different stages (preoperative, immediate postoperative and late postoperative).[7,19-22] As shown in the studies of Erbe et al[22] and Iannetti et al,[21] these methods demonstrated to be efficient, since they were manually performed by one single and trained examiner.

After applying the methodology, the results showed more horizontal relapse in the CG (without graft) than the observed in the TG (with grafting), i.e., more stability was obtained with the use of grafts. This fact was also observed by Hirano and Suzuki;[7] however, in their study, relapses occurred both horizontally and vertically and the only different approach was the use of autogenous bone graft to fill the gaps created by osteotomies, which may suggest the formation of an autograft mechanical barrier that is less efficient to restrict the movements of relapse.

At last, the present results corroborate the studies of Heliovaara et al[20] and Iannetti et al,[21] demonstrating the positive effects of performing bone grafting in order to minimize relapses in orthognathic surgery for cleft patients.

CONCLUSIONS

The use of allogeneic grafts in cleft patients undergoing Le Fort I maxillary osteotomy contributes to increase postoperative stability when compared to surgeries without bone grafting.

REFERENCES

1. Ankola AV, Nagesh L, Hegde P, Karibasappa GN. Primary dentition status and treatment needs of children with cleft lip and/or palate. J Indian Soc Pedod Prev Dent. 2005;23(2):80-82.

2. Nique T, Fonseca RJ, Upton LG, Scott R. Particulate allogeneic bone grafts into maxillary alveolar clefts in humans: a preliminary report. J Oral Maxillofac Surg. 1987;45(5):386-92.

3. Spina Vea. Classificação das fissuras lábio-palatinas. Sugestão de modificação. Rev Hosp Clin Fac Med São Paulo. 1972;27(1):5-7.

4. Bill J, Proff P, Bayerlein T, Weingaertner J, Fanghanel J, Reuther J. Treatment of patients with cleft lip, alveolus and palate: a short outline of history and current interdisciplinary treatment approaches. J Craniomaxillofac Surg. 2006;34 Suppl 2:17-21.

5. Schultes G, Gaggl A, Karcher H. Comparison of periodontal disease in patients with clefts of palate and patients with unilateral clefts of lip, palate, and alveolus. Cleft Palate Craniofac J. 1999;36(4):322-7.

6. Dahllof G, Ussisoo-Joandi R, Ideberg M, Modeer T. Caries, gingivitis, and dental abnormalities in preschool children with cleft lip and/or palate. Cleft Palate J. 1989;26(3):233-7; discussion 37-8.

7. Hirano A, Suzuki H. Factors related to relapse after Le Fort I maxillary advancement osteotomy in patients with cleft lip and palate. Cleft Palate Craniofac J. 2001;38(1):1-10.

8. Bailey LJ, Cevidanes LH, Proffit WR. Stability and predictability of orthognathic surgery. Am J Orthod Dentofacial Orthop. 2004;126(3):273-7.

9. Kerawala CJ, Stassen LF, Shaw IA. Influence of routine bone grafting on the stability of the non-cleft Le Fort 1 osteotomy. Br J Oral Maxillofac Surg. 2001;39(6):434-8.

10. Ayliffe PR, Banks P, Martin IC. Stability of the Le Fort I osteotomy in patients with cleft lip and palate. Int J Oral Maxillofac Surg. 1995;24(3):201-7.

11. Bishara SE, Chu GW, Jakobsen JR. Stability of the LeFort I one-piece maxillary osteotomy. Am J Orthod Dentofacial Orthop. 1988;94(3):184-200.

12. Proffit WR, Phillips C, Turvey TA. Stability following superior repositioning of the maxilla by LeFort I osteotomy. Am J Orthod Dentofacial Orthop. 1987;92(2):151-61.

13. Steinberg B, Padwa BL, Boyne P, Kaban L. State of the art in oral and maxillofacial surgery: treatment of maxillary hypoplasia and anterior palatal and alveolar clefts. Cleft Palate Craniofac J. 1999;36(4):283-91.

14. De Riu G, Meloni SM, Raho MT, Gobbi R, Tullio A. Delayed iliac abscess as an unusual complication of an iliac bone graft in an orthognathic case. Int J Oral Maxillofac Surg. 2008;37(12):1156-8.

15. Bothur S, Blomqvist JE, Isaksson S. Stability of Le Fort I osteotomy with advancement: a comparison of single maxillary surgery and a two-jaw procedure. J Oral Maxillofac Surg. 1998;56(9):1029-33; discussion 33-4.

16. Christian JM, Peterson LJ. Frozen femoral head allogeneic bone grafts for orthognathic surgery. J Oral Maxillofac Surg. 1982;40(10):635-9.

17. Scheffer P, Blanchard P, Attar A, Assa A. Cryopreserved allografts in orthognathic surgery]. Rev Stomatol Chir Maxillofac. 1988;89(4):220-8.

18. Precious DS. Treatment of retruded maxilla in cleft lip and palate: orthognathic surgery versus distraction osteogenesis: the case for orthognathic surgery. J Oral Maxillofac Surg. 2007;65(4):758-61.

19. Garrison BT, Lapp TH, Bussard DA. The stability of Le Fort I maxillary osteotomies in patients with simultaneous alveolar cleft bone grafts. J Oral Maxillofac Surg. 1987;45(9):761-65.

20. Heliovaara A, Ranta R, Hukki J, Rintala A. Skeletal stability of Le Fort I osteotomy in patients with isolated cleft palate and bilateral cleft lip and palate. Int J Oral Maxillofac Surg. 2002;31(4):358-63.

21. Iannetti G, Cascone P, Saltarel A, Ettaro G. Le Fort I in cleft patients: 20 years' experience. J Craniofac Surg. 2004;15(4):662-9

22. Erbe M, Stoelinga PJ, Leenen RJ. Long-term results of segmental repositioning of the maxilla in cleft palate patients without previously grafted alveolo-palatal clefts. J Craniomaxillofac Surg. 1996;24(2):109-17.

23. Louis PJ, Waite PD, Austin RB. Long-term skeletal stability after rigid fixation of Le Fort I osteotomies with advancements. Int J Oral Maxillofac Surg. 1993;22(2):82-6.

Permissions

All chapters in this book were first published in DPJO, by Dental Press International; hereby published with permission under the Creative Commons Attribution License or equivalent. Every chapter published in this book has been scrutinized by our experts. Their significance has been extensively debated. The topics covered herein carry significant findings which will fuel the growth of the discipline. They may even be implemented as practical applications or may be referred to as a beginning point for another development.

The contributors of this book come from diverse backgrounds, making this book a truly international effort. This book will bring forth new frontiers with its revolutionizing research information and detailed analysis of the nascent developments around the world.

We would like to thank all the contributing authors for lending their expertise to make the book truly unique. They have played a crucial role in the development of this book. Without their invaluable contributions this book wouldn't have been possible. They have made vital efforts to compile up to date information on the varied aspects of this subject to make this book a valuable addition to the collection of many professionals and students.

This book was conceptualized with the vision of imparting up-to-date information and advanced data in this field. To ensure the same, a matchless editorial board was set up. Every individual on the board went through rigorous rounds of assessment to prove their worth. After which they invested a large part of their time researching and compiling the most relevant data for our readers.

The editorial board has been involved in producing this book since its inception. They have spent rigorous hours researching and exploring the diverse topics which have resulted in the successful publishing of this book. They have passed on their knowledge of decades through this book. To expedite this challenging task, the publisher supported the team at every step. A small team of assistant editors was also appointed to further simplify the editing procedure and attain best results for the readers.

Apart from the editorial board, the designing team has also invested a significant amount of their time in understanding the subject and creating the most relevant covers. They scrutinized every image to scout for the most suitable representation of the subject and create an appropriate cover for the book.

The publishing team has been an ardent support to the editorial, designing and production team. Their endless efforts to recruit the best for this project, has resulted in the accomplishment of this book. They are a veteran in the field of academics and their pool of knowledge is as vast as their experience in printing. Their expertise and guidance has proved useful at every step. Their uncompromising quality standards have made this book an exceptional effort. Their encouragement from time to time has been an inspiration for everyone.

The publisher and the editorial board hope that this book will prove to be a valuable piece of knowledge for researchers, students, practitioners and scholars across the globe.

List of Contributors

Mariana Trevizan
Universidade de São Paulo, Faculdade de Odontologia de Ribeirão Preto, Programa de Pós-Graduação de Odontopediatria (Ribeirão Preto/SP, Brazil)

Alberto Consolaro
Universidade de São Paulo, Faculdade de Odontologia de Ribeirão Preto, Programa de Pós-Graduação de Odontopediatria (Ribeirão Preto/SP, Brazil)
Universidade de São Paulo, Faculdade de Odontologia de Bauru (Bauru/SP, Brazil)

Paulo Nelson Filho
Universidade de São Paulo, Faculdade de Odontologia de Ribeirão Preto, Departamento de Clínica Infantil (Ribeirão Preto/SP, Brazil)

Solange de Oliveira Braga Franzolin
Universidade do Sagrado Coração, Departamento de Odontologia (Bauru/SP, Brazil)

Omar Gabriel da Silva Filho
MSc in Orthodontics, State University of São Paulo (UNESP)

Orlando Motohiro Tanaka
Professor, Pontifícia Universidade Católica do Paraná (PUC-PR), School of Health and Biosciences, Graduate Dentistry Program in Orthodontics, Curitiba, Paraná, Brazil

Calliandra Moura Pereira de Lima
Specialist in Orthodontics, State University of Maringá (UEM/Brazil). MSc student in Health, Federal University of Santa Maria (UFSM/Brazil)

Laurindo Zanco Furquim
PhD in Oral Patology, Bauru Dental School. Head Professor of Orthodontics, UEM/Brazil

Adilson Luiz Ramos
PhD in Orthodontics, São Paulo State University (UNESP/Brazil). Head Professor of Orthodontics, UEM/Brazil

Denise Yagura
Graduated in Dentistry, School of Dentistry of Barretos. Specialist in Orthodontics. Londrina State University (UEL)

Paulo Eduardo Baggio
Associate Professor, Graduate Program Director in Orthodontics, UEL

Luiz Sérgio Carreiro and Ricardo Takahashi
Associate Professor, UEL

Luiz Filiphe Gonçalves Canuto
Post-Doctor in Orthodontics, FOB-USP. Professor, Specialization Course in Orthodontics, ABO-PE and FACSETE

Marcos Roberto de Freitas
Professor, Orthodontics, FOB-USP

Karina Maria Salvatore de Freitas
PhD in Orthodontics, FOB-USP. Post-Doctor in Orthodontics, Toronto Dentistry University

Rodrigo Hermont Cançado
Adjunct Professor, Uningá. Professor, Specialization Course in Orthodontics, UFVJM

Leniana Santos Neves
Professor, Specialization Course in Orthodontics, UFVJM

Daniela de Cassia Faglioni Boleta-Ceranto
Full professor, Paranaense University (UNIPAR)

Ricardo Sampaio de Souza
Full professor, Department of Orthodontics, UNIPAR

Sandra Silverio-Lopes
Professor, Graduate program, Brazilian Institute of Therapy and Education (IBRATE)

Nathalie Canola Moura
Specialist in Orthodontics, UNIPAR

Luiz Filiphe Gonçalves Canuto
Professor of graduate program in Orthodontics at the Brazilian Dental Association / Pernambuco (ABO-PE)

Karina Maria Salvatores de Freitas
Professor of the graduate program in Orthodontics at UNINGÁ

Marcos Roberto de Freitas
Full professor of Pediatric Dentistry, Orthodontics and Public Health at USP, Bauru Dental School

Rodrigo Hermont Cançado
Associate professor at UNINGÁ

Caroline Pelagio Raick Maués
DDS in Dentistry, Fluminense Federal University (UFF)

Rizomar Ramos do Nascimento
Specialist in Orthodontics, UFF

Oswaldo de Vasconcellos Vilella
Professor, Postgraduate program in Orthodontics, UFF

Mauren Bitencourt Deprá and Josiane Xavier de Almeida
Graduate Student, School of Dentistry – PUCPR

Taís de Morais Alves da Cunha and Luis Filipe Siu Lon
MSc in Orthodontics, Orthodontic Department, School of Dentistry - PUCPR

Luciana Borges Retamoso
PhD Student, Department of Dental Materials - PUCRS

Orlando Motohiro Tanaka
Professor - Orthodontics – PUCPR

Bruno D'Aurea Furquim
PhD Student in Oral Rehabilitation, School of Dentistry of Bauru, University of São Paulo (FOB-USP)

José Fernando Castanha Henriques and Guilherme Janson
Full and Head Professor, University of São Paulo (USP)

Danilo Furquim Siqueira
PhD in Orthodontics, FOB-USP. Professor, UNICID

Laurindo Zanco Furquim
PhD in Oral Pathology, FOB-USP. Associate Professor, State University of Maringá (UEM)

Matheus Melo Pithon
Professor of Orthodontics, Universidade Estadual do Sudoeste da Bahia (UESB), Jequié, Bahia, Brazil

Caio Souza Ferraz
Undergraduate student in Dentistry, Universidade Estadual do Sudoeste da Bahia (UESB), Jequié, Bahia, Brazil

Francine Cristina Silva Rosa
Professor of Microbiology, Universidade Federal da Bahia (UFBA), Vitória da Conquista, Bahia, Brazil

Luciano Pereira Rosa
Professor of Radiology, Universidade Federal da Bahia (UFBA), Vitória da Conquista, Bahia, Brazil

Guilherme Thiesen
MSc in Orthodontics and Facial Orthopedics, PUCRS. Professor of Orthodontics, UNISUL and UNIASSELVI

Guilherme Pletsch
Specialist in Orthodontics, UNISUL

Michella Dinah Zastrow
MSc in Radiology, UFSC. Professor of Radiology and Stomatology, UNISUL

Caio Vinicius Martins do Valle
MSc in Orthodontics, Bauru School of Dentistry – São Paulo University (FOB-USP). Coordinator of the Specialization Course in Orthodontics, UNIASSELVI. PhD Student in Oral Rehabilitation, FOB-USP

Karyna Martins do Valle-Corotti
MSc and PhD in Orthodontics, FOB-USP. Associate Professor, Department of Orthodontics, São Paulo City University (UNICID). Professor of the MSc Program in Orthodontics, UNICID

Mayara Paim Patel
MSc and PhD in Orthodontics, FOB-USP. Professor of the Specialization Course in Orthodontics, Dentistry and Health Catarinense Institute

Paulo Cesar Rodrigues Conti
Head Professor of the Prosthesis Department, FOB-USP. Honorary member of the Ibero Latin American Academy of Craniomandibular Dysfunction and Orofacial Pain

Carla Maria Melleiro Gimenez
PhD in Orthodontics, FOA-UNESP

Francisco Antonio Bertoz
Head Professor, Department of Pediatric Dentistry, FOA-UNESP

Marisa Aparecida Cabrini Gabrielli, Oswaldo Magro Filho, Idelmo Garcia and Valfrido Antonio Pereira Filho
Assistant Professor, Oral and Maxillofacial Surgery, FOA-UNESP

Júlia Olien Sanches and Betina Grehs
Undergraduate student, Araraquara Dental School, São Paulo State University (UNESP)

Lourdes Aparecida Martins dos Santos-Pinto
Full Professor, Children's Clinic Department, Araraquara Dental School (UNESP)

Ary dos Santos-Pinto
Associate Professor, Children's Clinic Department, Araraquara Dental School (UNESP)

Fabiano Jeremias
Graduate student, Araraquara Dental School (UNESP)

André Weissheimer
PhD Student in Orthodontics, PUC-RS

Arno Locks
Professor of Orthodontics, UFSC

Luciane Macedo de Menezes
Professor of Orthodontics, PUC-RS

Adriano Ferreti Borgatto
Professor of Statistics, UFSC

Carla D'Agostini Derech
Professor of the Specialization Course in Orthodontics, UFSC

Fernanda Pinelli Henriques and Daniela Cubas Pupulim
PhD resident, Universidade de São Paulo, School of Dentistry, Bauru, São Paulo, Brazil

Guilherme Janson and Jose Fernando Castanha Henriques
Full professor, Universidade de São Paulo, School of Dentistry, Bauru, São Paulo, Brazil

Lorena Marques Ferreira de Sena and Arthur Costa Rodrigues Farias
Post-graduation program, Department of Dentistry, Universidade Federal do Rio Grande do Norte, Natal, RN, Brazil

Lislley Anne Lacerda Damasceno e Araújo
Federal University of Rio Grande do Norte, Department of Dentistry, Natal, RN, Brazil

Hallissa Simplício Gomes Pereira
Adjunct professor in Orthodontics, Department of Dentistry, Universidade Federal do Rio Grande do Norte, Natal, RN, Brazil

Lara Carvalho Freitas Sigilião
Dentist, Brazilian Navy, Rio de Janeiro, Rio de Janeiro, Brazil

Mariana Marquezan
Postdoc resident in Orthodontics, Universidade Federal do Rio de Janeiro (UFRJ), Rio de Janeiro, Rio de Janeiro, Brazil

Carlos Nelson Elias
Professor, Instituto Militar de Engenharia (IME), Rio de Janeiro, Rio de Janeiro, Brazil

Antônio Carlos Ruellas and Eduardo Franzotti Sant'Anna
Professor, Universidade Federal do Rio de Janeiro (UFRJ), Rio de Janeiro, Rio de Janeiro, Brazil

Juliana Volpato Curi Paccini
MSc, Universidade Cidade de São Paulo (UNICID), Department of Orthodontics, São Paulo, São Paulo, Brazil

Flávio Augusto Cotrim-Ferreira and Flávio Vellini Ferreira
Professor, Universidade Cidade de São Paulo (UNICID), Department of Orthodontics, São Paulo, São Paulo, Brazil

Karina Maria Salvatore de Freitas, Rodrigo Hermont Cançado and Fabrício Pinelli Valarelli
Professor, Faculdade Ingá, Department of Orthodontics, Maringá, Paraná, Brazil

Jamille Barros Ferreira
Master's degree in Orthodontics, Universidade Federal Fluminense, Niterói / RJ, Brazil

Licínio Esmeraldo da Silva
Professor, Statistics Department, Universidade Federal Fluminense, Niterói / RJ, Brazil

Márcia Tereza de Oliveira Caetano, Andrea Fonseca Jardim da Motta and Adriana de Alcantara Cury-Saramago
Professor, Dental Clinics Department, Universidade Federal Fluminense, Niterói / RJ, Brazil

José Nelson Mucha
Full professor, Dental Clinics Department, Universidade Federal Fluminense, Niterói / RJ, Brazil

Cristiane Cherobini Dalla Corte
Specialist in Orthodontics, Centro Universitário Franciscano (UNIFRA), Santa Maria, Rio Grande do Sul, Brazil

Bruno Lopes da Silveira
Professor, Universidade Federal de Santa Maria (UFSM), Department of Restorative Dentistry, Santa Maria, Rio Grande do Sul, Brazil

Mariana Marquezan
Postdoc resident, Universidade Federal do Rio de Janeiro (UFRJ), Department of Pediatric Dentistry and Orthodontics, Rio de Janeiro, Rio de Janeiro, Brazil Dentist, Universidade Federal de Santa Maria (UFSM), Department of Restorative Dentistry, Santa Maria, Rio Grande do Sul, Brazil

Roberto Carlos Bodart Brandão
Adjunct professor of Orthodontics, Federal University of Espírito Santo (UFES)

Larissa Bustamente Capucho Brandão
Specialist in Orthodontics, Fluminense Federal University (UFF)

Anna Júlia de Oliveira Façanha
Specialist in Orthodontics, Hospital for Rehabilitation of Craniofacial Anomalies – São Paulo University (HRAC-USP)

Tulio Silva Lara
Professor of Interceptive Orthodontics (HRAC-USP)

Daniela Gamba Garib
Full professor, School of Dentistry — University of São Paulo/Bauru. Professor of Orthodontics (HRAC-USP)

Edilene Kawabata and Vera Lucia Dantas
Specialist in Orthodontics, Associação Brasileira de Ortodontia, Belém, Pará, Brazil

Carlos Brito Kato
Professor in Orthodontics, Associação Brasileira de Ortodontia, Belém, Pará, Brazil

David Normando
Adjunct professor, Universidade Federal do Pará (UFPA), School of Dentistry, Belém, Pará, Brazil

Daniela Ferreira de Carvalho Notaroberto
Universidade do Estado do Rio de Janeiro, Programa de Pós-graduação em Odontologia, Departamento de Odontologia Preventiva e Comunitária (Rio de Janeiro/RJ, Brazil)

Mariana Martins e Martins
Universidade Federal Fluminense, Faculdade de Odontologia, Disciplina de Ortodontia (Niterói/RJ, Brazil)

Maria Teresa de Andrade Goldner, Alvaro de Moraes Mendes and Cátia Cardoso Abdo Quintão
Universidade do Estado do Rio de Janeiro, Departamento de Odontologia Preventiva e Comunitária, Disciplina de Ortodontia (Rio de Janeiro/RJ, Brazil)

Armando Yukio Saga
Professor, Pontifícia Universidade Católica do Paraná (PUC-PR), School of Health and Biosciences, Residency in Orthodontics, Curitiba, Paraná, Brazil

Hiroshi Maruo
Professor, Associação Brasileira de Odontologia (ABO-PG), Ponta Grossa, Paraná, Brazil

Marco André Argenta
Adjunct professor, Universidade Federal do Paraná (UFPR), Department of Civil Engineering, Graduate Program in Numerical Methods, Curitiba, Paraná, Brazil

Ivan Toshio Maruo
Professor, Pontifícia Universidade Católica do Paraná (PUC-PR), Residency in Orthodontics, and Associação Brasileira de Odontologia (ABO-PR), Curitiba, Paraná, Brazil

Kelston Ulbricht Gomes
PhD in Oral and Maxillofacial Surgery, Pontifical Catholic University of Paraná (PUC-PR)

Wilson Denis Benato Martins and Marina de Oliveira Ribas
Professor of Dentistry at PUC-PR

Index

www.ingramcontent.com/pod-product-compliance
Lightning Source LLC
Chambersburg PA
CBHW080633200326
41458CB00013B/4617

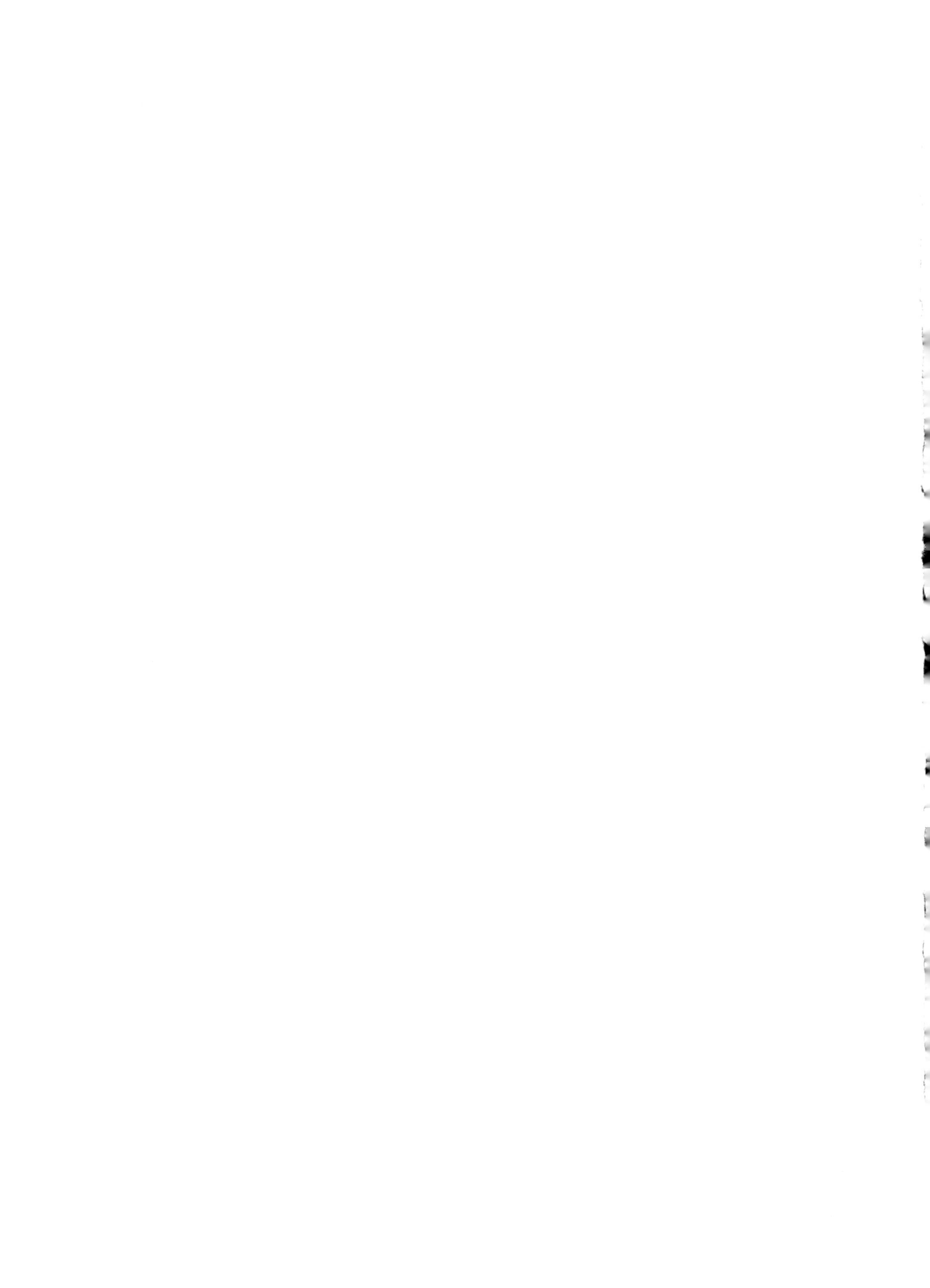